ESSENTIALS OF
HEALTH
PROMOTION

Sara Miller McCune founded SAGE Publishing in 1965 to support the dissemination of usable knowledge and educate a global community. SAGE publishes more than 1000 journals and over 800 new books each year, spanning a wide range of subject areas. Our growing selection of library products includes archives, data, case studies and video. SAGE remains majority owned by our founder and after her lifetime will become owned by a charitable trust that secures the company's continued independence.

Los Angeles | London | New Delhi | Singapore | Washington DC | Melbourne

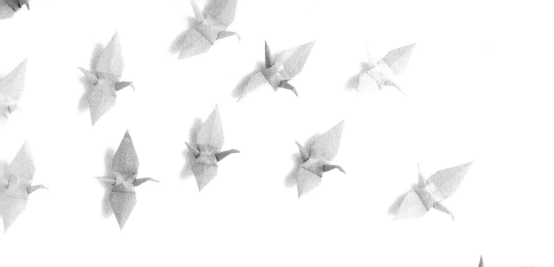

ESSENTIALS OF
HEALTH
PROMOTION

JAMES WOODALL
RUTH CROSS

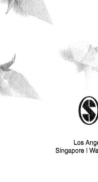

⑤SAGE

Los Angeles | London | New Delhi
Singapore | Washington DC | Melbourne

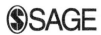

Los Angeles | London | New Delhi
Singapore | Washington DC | Melbourne

SAGE Publications Ltd
1 Oliver's Yard
55 City Road
London EC1Y 1SP

SAGE Publications Inc.
2455 Teller Road
Thousand Oaks, California 91320

SAGE Publications India Pvt Ltd
B 1/I 1 Mohan Cooperative Industrial Area
Mathura Road
New Delhi 110 044

SAGE Publications Asia-Pacific Pte Ltd
3 Church Street
#10-04 Samsung Hub
Singapore 049483

Editor: Alex Clabburn
Assistant editor: Ruth Lilly
Production editor: Tanya Szwarnowska
Copyeditor: Neil Dowden
Proofreader: Genevieve Friar
Indexer: Adam Pozner
Marketing manager: George Kimble
Cover design: Sheila Tong
Typeset by: C&M Digitals (P) Ltd, Chennai, India
Printed in the UK

Library of Congress Control Number: 2021935183

British Library Cataloguing in Publication data

A catalogue record for this book is available from the British Library

ISBN 978-1-5264-9624-9
ISBN 978-1-5264-9623-2 (pbk)

At SAGE we take sustainability seriously. Most of our products are printed in the UK using responsibly sourced papers and boards. When we print overseas we ensure sustainable papers are used as measured by the PREPS grading system. We undertake an annual audit to monitor our sustainability.

CONTENTS

ABOUT THE AUTHORS

Dr James Woodall is a Reader and Head of Subject in Health Promotion and Dr Ruth Cross is a Course Director in Health Promotion both at Leeds Beckett University. They have considerable experience in teaching health promotion at undergraduate and postgraduate levels in the UK and internationally. They both are active researchers and have published extensively in the field of health promotion, as well as holding editor-in-chief positions for well-respected academic journals.

INTRODUCTION

Essentials of Health Promotion is a core textbook for students studying health promotion, public health and health studies degrees at undergraduate level. It is also an ideal companion for those working in health promotions roles. This book provides an accessible, contemporary, practical and easy-to-read guide to health promotion written by Dr James Woodall and Dr Ruth Cross, two established authors in the field from Leeds Beckett University, UK. The book is designed to be versatile and comprehensive so as to be an essential health promotion course text that will satisfy practitioners, students and lecturers at all levels of their undergraduate education. The book is designed to provide both the theory and practical skills for success – providing depth and breadth of content for all of those working and studying in health promotion. *Essentials of Health Promotion* aims to simplify complex concepts and ideas but to enable a comprehensive view of contemporary health promotion.

The book is divided into six sections covering the essentials that you will need to know – we have summarised these sections as the 'what', 'why', 'when', 'who', 'where' and 'how' of health promotion. Health promotion is introduced in the early sections (the 'what' and 'why') with this material ideally suited to those new to health promotion. The mid-sections ('when' and 'who') and the final two sections ('where' and 'how') of the book seek to prepare students for the realities of health promotion practice and the necessary skills to succeed both academically and professionally. The book offers a fresh perspective on health promotion taking into account historical ideas and practices, but also goes beyond other texts in the field by focusing on contemporary developments in health promotion; for example, 'virtual' environments and demonstrating the current professional competencies deemed necessary for practice.

The book has several features that run throughout the chapters that readers may find useful. Case studies from around the world are embedded in chapters to provide some context or illustration of key theories or concepts. The book also has many reflective exercises that can be used to encourage thought or contemplation. These can ideally be used in seminars or in classroom situations. To cater for those with a more advanced understanding of health promotion there are 'go further' activities which will encourage more in-depth, critical thinking.

SECTION 1: WHAT IS HEALTH PROMOTION?

In order to understand health promotion, it is necessary to first explore meanings of health in Chapter 1. This chapter introduces health through a medical and social model and also considers positive and negative aspects of health, incorporating ideas such as disease and well-being. The section will provide, but not dwell upon, the historical context of the origins of health promotion in order to understand how modern health promotion emerged – this will be covered in Chapter 2. This chapter also outlines the relationships between health promotion and other disciplines, like public health. The broad range of activities and strategies under the banner of 'health promotion' will be discussed in Chapter 3. This will be done through drawing on theoretical and conceptual models – explained in an accessible way – using examples from a range of health topics. A socio-ecological view of health promotion will be forwarded, suggesting that health promotion needs to operate at individual (micro), community (meso) and national/international levels (macro) to be effective.

SECTION 2: WHY HEALTH PROMOTION?

In Section 1, health promotion is defined and outlined. Section 2, though, will outline why health promotion remains an important discipline in addressing health and contemporary health challenges. In Chapter 4 the utility of health promotion approaches to tackle contemporary health issues such as climate change, obesity and disease outbreaks and emergencies will be explained using current research examples and case studies. Chapter 5 will explain why some people live longer and experience better health than others using theoretical insights. The reason why health promotion is well placed to address these social injustices will be outlined. The section will focus on the values that are associated with health promotion and how these underpin 'why' health promotion remains relevant and useful. Values such as empowerment, partnership, control and choice will be highlighted with a broader recognition of the importance of working with, not on, individuals and communities explicitly addressed in Chapter 6.

SECTION 3: WHEN IS HEALTH PROMOTION RELEVANT?

This section focuses on 'when' the introduction of health promotion approaches is relevant. To do so, the section broadly focuses on health needs assessment and epidemiological principles. Chapter 7 outlines the process of health needs assessment which is considered the initial part of considering the value and appropriateness of any health promotion intervention – it covers the approach to gathering health needs information and how to assess this. Within the health needs assessment process, the value of lay perspectives are often overshadowed by professional points of view. In Chapter 8, the value of listening to lay views in health promotion will be described and examples given where such strategies have created more effective interventions and programmes. Finally, Chapter 9 focuses on a key contributing discipline to health promotion – epidemiology. The chapter will explain key concepts and ideas in epidemiology, highlighting both the value of descriptive and analytical epidemiology.

SECTION 4: WHO IS RESPONSIBLE FOR HEALTH PROMOTION?

Up to this point, it will be clear to the reader that health promotion is a broad and versatile discipline that can contribute fully to improving health. This position, though, raises questions about responsibility for health promotion and whether health promotion should be the choice of individuals or whether governments and global organisations should take control.

This raises questions about 'free will' and the role of the state in becoming involved in health choices. Section 4 plays out the 'structure'/'agency' debate – generally overlooked in health promotion – and will explore who then is responsible for delivering health promotion – looking at the role of the individual (Chapter 10) and the role of the state (Chapter 11). This will take a global, national, local and individual perspective showing the importance of the World Health Organization, governmental and non-governmental organisations, local communities and individuals, and the value of partnership working and collaborative working (Chapter 12).

SECTION 5: WHERE IS HEALTH PROMOTION DELIVERED?

The importance of setting and context will be discussed in addressing the key question of 'where' health promotion should be delivered. Starting with the theoretical overview of the approach in Chapter 13, the section then focuses on the settings approach to health promotion and in doing so draws on practical examples from a range of environments such as schools, workplaces and prisons in Chapter 14. Uniquely, the section takes time to explore in Chapter 15 'virtual settings' and how health promotion can be delivered via social media and through virtual communities.

SECTION 6: HOW IS HEALTH PROMOTION PRACTISED?

Translating the 'what', 'why', 'when', 'where' and 'who' of health promotion is very challenging. Section 6, therefore, focuses on the 'how' of health promotion. Chapter 16 will draw on established competency frameworks for practising health promotion, but will offer a more candid view of the challenges, realities and pitfalls of health promotion practice. The skills and attributes needed to practise health promotion will be outlined with a 'toolkit' developed and described to enable effective practice. This includes searching and appraising the evidence (Chapter 17) and planning and designing health promotion programmes (Chapter 18). Finally, the skills necessary for health promotion research and evaluation and communicating effectively are outlined in Chapters 19 and 20.

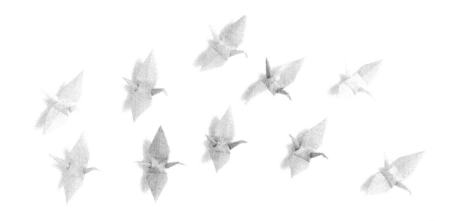

SECTION 1

WHAT IS HEALTH PROMOTION?

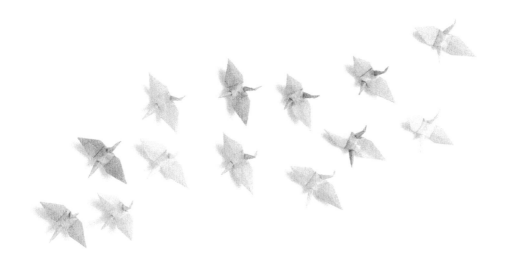

WHAT IS 'HEALTH'?

1

INTRODUCTION

Health means different things to different people at different times in different contexts. This chapter outlines the concept of health and the importance of understanding how health might be defined in order to promote it. If we do not have an appreciation of what health *is*, it is difficult to undertake effective health *promotion*. This chapter explores various dimensions of health including physical, mental, spiritual and social dimensions. A range of key concepts will be discussed including biomedical perspectives on health, the social model of health and the value of lay understandings of health. We will describe different aspects of disease and illness as well as considering health in more positive ways such as wellness, well-being and happiness. Salutogenic perspectives on health are briefly considered and, finally, the World Health Organization's conceptualisation of health is outlined.

PHYSICAL HEALTH

Health is often viewed as being located within the physical realm. This is because we inhabit physical bodies which can get sick, injured or hurt, or feel well and be physically fit. Physical health is important because it enables us to function and do what we want to do in life. Viewing health physically often means a focus on illness or disease or disability – namely on singling out physiological abnormalities. If we are not sick or injured we are deemed to be well or 'healthy'. But is it that simple? As Warwick-Booth et al. (2021) point out, a person might be physically unwell or have disabilities yet still report feeling healthy. Conversely, a person might be fully physically 'well' and yet feel unhealthy in some way, for example feeling mentally unwell. Historically, particularly in Western contexts, health has been more readily linked to our physical well-being. However, more recently (in the past few decades) there has been a greater appreciation of other dimensions of health.

MENTAL HEALTH

Defining mental health is more complicated than defining physical health (Green et al., 2019) and yet it is, arguably, more important. Often when we talk about mental health we are actually referring to mental *ill* health. Put simply, mental health is concerned with thoughts and feelings. The mental and emotional dimensions of health are therefore related. The World Health Organization defines mental health as 'a state of well-being in which every individual realizes his or her own potential, can cope with the normal stresses of life, can work productively and fruitfully, and is able to make a contribution to her or his community' (WHO, 2014: n.p.). Prince et al. (2007) argue that there can be no health without mental health. Mental health is inextricably linked to physical health. If we experience undue psychological stress it will manifest in physical symptoms. Likewise, when we are sick it can have an impact on our psychological state. Further, the importance of mental health is illustrated when we consider the global burden of disease. Mental health problems contribute significantly to disease and disability patterns worldwide. In early 2020, it was estimated that depression affected approximately 264 million people globally, a major contribution to the global burden of disease (WHO, 2020a). In late 2020 the detrimental impact of the coronavirus pandemic on global mental health was very clear and led to an increase in, for example, anxiety, stress and depressive symptoms resulting in part from requirements to socially isolate or quarantine (Torales et al., 2020).

SPIRITUAL HEALTH

Green et al. (2019: 17) note that 'many people have asserted that any serious consideration of positive health must include the spiritual dimension'. Spiritual health is related to mental health. Spiritual health is increasingly being viewed as an integral aspect of human health and human experience (Nunes et al., 2018; Ramezani et al., 2014). We have begun to develop a greater appreciation of the spiritual dimension of health and the importance of this. However, an agreed definition of spiritual health has so far eluded us (Vader, 2006). Similarly to mental health, spiritual health also has a cognitive element (thoughts) and an affective element (feelings or emotions). It has been linked with religious beliefs but more recently with faith. Fisher et al. (2000) put forward four domains of spiritual health concerned with the self, community, environment and God and, since then, the number of studies concerned with spiritual health has increased. However, as Hsaio et al. (2010) point out, there is still a relative lack of spirituality health-related research in non-Western countries. In their study on spiritual health in nursing students, Hsaio et al. (2010) found that spiritual health was related to a greater ability to manage stress, reduced symptoms of depression and enhanced health-promoting behaviours. Whilst there are many different definitions of mental health and spiritual health (Jaberi et al., 2017) the importance of both as distinct dimensions of health is clear.

CASE STUDY 1.1: SPIRITUALITY AND HEALTH IN NEPAL

Spirituality is a very important part of Nepalese culture. Hinduism and Buddhism are the two main religions in Nepal. Ancient cultures and beliefs are still very much apparent in the twenty-first century to any Western visitor to Everest. Those wanting to climb the mountain must observe a number of customs and traditions including taking part in a blessing ceremony, praying and offering small sacrifices at altars in order to bring good karma before they can make any attempt to ascend to the summit of Everest. The Nepalese believe that if these rituals do not take place then bad luck and misfortune will ensue. Prayer flags dot the landscape as a testimony to the magnitude and strength of these beliefs. 'There is a very important Puja (blessing) ceremony for every Everest expedition. It is held at Base Camp on a date decided by a local Lama. In the ceremony, the Lama asks the mountain gods' permission for the climbers to climb, forgiveness for any damage caused by the climbing and for the safety of everyone involved.' This case study also illustrates a cultural dimension to health.

Sources: www.iexplore.com, www.welcomenepal.com, Fogle and Fogle (2018: 70)

SOCIAL HEALTH

Social health is concerned with the nature of our relationships and connections with other people and our wider communities as well as the health of society at large. It is another complex, not-easily defined dimension to health which is highly important to experiences of health (Green et al., 2019). It has two main facets – the social health of the individual and the social health of society. An unhealthy individual may be described as 'sick'; likewise, an unhealthy society may be described as a 'sick society'. A sick society is characterised by a lack of cohesion, a lack of participation and alienation of its citizens, among other things. An individual might be said to be experiencing social ill health if they lack meaningful connections with other people. Social isolation and loneliness are significant problems for older people in some countries (i.e. the United Kingdom and the United States of America) and are associated with increased risk of mortality (Steptoe et al., 2013). It is evident from research and the wider literature that social connection and social support are associated with better health (Seppala et al., 2013; Small et al., 2011). The limits placed on social interaction during the global coronavirus pandemic of 2020 have had many negative effects on social health such as increased isolation and loss of social networks and support (Millman et al., 2020).

REFLECTIVE EXERCISE 1.1

So far we have considered four different dimensions of health – physical, mental, spiritual and social. Take a few minutes to reflect on your own understanding of health. What does health mean to you? Do the dimensions of health that have been discussed resonate with your own ideas and experiences? If yes, how? If no, why not? Are there any dimensions missing? What would these be?

THE BIOMEDICAL PERSPECTIVE

The biomedical model of health has historically dominated Western understandings of health. This is also referred to as the 'medical model' of health. The medical model has its roots in scientific perspectives and views health in terms of pathology, illness, disease, diagnosis, treatment and cure (Warwick-Booth et al., 2021). Importantly, the medical model separates the physical body from social or psychological aspects of health and does not take into account the other dimensions of health that we have discussed. Health is viewed as being located within the individual (body) and is conceptualised as the absence of illness or defect. If someone is not sick, then they are viewed as healthy. The medical model is highly influential, particularly in the Western world, and particularly within the past 200 years or so. This is not necessarily the case in other contexts. Whilst we might be very glad to receive medical intervention if we had appendicitis or broke a leg, the medical model of health is a very limited way of viewing human health experience. It is difficult to fully appreciate the complexities of health if we view it as solely located in, and defined by, our physical bodies. This is where the social model of health comes to the fore. Health promotion therefore privileges the social model of health over the medical model of health (Cross et al., 2021).

THE SOCIAL PERSPECTIVE AND HOLISTIC HEALTH

Whilst we have considered different dimensions of health separately in this chapter it should be apparent that it is not that easy to neatly draw lines between these. There are overlaps between the different dimensions and the relationships between them are complex. The social perspective on health takes these complexities into account and acknowledges that understandings of health are broad and multi-faceted (Dixey Cross, Foster and Woodall, 2013). Also referred to as the 'social model' of health, the social perspective views health as *holistic*. A holistic view of health takes an integrated approach considering all of the different dimensions of health and the person as a 'whole' not simply a biological body (Warwick-Booth et al., 2021). A holistic approach to health underpins many of the complementary and so-called 'alternative' approaches to health such as acupuncture and aromatherapy. Importantly, the social model of health takes into account lay perspectives which are discussed later in this chapter. The social model of health also moves beyond the individual person and considers the wider, social determinants of health. This is a key concept in health promotion. In the social model of health, the factors that influence health are taken into account. Table 1.1 outlines a number of other key differences between the medical and social models of health.

REFLECTIVE EXERCISE 1.2

What do you think is meant by the wider or social determinants of health? It might help to think about the factors that influence your health, or impact on it in some way. Reflect on the nature of your everyday life. How does what you do, where you go, who you interact with and how, and what you experience impact on your health? If you would find it easier you can think specifically about one aspect of your life, such as eating, working or studying.

The focus on the wider, social determinants of health is one of the key things that distinguishes the social model of health from the medical model of health. As you will have appreciated from undertaking Reflective Exercise 1.2, many different factors influence our health in some way. A number of models and theories have been developed in order to try to make sense of these factors; for example, Dahlgren and Whitehead's (1991) 'rainbow' model of health determinants (see Figure 1.1).

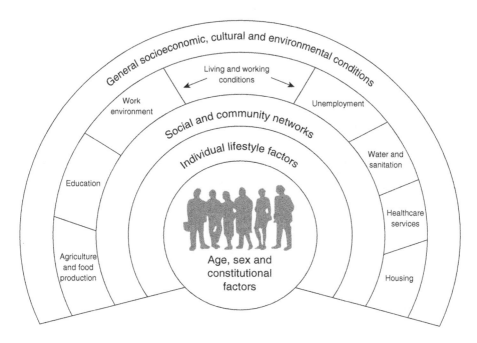

Figure 1.1   Dahlgren and Whitehead's (1991) 'rainbow' model

Source: Dahlgren and Whitehead (1991) Reproduced by kind permission of The Stokholm Institute of Future Studies

In the rainbow model, Dahlgren and Whitehead identify different layers of influence starting at the centre of the model with factors that cannot be altered such as our genetic make-up and our age. Each layer describes, in turn, individual lifestyle factors (such as behaviours), social and community factors (such as families and friends), our living and working conditions (such as where we live and the jobs that we do) and, in the outer layer, the general socio-economic, cultural and environmental conditions that impact on our health experience. This model does not, however, account for everything that influences our health and, since it was devised 30 years ago, our world has changed enormously. For a more detailed critique of Dahlgren and Whitehead's model see Warwick-Booth et al. (2021). Solar and Irwin (2010) have developed a more recent conceptual framework of social determinants of health (see Figure 1.2). This is much more complex than Dahlgren and Whitehead's model and takes into account a number of additional factors such as the political context of health.

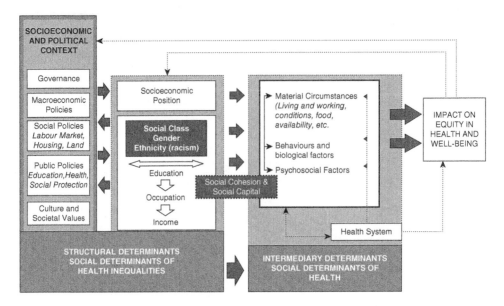

Figure 1.2   Solar and Urwin's (2010) conceptual framework of social determinants of health

Source: Reproduced from O. Solar and A. Irwin (2010) A Conceptual Framework for Action on the Social Determinants of Health. Social Determinants of Health Discussion Paper 2 (Policy and Practice). By kind permission of the World Health Organization.

Consideration of the wider, social determinants of health is necessary in order to explore and address inequalities in health. This is a central plank of health promotion. Chapter 5 is dedicated to discussing inequalities in health in more detail.

Table 1.1   A comparison of the medical model of health with the social model of health

Medical Model	Social Model
Narrow or simplistic understanding of health.	Broad or complex understanding of health.
Medically biased definitions focusing on the absence of disease or disability.	More holistic definitions of health taking a wider range of factors into account such as mental and social dimensions of health.
Does not take into account the wider influences on health (outside of the physical body).	Takes into account wider influences on health such as the environment and the impact of inequalities.
Influenced by scientific and expert knowledge.	Takes into account lay knowledge and understandings.
Emphasises personal, individual responsibility for health.	Emphasises collective, social responsibility for health.

Source: Warwick-Booth et al. (2021), reproduced by kind permission of Polity Books

LAY UNDERSTANDINGS OF HEALTH

As you will have seen from Table 1.1., the social model of health privileges lay understandings of health in contrast with the medical model in which expert, scientific views dominate. Many things influence our understanding of what health *is*: our gender, our age, our health status, our culture, our ethnicity, our social class, how we live, our personal experiences, what we do (occupation) and where we live (accommodation, location and country of residence). A substantial amount of research has been done that explores lay beliefs and understandings about health at different times in different contexts. Whilst understandings do vary according to a number of different factors, there are some common themes across the literature. Much of the research points to the importance that people in different contexts place on being able to *function* or to carry out the activities in daily life that enable a person to live, work and enjoy their leisure time (Blaxter, 2010; Stainton-Rogers, 1991). Health is often equated with being fit (Wright et al., 2006) or with not being ill (Blaxter, 2010), ideas which resonate with the medical model of health. It is also viewed as a *resource* for living (Bopp et al., 2012). However more complex, sophisticated understandings are also apparent such as health being about a kind of balance or equilibrium (Omonzejele, 2008; Robertson, 2006) and about having a sense of well-being or happiness (Bishop and Yardley, 2010; Cloninger and Zohar, 2011). In a study exploring young women's ideas about health, Cross (2013) found that they equated being healthy with being slim, doing the 'right' thing (i.e. exercising, eating well, not drinking too much) and looking after yourself. More recent research in South Africa exploring constructs of health in young adults found that ideas of personal freedom were important in expressing understanding about what health is (De Jong et al., 2019). Clearly, as Green et al. (2019: 11) argue, 'lay interpretations [of health] are complex and multidimensional'.

WELLNESS, WELL-BEING AND HAPPINESS

Wellness, well-being and happiness are connected. They are also fundamentally related to what it means to be or to feel 'healthy'. Subjective experiences of health, including ideas about well-being and happiness, are receiving increasing attention. Across the world, the importance of subjective experience is being recognised more and more in terms of evaluating health outcomes. Wellness is relatively easy to define and is clearly the absence of illness. However, it is not as easy to define what is meant by 'well-being'. Well-being is influenced by a number of different factors. What well-being means to one person may not be the same as to the next. Well-being is often closely associated with mental health (Gu et al., 2015). Elements of well-being include having one's basic psychological needs met, experiencing positive emotions, engaging with others, having meaningful relationships and accomplishing things (Johnson et al., 2016). Grant et al. (2007) identify three dimensions of well-being – psychological, physical and social. Interestingly these are all also dimensions of health so the connection between well-being and health is clear.

Happiness, on the other hand, is perhaps easier to define. Simply put, it is a human state that exists in opposition to sadness. We tend to put a high value on being happy and many people actually equate feeling happy with feeling, or being, healthy. There is an expanding field of research exploring the relationship between health and happiness; for example, Angner et al. (2009) whose work examined health and happiness among older people. They found that subjective measures of health (notions of well-being) were much better predictors of happiness than objective measures (illness and infirmity). In a Thai study, mental health and social support were strongly correlated with happiness (Yiengprugsawan et al., 2012). Similar results can be found across the literature on happiness and health.

GO FURTHER 1.1

Given the increased focus on notions of happiness and well-being in the research and literature on health, what would you identify as some of the challenges in measuring these concepts? If you were going to find out how happy the people who live in your neighbourhood or community are, what would you do? What type of questions would you ask? What would you look for?

The increased focus on wellness, well-being and happiness has resulted in new measures of health. There is now a proliferation of different scales designed to measure subjective experiences of health and happiness (see, for example, information available on Harvard's Center for Health and Happiness website: www.hsph.harvard.edu/health-happiness). The World Economic Forum (2015) has recognised the importance of finding better measures of lived experience than simply looking at how much money someone has. Box 1.1 illustrates how subjective well-being might be determined.

BOX 1.1 MEASURING SUBJECTIVE WELL-BEING

The UK Office for National Statistics (ONS) now include the following questions in the national household survey:

- Overall, how satisfied are you with your life nowadays?
- Overall, how happy did you feel yesterday?
- Overall, how anxious did you feel yesterday?
- Overall, to what extent do you feel the things you do in your life are worthwhile?

Source: World Economic Forum (2015)

Notably, in Bhutan, the government now measures national 'success' using a Gross National Happiness Index instead of the more commonly used gross national product. We also have the Happy Planet Index which evaluates how 'well' countries are doing in relation to each other by measuring factors such as subjective well-being and sustainability (see Case Study 1.2).

CASE STUDY 1.2: COSTA RICA AND THE HAPPY PLANET INDEX

In 2018 the small Central American country of Costa Rica had the highest ranking globally on the Happy Planet Index. The Happy Planet Index explores how well countries are doing in 'achieving long, happy, sustainable lives'. Despite having a comparatively lower income than many richer countries and experiencing relatively high levels of in-country income inequality, Costa Ricans report higher levels of well-being and happiness. In addition, the average life expectancy of Costa Ricans is higher than in the USA (the richest country in the world). Interestingly, Costa Rica has no armed forces. Since 1948 funds have been diverted instead to providing health, compulsory primary and secondary education, and pensions. In addition, universal access to social services, environmental protection and conservation are very high priorities in Costa Rica. Costa Rica consistently ranks as one of the happiest countries in the world.

Sources: www.happyplanetindex.org, www.huffingtonpost.co.uk,
www.theguardian.com

Quality of life is another important and related concept. Most people would agree that it is quality of life that is important, as compared with quantity of life (or number of years lived). We will return to these ideas more in Section 3 of this book.

Labonté (1998, cited in Orme et al., 2003: 287) offers a model of health that places well-being at the centre (see Figure 1.3). As you will see, Labonté's model has the three overlapping spheres or dimensions of health that were discussed earlier in this chapter – mental, physical and social health.

Each dimension connects and shares features with the others. This model however, does not take into account other important dimensions of health such as the spiritual dimension. All of these concepts point to the idea of health as a positive state of being and also as an asset for life. This leads us to consider the theory of salutogenesis.

SALUTOGENIC PERSPECTIVES

Another important concept in health promotion is *salutogenesis*. In the medical model of health, the focus is on 'pathogenesis' or what causes illness and disease. In contrast, salutogenesis focuses on what causes or creates health. Antonovsky (1996) developed this idea as a challenge to the pathogenic nature of the medical model discussed earlier

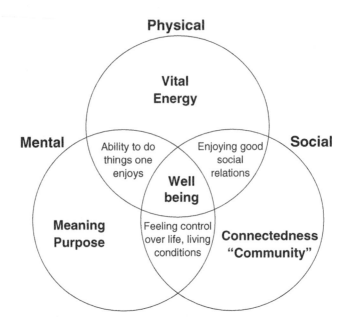

Figure 1.3 Labonté's (1998) model of health

Source: Labonté (1998) reproduced by kind permission of Ronald Labonté

and argued that we should be focusing on wellness, not illness. He advocated for an understanding of health as a continuum arguing that we can never fully achieve a 100 per cent healthy state but rather that, because we are biological beings, we are continually moving somewhere between states of ill health and health (Antonovsky called this the 'health-ease-dis-ease continuum'). In addition, Antonovsky developed ideas around what he called a 'sense of coherence' which comprises three main elements – comprehensibility, meaningfulness and manageability. In short, comprehensibility is about how we understand our worlds and make sense of them, meaningfulness is about how we feel about these and manageability is about the extent to which we can cope with what life throws at us (Sidell, 2010). More positive, agentic, asset-based ideas about health can be described as being 'salutogenic' in nature. We will return to ideas about agency and assets later in this book.

THE WORLD HEALTH ORGANIZATION'S PERSPECTIVE ON 'HEALTH'

The most useful and comprehensive model of health that we have come across is Green et al.'s (2019) 'working model of health' – see Figure 1.4. This model recognises the importance of numerous different factors (or variables) for understanding what health is. It accounts for the many different dimensions and perspectives of health that we have considered in this chapter and takes other things into consideration as well. It is necessarily complex and multifaceted reflecting the challenges of arriving at a universally accepted definition. Note how the model includes positive and negative ideas about health, health at both the individual and societal levels, and also highlights the importance of mental and social health.

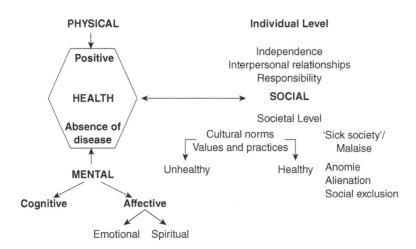

Figure 1.4   A working model of health

Source: Green et al. (2019: 15)

A number of definitions of health exist but we are not going to detail them all here. Instead we will focus on those provided by the World Health Organization since it has led the agenda on health promotion over the past few decades (see Chapter 2 for more details). The World Health Organization's (1948) original definition of health as 'a state of complete physical, mental and social well-being and not merely the absence of disease and infirmity' (WHO, 1948 cited in WHO, 2006) has been heavily criticised as being utopian, unattainable and for not considering other dimensions of health (Huber, 2011). However, the WHO's conceptualisation of 'health' has not remained static. In 1977 WHO acknowledged that health was 'the ability to conduct a socially and economically productive life' – a key goal of the 'Health for All by the Year 2000' global strategy (WHO, 1977). With the birth of the Ottawa Charter for Health Promotion in 1986 there was a further refinement whereby it was acknowledged that 'health is created in the context of everyday life and environment, where people live, love, work, and play' (WHO, 1986). Svalastog et al. (2017) point out that this development introduced 'an active and interactive understanding of health'. More recently there have been discussions about adding the spiritual dimension of health to WHO's definition of health but, although the importance of this dimension is acknowledged, the definition has not yet been revised (Chirico, 2016; Nahr et al., 2011). The World Health Organization's health promotion agenda will be discussed in more detail in the next chapter (Chapter 2).

GO FURTHER 1.2

As illustrated by the discussion in this chapter, defining health is very difficult. If you were asked to define what health is, how would you do that? How might the World Health Organization's definition be improved? What do you think are the most important aspects that need to be included?

SUMMARY

This chapter has considered the overarching question, 'What is health?' It has explored several different dimensions of health including physical health, mental health, spiritual health and social health. It has compared and contrasted the medical and social model of health and highlighted the importance of lay perspectives for health promotion. The theory of salutogenesis has been introduced and the World Health Organization's position on what health is has been outlined. This chapter highlights how complex health is and many of the different ways that we can think about health. In addition, we have started to explore what impacts on, creates and maintains health. The next chapter provides more detail about the historical context of the development of health promotion.

SUGGESTED READING

Blaxter, M. (2010) *Health*. 2nd edn. Cambridge, Polity Press.

Solar, O. and Irwin, A. (2010) A conceptual framework for action on the social determinants of health. *Social Determinants of Health Discussion Paper 2* (Policy and Practice). Geneva, WHO.

Warwick-Booth, L., Cross, R. and Lowcock, D. (2021) What is health? In *Contemporary Health Studies: An Introduction*. 2nd edn. Cambridge, Polity.

HEALTH PROMOTION

2

A HISTORICAL OVERVIEW

INTRODUCTION

The previous chapter explored what health is. This chapter will start to outline what *health promotion* is. To begin we consider how health promotion has developed over time drawing on the World Health Organization's agenda which has significantly influenced the evolution of health promotion at a global level. The importance of the Ottawa Charter for Health Promotion will be outlined and the subsequent development of health promotion through key World Health Organization health promotion conferences and their associated documents will also be presented bringing us to reflect on the current state of health promotion worldwide. We will also consider how health promotion fits with other fields such as health education, environmental health, primary healthcare and public health.

THE 'BIRTH' OF HEALTH PROMOTION

Most health promotion scholars point to the publication of the Lalonde Report in Canada in 1974 as the time when the idea of health promotion initially came about (Glouberman and Millar, 2003). This was the first time that the more traditional approach to health – that of simply using medical intervention to address health issues – was challenged by a Western democracy (Cross, Rowlands and Foster, 2021). The report was entitled 'A new perspective on the health of Canadians' (Lalonde, 1974). In it, Lalonde suggested a new way of looking at health which he called the *health field concept* (see Figure 2.1).

The report called for more attention to be paid to the *prevention* of ill health and therefore to the role that the environment and lifestyles have to play in health outcomes, not just medical and healthcare services. As you will see in Figure 2.1, the health field concept has four main elements – human biology, environment, lifestyle and healthcare organization. Box 2.1 provides further details about each one.

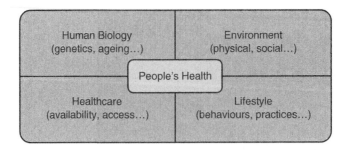

Figure 2.1 The health field concept

Source: Lalonde (1974)

BOX 2.1 THE FOUR MAIN ELEMENTS OF THE HEALTH FIELD CONCEPT

Human biology: All aspects of health, physical and mental, developed within the human body as a result of our basic biology and organic make-up. Very little can be done to change these factors.

Environment: All matters related to health external to the human body and over which the individual has little or no control, including the physical and social environment.

Lifestyle: The aggregation of personal decisions, over which the individual has some control including self-imposed risks created by unhealthy lifestyle choices which might contribute to, or cause, illness or death; for example, unhealthy behaviours like drinking too much alcohol or not doing enough exercise.

Healthcare: The quantity, quality, arrangement, nature and relationships of people and resources in the provision of healthcare.

Sources: Adapted from Green et al. (2019), Groff and Goldberg (2000) and Lalonde (1974)

Each of these four elements indicate factors that influence health, but they may also provide direction for policy and practice as to how health can be improved (Warwick-Booth et al., 2021). The primary significance of the health field concept is that the wider, social determinants of health were highlighted for the first time.

Attention to the wider, social determinants of health has continued through the global agenda on health promotion led by the World Health Organization. Several important milestones in the development of health promotion have subsequently been achieved.

Table 2.1 summarizes the key global conferences that have taken place over the past 40 years and highlights the main outcomes from each one. The Alma Ata conference on primary healthcare in 1978 is viewed as a major milestone in the development of health promotion because of its focus on promoting health for everyone through primary healthcare, and on the social determinants of health (Bhutta et al., 2018). We can now appreciate that the Alma Ata conference's somewhat utopian vision of 'Health for All by the Year 2000' was not realised. However, the principles underpinning the declaration are as pertinent as ever because, whilst we have made huge gains in some areas, such as wealth and health, inequalities still persist as do preventable illness, disabilities and deaths (Yamey et al., 2018).

Table 2.1 Summary of the key global conferences on health promotion

Conference	Outcome
1977 – Meeting of the World Health Organization at the 30th World Health Assembly	• Launch of 'Health for All by the Year 2000'

1978 – Alma-Ata Declaration (seen as the means to achieve 'Health for All'; resulted in the *Declaration of Alma-Ata*)	• Focus on primary health care
	Key issues:
	  – Social justice
	  – Addressing health in equalities
	  – Government responsibility

1986 – First International Conference on Health Promotion in Ottawa, Canada (resulted in the *Ottawa Charter*)	• Five key areas of action:
	  – Building healthy public policy
	  – Creating supportive environments
	  – Strengthening community action
	  – Developing personal skills
	  – Reorienting health services
	• To be achieved by:
	  – Advocacy
	  – Enabling
	  – Mediation

1988 – Second International Conference on Health Promotion in Adelaide, Australia	• Focus on healthy public policy • Alliances for health
1991 – Third International Conference on Health Promotion in Sundsvall, Sweden (resulted in the *Sundsvall Statement on Supportive Environments for Health*)	• Focus on supportive environments for health

1997 – Fourth International Conference on Health Promotion in Jakarta, Indonesia (resulted in the *Jakarta Declaration on Leading Health Promotion into the 21st Century*)	• Reinforced health as a basic human right
	• Identified *settings* as key to promoting health
	• Set out the following priorities:
	  – Promote social responsibility for health
	  – Increase investments for health development
	  – Consolidate and expand partnerships for health
	  – Increase community capacity and empower the individual
	  – Secure an infrastructure for health promotion

(Continued)

Table 2.1   (Continued)

Conference	Outcome

2000 – Fifth International Conference on Health Promotion in Mexico City, Mexico	• Highlighted the need to:
	  – invest in health
	  – create an infrastructure for health promotion
	  – reduce inequity

2005 – Sixth International Conference on Health Promotion in Bangkok, Thailand (resulted in the *Bangkok Charter for Health Promotion in a Globalized World*)	• Emphasised policy and partnership • Emphasised the need to address determinants of health

2009 – Seventh International Conference on Health Promotion in Nairobi, Kenya (resulted in *The Nairobi Call to Action*)	• Five sub-themes:
	  – Build capacity for health promotion
	  – Strengthen health systems
	  – Partnerships
	  – Inter-sectoral action
	  – Community empowerment
	And a focus on:
	  – Health literacy
	  – Health behaviours

2013 – Eighth International Conference in Helsinki, Finland (resulted in *The Helsinki Statement of Health in All Policies*)	• Emphasised the 'Health in All Policies' agenda • Called for cross-governmental action and political will
2016 – Ninth International Conference on Health Promotion in Shanghai, China (resulted in the *Shanghai Declaration*)	• Focused on promoting health in the 2030 Agenda for Sustainable Development • Reinforced the importance of structural factors and wider determinants of health

Source: Adapted from Cross, Rowlands and Foster (2021)

THE OTTAWA CHARTER

The Ottawa Charter (WHO, 1986) is viewed as the cornerstone of health promotion. The charter came out of the first international conference on health promotion and provides a definition of health promotion as follows: 'Health promotion is the process of enabling people to increase control over, and to improve, their health' (WHO, 1986: 1). In addition to the definition of health promotion, the Ottawa Charter highlights a number of prerequisites for health. It stated that, in order for health to be improved or promoted, the following conditions and resources are fundamental – peace, shelter, education, food, income, a stable eco-system, sustainable resources, and social justice and equity (WHO, 2009a). The charter emphasised the importance of tackling the social determinants of health together with enabling people to achieve healthier lives (Svalastog et al., 2017). The charter also outlines five areas of action that are necessary for health promotion (see Table 2.1). Each area of action is equally important and these reinforce the fact that health is not simply created by the provision of healthcare (Cross, Rowlands and Foster, 2021). In addition to the five areas of action, the charter proposed three processes central to health promotion – advocacy, enabling and mediation. Advocacy is concerned with bringing about the conditions in which health can flourish. Enabling is about helping everyone to achieve their health potential and to be able to take control over their own health. Mediation is about ensuring that joined-up action takes place involving all concerned in promoting health as well as making sure that everyone's interests are taken into account.

KEY HEALTH PROMOTION CONFERENCES

As you will see from Table 2.1 a number of subsequent and influential World Health Organization-led conferences have taken place since the Ottawa Charter came into being. Each conference has furthered some of the key ideas and themes that first appeared in the Ottawa Charter. Among the five areas for action, the Ottawa Charter highlighted the importance of building healthy public policy for health. The second conference in Adelaide, Australia, in 1988 specifically built on this aspect, focusing on developing policy for health and on creating alliances for health (WHO, 1988). The significance of healthy public policy was further cemented in the World Health Organization's 'Health in All Policies' approach. The creation of supportive environments through healthy public policy is intended to make the healthier choice the easier choice (Green et al., 2019). This approach recognises that 'health promotion is not just the responsibility of the health sector but goes beyond healthy lifestyles to well-being and supportive environments' (WHO, 2011). Therefore health has to be considered across all policy dimensions, not solely reflected in the provision of health-care services. At the eighth international conference which took place in Helsinki in 2013 healthy public policy was again the focus where inter-sectoral action was also identified as a key requirement for promoting health. The 'Health in All Policies' approach was reiterated at this conference alongside a call for increased political will (WHO, 2013).

GO FURTHER 2.1

Think back to the dimensions and definitions of health that we considered in Chapter 1. What implications do these have for healthy public policy? What other policy areas need to incorporate consideration of health outside of healthcare provision? Choose one public health issue from the following:

- HIV/AIDS
- Road traffic accidents
- Malaria
- Mental health
- Reproductive health

See if you can find a local or national policy relating to the public health issue you have chosen. Read the policy and see if you can identify any elements of supportive environments and/or tackling the wider, social determinants of health.

Having undertaken Go Further 2.1 you should now have an appreciation of the scope of policy areas that are related to health. As we discussed in Chapter 1, health is influenced by many different factors and so it is necessary for policy to reflect that. Hence we need to build healthy public policy across all sectors (for example, in education, housing, employment, transport, sustainable environments and technology).

The 'create supportive environments' area of action was the main theme of the Sundsvall conference which took place in Sweden in 1991. The conference focused on four dimensions of supportive environments – the social dimension, the political dimension, the economic dimension and the gender dimension – and highlighted how 'a supportive environment is of paramount importance for health' (WHO, 1991: n.p.). At the conference a number of environmental concerns were highlighted as being detrimental to health including food insecurity, population growth, conflict and the depletion of natural resources. It resulted in the *Sundsvall Statement on Supportive Environments for Health* (WHO, 1991) which emphasised the importance of sustainable development and of social action. Sustainability has been, and still is, a key theme in the World Health Organization's health promotion agenda.

The next conference, in Jakarta, revisited some of the central ideas within the Ottawa Charter, namely what progress had been made on the social determinants of health. It resulted in *The Jakarta Declaration on Leading Health Promotion into the 21st Century* (WHO, 1997a). Similarly to previous conferences this one reiterated the idea that health is a basic human right but also that health is very necessary for a country's progress and development (Green et al., 2019). It also highlighted the new challenges that health promotion faced such as advancing technology, increased threats to the environment and an increasingly connected world, and called for strong partnerships to promote health. Importantly this was the first conference to emphasise 'settings for health'. In Section 5 of this book we discuss settings in more detail.

In Mexico, in 2000, the fifth international conference focused on 'bridging the equity gap' (WHO, 2000). The *Mexico Ministerial Statement for the Promotion of Health* (WHO, 2000) highlighted the importance of good health as an asset for life and as necessary for social and economic development, re-emphasised governmental responsibility for health, and reinforced the imperative to tackle the social, economic and environmental determinants of health. The statement concluded that 'health promotion must be a fundamental component of public policies and programmes in all countries in the pursuit of equity and better health for all' (WHO, 2000: 17). Importantly, the conference noted that there was 'ample evidence that good health promotion strategies of promoting health are effective' (WHO, 2000: 21).

The *Bangkok Charter for Health Promotion in a Globalized World* (WHO, 2005) came out of the sixth international conference in Thailand and, again, re-emphasised the key themes of the previous conferences, this time giving more attention to inequalities between countries, new patterns of communication and environmental change. This called for four commitments from the international community, to make health promotion:

- Central to the global development agenda
- A core responsibility for all of government

- A key focus of communities and civil society; and
- A requirement for good corporate practice

(WHO, 2009a: 26)

The Nairobi conference in 2009 was significant in that it was the first of the international conferences to take place in Africa. This seventh international conference on health promotion resulted in the *Nairobi Call for Action* (WHO, 2009b). The call for action aimed to address the implementation gap in health and development through health promotion (Catford, 2010) and identified a number of key strategies and commitments that were required for this to happen as follows (Sparks, 2010):

- Strengthen leadership and workforces
- Mainstream health promotion
- Empower communities and individuals
- Enhance participatory processes
- Build and apply knowledge

The 'Health in All Policies' approach was emphasised at the eighth conference on health promotion held in Helsinki, Finland in 2013. The importance of healthy public policy and intersectoral action, as iterated in the Ottawa Charter, was further cemented at this conference which also called for increased political will from the global community to tackle health challenges (WHO, 2013). The resulting statement highlighted the importance of 'health for all' as the 'cornerstone for development' (WHO, 2013: 1). The ninth international conference on health promotion resulted in the *Shanghai Declaration* (WHO, 2016). The declaration focuses on what is needed in order to achieve the 2030 Agenda for Sustainable Development which is reflected in the 17 Sustainable Development Goals. The Shanghai Declaration stated the following:

> We reaffirm health as a universal right, an essential resource for everyday living, a shared social goal and a political priority for all countries. The United Nations Sustainable Development Goals (SDGs) establish a duty to invest in health, ensure universal health coverage and reduce health inequities for people of all ages. We are determined to leave no one behind.

(WHO, 2017a: 7)

The declaration emphasised the political nature of health and called for political leadership and co-ordinated action in order to achieve health and to meet the Sustainable Development Goals. It also reinforced the idea that health is a shared responsibility.

THE SUSTAINABLE DEVELOPMENT GOALS

It is worth discussing the Sustainable Development Goals (SDGs) in a little more detail at this point. These replaced the Millennium Development Goals (MDGs) in 2015. The eight MDGs were established in 2000 with a target date of 2015 (see Box 2.2).

BOX 2.2 THE MILLENNIUM DEVELOPMENT GOALS

1.   Eradicate both extreme poverty and hunger
2.   Achieve universal primary education
3.   Promote gender equality
4.   Reduce child mortality
5.   Reduce maternal mortality
6.   Combat HIV/AIDS, malaria and other diseases
7.   Ensure environmental sustainability
8.   Global partnerships for health

The MDGs were created as a means for UN member states to tackle poverty and inequality, and to improve health, and have been very influential in terms of global policy development (Warwick-Booth and Cross, 2018b). The outcomes of the MDGs have varied; however, they are generally viewed as being positive for global health and it is believed that millions of people worldwide experienced less poverty and better health because of the targets that were associated with them, particularly in poorer countries (see Case Study 2.1). However, despite these achievements, the MDGs attracted some criticism such as being too broad (Warwick-Booth and Cross, 2018b), neglecting human rights (Mepham, 2014), and as not being sensitive enough to country-level contexts influencing outcomes, particularly in Africa (Cohen et al., 2014).

CASE STUDY 2.1: ETHIOPIA AND THE MILLENNIUM DEVELOPMENT GOALS

Like many African countries, Ethiopia achieved a number of health-related MDGs (see MDGs 4, 5 and 6 in Box 2.2). For example, a 67 per cent reduction in under-five mortality, a 71 per cent decline in maternal mortality, a 90 per cent decline in new HIV infections, 73 per cent decrease in malaria-related deaths and more than a 50 per cent decline in deaths due to tuberculosis. These successes were attributed to comprehensive cross-sector governmental strategies, disease control programmes and the strengthening of the health system. However, importantly, it was also noted that the improvements in health could not have been achieved without progress in the other MDGs, namely poverty reduction, education, access to safe drinking water, and peace and stability in the country. It was also noted that 'the gains were not equitable, with differences between urban and rural areas, among regions and socioeconomic strata'. These differences were attributed to disparities in healthcare service provision and more development, in general, in urban areas.

Source: Assefa et al. (2017: n.p.)

The Sustainable Development Goals are a new set of targets that are now guiding all UN member states' policy and practice until 2030. The 17 goals specify what (ideally) needs to be achieved in order to improve global health and well-being – see Box 2.3.

BOX 2.3 THE SUSTAINABLE DEVELOPMENT GOALS

1. End poverty in all its forms everywhere
2. End hunger, achieve food security and improve nutrition, and promote sustainable agriculture
3. Ensure healthy lives and promote well-being for all at all ages
4. Ensure inclusive and equitable quality education and promote lifelong learning opportunities for all
5. Achieve gender equality and empower all women and girls
6. Ensure availability and sustainable management of water and sanitation for all
7. Ensure access to affordable, reliable, sustainable and modern energy for all
8. Promote sustained, inclusive and sustainable economic growth, full and productive employment and decent work for all
9. Build resilient infrastructure, promote inclusive and sustainable industrialization, and foster innovation
10. Reduce inequality within and among countries
11. Make cities and human settlements inclusive, safe, resilient and sustainable
12. Ensure sustainable consumption and production patterns
13. Take urgent action to combat climate change and its impacts
14. Conserve and sustainably use the oceans, seas and marine resources for sustainable development
15. Protect, restore and promote sustainable use of terrestrial ecosystems, sustainably manage forests, combat desertification, drought and floods, and strive to achieve a land-degradation neutral world
16. Promote peaceful and inclusive societies for sustainable development, provide access to justice for all and build effective, accountable and inclusive institutions at all levels
17. Revitalize the global partnership for sustainable development

Source: https://sustainabledevelopment.un.org

Only one goal, number 3, specifies the word 'health'; however, it should be apparent that all of the SDGs have a bearing on health in some way. Notably the word 'sustainable' appears many times in the list of goals. The focus on this is really important given the state that our planet is currently in – sustainability is vital. Unsurprisingly the SDGs have also been criticised, for having too many associated targets (Brende and Hoie, 2015), for being too idealistic (Horton, 2014), for being inconsistent, and too difficult to monitor or measure (Swain, 2017). Nevertheless, the SDGs provide a framework for developmental progress over the next decade; see Case Study 2.2 for how this is the case in South Asia.

CASE STUDY 2.2: THE SDGS IN SOUTH ASIA

The SDG agenda is of particular importance to South Asia because this region has 36 per cent of the world's poor and almost 50 per cent of the world's undernourished children. In order to make progress towards the SDGs, as in any region, political will is necessary. In addition, the SDGs need to be subsumed into regional and national development plans and budgets. Goal 5 is of particular importance in this context – gender equality. Women make up half the population so not addressing gender inequality can slow down progress and hinder development. For example, 'if we were to tackle bettering women's access to sexual and reproductive health, rights and services, this would also directly link to reductions in maternal mortality and supporting the end of communicable diseases such as HIV and AIDS (SDG 3). When women and girls have autonomy over their health, it has positive effects on education (SDG 4), sanitation and hygiene (SDG 6), and employment (SDG 8)' (Tsumori, 2018).

Sources: www.unescap.org, www.asia-pacific.undp.org

HEALTH PROMOTION VALUES

The series of World Health Organization conferences has highlighted several central planks of health promotion that are often referred to as 'values'. We believe that the most important of these are empowerment and equity (Green et al., 2019). You will note that each of these values recur throughout the discussion in this book and specifically in Chapter 6. A number of other values appear as themes throughout the World Health Organization's agenda and underpin what health promotion is about. These include health as a right, participation, community engagement, partnerships and social justice. Again, you will see these recurring in this book. In addition, the focus on tackling health inequalities, on addressing the wider, social determinants of health, on ethical practice, and using evidence of effectiveness are also fundamental to health promotion. Health promotion also privileges the social model of health, as we saw in Chapter 1.

REFLECTIVE EXERCISE 2.1

We have spent some time exploring the development of health promotion and outlined what health promotion is according to the definition from the Ottawa Charter (WHO, 1986). Before you read on take some time to consider how health promotion differs from, or is similar to, *health education, environmental health* and *public health*. Use the internet to find out more about each of these and try to determine what might make health promotion distinct in relation to each one.

HEALTH EDUCATION

The World Health Organization's (1986) definition of health promotion presented earlier as found in the Ottawa Charter is seminal. Consequently, we will not discuss definitions of health promotion any further. However, we do need to take into consideration a number of other terms and how they may, or may not, relate to health promotion. Let's start with *health education*. For many, historically at least, the term health education has been synonymous with the term health promotion; however, whilst they are no doubt related, there are distinct differences between the two (Green et al., 2019). Green et al. (2019: 36) define health education as 'any planned activity designed to produce health- or illness-related learning'. Naidoo and Wills (2016: 64) note that health education includes:

- raising awareness of health issues and factors contributing to ill health;
- providing information;
- motivating and persuading people to make changes in their lifestyle for their health;
- equipping people with the skills and confidence to make those changes.

Health education is, therefore, a necessary and important component of health promotion. But, health promotion is much more complex and diverse than this (Warwick-Booth et al., 2021). It is not just about acquiring knowledge or skills. In the next chapter (Chapter 3) we will consider this in more detail.

WHAT OF ENVIRONMENTAL HEALTH, PRIMARY HEALTH-CARE AND PUBLIC HEALTH?

Environmental health, primary healthcare and public health are also terms that appear to reflect what health promotion is; however, each of these is not quite the same and can be distinguished from health promotion in some way. 'Environmental health refers to the physical environment in which people live, and the importance of good-quality housing, transport, sanitation and pure-water facilities' (Naidoo and Wills, 2016: 5). Clearly environmental health is very important for health and well-being; however, it has a specific focus on our physical environment so, in that sense, it is more concerned with the physical dimension of health. As such it does not take into account the complexities of the other dimensions of health that we discussed in Chapter 1, nor does it factor in social determinants of health and well-being.

Primary healthcare is also extremely important for promoting health and was advocated by the Declaration of Alma Ata Declaration (WHO, 1978) as the main way to achieve health. Primary healthcare is different to primary medical care, and in the Alma Ata Declaration it was 'envisaged as embracing all the services that impact in health, including, for example, education, housing and agriculture' (Green et al., 2019: 21). Naidoo and Wills (2016: 128) outline the principles that characterise primary healthcare as follows:

- a holistic understanding of health as well-being, rather than the absence of disease;
- recognition that the presence of good health is dependent upon multiple determinants – health services are important, but so too are housing, education, agriculture and other services;
- health services reflect local needs and involve communities and individuals at all levels of planning and provision of services;
- services and technology are affordable, accessible and acceptable to communities;
- health services strive to address inequity and prioritize services to the most needy.

There are a number of commonalities between primary healthcare and health promotion, as you will have seen from the above list. However, health promotion is broader than this.

Health promotion is also often equated with public health and, as Green et al., (2019) argue, for some people there is no difference between the two. However, in this book we do make a distinction between health promotion and public health because we consider this distinction to be important. For us, health promotion operates from a distinct ideological position as indicated by the values outlined earlier in this chapter and discussed later in Chapter 6. However, there is no doubt that health promotion and public health are related. For some, health promotion is a defined part of public health yet sits under its wide umbrella (Raeburn and MacFarlane, 2003). For others, health promotion is set apart from public health due to the former's focus on the social model of health and the latter's concern with the preventative medical model of health. For others still, like us, the value base of health promotion clearly sets it apart from public health (Tilford et al., 2003). Naidoo and Wills's (2016: 57) definition of public health further clarifies the distinction – 'public health involves activities based on a biomedical understanding of health, focused on the identification of health-related needs and population-based actions such as immunization and screening'. In Chapter 3 we will discuss the important part that such efforts play in approaches to promoting health.

The use and popularity of different terms ebb and flow according to time and context. Currently in some parts of the world (here in the UK, for example) the term 'health promotion' is relatively out of vogue (Duncan, 2013) and a public health paradigm is dominating; however, this is not the case elsewhere (Warwick-Booth et al., 2018). Arguably it doesn't matter what term we use as long as we are working towards the same end – improving people's health and lives – but for the purposes of this book we are favouring *health promotion* as it is defined in the Ottawa Charter (1986) cited previously in this chapter.

GO FURTHER 2.2

This chapter charts the development of health promotion in line with the World Health Organization's agenda. All of the documents that have been produced at each successive conference are available at www.who.org. Take some time to access and read some of the original documents. Although the WHO's agenda has been widely received there have been some significant criticisms of it in the health promotion academic literature. See if you can find out what these are. Start with the Ottawa Charter which has been revisited and re-evaluated by different scholars 25 years and 30 years after it was written. A quick Google search will be a good place to begin.

SUMMARY

This chapter has traced the historical development of health promotion drawing on the World Health Organization's agenda. It has outlined the key global conferences that have taken place since the mid-1970s until the present day highlighting the central importance of the Ottawa Charter (1986) which laid the foundations for contemporary health promotion policy and practice. The Ottawa Charter's definition of health promotion has been presented and the chapter has considered what is unique about health promotion and how it differs from health education, environmental health, primary healthcare and public health. As illustrated, the influence of the World Health Organization on the global development of health promotion is significant and that influence continues today. The next chapter will discuss different approaches to promoting health.

SUGGESTED READING

Cross, R., Rowlands, S. and Foster, S. (2021) The foundations of health promotion. In R. Cross, L. Warwick-Booth, S. Rowlands, J. Woodall, I. O'Neil and S. Foster, *Health Promotion: Global Principles and Practice*. 2nd edn. Wallingford, CABI. pp. 1–44.

Green, J., Cross, R., Woodall, J. and Tones, K. (2019) Health and health promotion. In *Health Promotion: Planning and Strategies*. 4th edn. London, Sage. pp. 9–67.

Naidoo, J. and Wills, J. (2016) Defining health promotion. In *Foundations for Health Promotion*. 4th edn. London, Elsevier. pp. 57–74.

HEALTH PROMOTION APPROACHES

3

INTRODUCTION

This chapter presents and discusses a number of different approaches to promoting health. It will outline the difference between individual and structural approaches to promoting health, upstream and downstream approaches, and top-down versus bottom-up approaches. Each approach will be discussed with reference to relevant examples relating to health promotion, and in terms of the advantages and disadvantages of using such approaches. In addition, a number of theoretical models of health promotion will be introduced and explained including Tannahill's model, Beattie's model, Caplan and Holland's model and the Red Lotus model. Finally, the chapter will provide an overview of the socio-ecological view of health promotion and relate this to health promotion practice.

APPROACHES TO PROMOTING HEALTH

A cursory glance at the health promotion literature will reveal that there are many different ways of promoting health.

REFLECTIVE EXERCISE 3.1

Reflect on what you have learned already about health and health promotion from reading Chapters 1 and 2. How might health be promoted? What kind of things can we do to promote health, at the individual level, at the community level, at societal level, or at a global level even? Can you think of any examples of health promotion campaigns? If not, why not use the internet to find some. What approaches (or methods) are used in the campaign/s that you have found?

Undertaking Reflective Exercise 3.1 will have exposed you to a number of ways that health can be promoted. Health promotion approaches describe what we do to promote health or, essentially, the different methods or activities that we use. Naidoo and Wills (2016) offer an oft-used framework on approaches to health promotion that is useful here. Their framework or 'typology' details five different approaches to promoting health. Different elements of this typology overlap with the approaches that we are discussing in this chapter. See Table 3.1 for further details about the five approaches framework.

Table 3.1 Naidoo and Wills's five approaches framework or typology

Approach	Examples
Medical or Preventative Activity that aims to reduce illness, disability and deaths targeted at whole populations or high-risk groups using medical intervention.	• Screening for high-blood pressure • Immunisation • Pharmaceutical interventions
Behaviour Change Activity that encourages people to behave in more healthy ways.	• Smoking cessation programmes • Healthy eating campaigns • Weight-loss programmes
Educational Activity that provides knowledge, information and the skills needed to make an informed, healthier choice.	• Providing information leaflets • One-to-one counselling • Internet campaigns
Empowerment Activity that enables people to take control over their health and lives.	• Client-centred approaches • Community development
Social Change Activity that focuses on the socio-environmental or policy level (sometimes also called 'radical health promotion').	• Developing healthy public policy • Providing green leisure spaces • Restricting the number of fast-food outlets in a neighbourhood

Source: Adapted from Naidoo and Wills (2016: 76–81)

INDIVIDUAL AND STRUCTURAL APPROACHES

It is important to distinguish between individual and structural approaches to health. These are viewed as being polar opposite in nature but in practice are often used in combination (Hubley et al., 2021). By 'individual' we mean any activity that is aimed at the individual person or persons (also referred to as 'individualist' or 'individualistic'). We need to be very careful when using individual approaches to promoting health as this can lead to victim-blaming (Green et al., 2019). It is very easy to make a simple judgement that someone is not behaving in a healthy enough way; however, there may be a number of reasons why that is the case such as not having access to resources, or not having the necessary skills and knowledge to do things differently. The aim of individual approaches is to encourage individuals to change their behaviour in some way. As such the behaviour change approach in Table 3.1 is an example of individual approaches to health promotion. There are many challenges with using individual approaches. Firstly, behaviour change is a very complex process and takes time (Connor and Norman, 2015). Secondly, such approaches assume that health is the property, and therefore responsibility, of the individual (Naidoo and Wills, 2016). Thirdly, they fail to account for the complexity of the factors that impact on behaviour choices and behavioural outcomes (Cross et al., 2017). Fourthly, behaviour is determined by a number of different things including internal factors (such as self-esteem) and external factors (such as our environment) (Connor and Norman, 2017). Individual approaches tend to neglect external factors. Finally, individual approaches operate under the assumption that it is actually possible for people to make real changes to their lives and to their health. After reading Chapters 1 and 2 you will appreciate that it is not that simple. This is where structural approaches come in.

By structural approaches to promoting health we mean any activity that is aimed at changing the structures in society in which we live our lives in order to improve health outcomes and health experience for people (also referred to as structuralist). 'Structure' is a sociological term which refers to the ways in which societies are organised and the ways in which components or 'structures' of society, and the people within it, interact with one another; for example, class, gender, ethnicity, politics and culture (Hubley et al., 2021) – Chapter 11 discusses this further. Structural approaches put the focus on societal systems or forces that mitigate against positive health and cause disadvantage. Structural approaches therefore challenge the distribution of power. The social change approach in Table 3.1 is an example of structural approaches to health promotion. Given the criticisms of individual approaches cited earlier structural approaches to health promotion are more aligned to the values of health promotion that were briefly mentioned in Chapter 2 and that will be expounded upon in Chapter 6. The following case study illustrates individual versus structural approaches with reference to open defecation.

CASE STUDY 3.1: OPEN DEFECATION

It is estimated that more than 1 billion people worldwide practise open defecation (WHO, 2012). Open defecation refers to defecating in the open (i.e. fields, bushes, rivers) and typically occurs when people do not have access to toilets. *Individual approaches* to reducing open defecation would include teaching people about the effects of it (i.e. spread of disease, contamination of food sources) and encouraging changes in personal sanitation habits. *Structural approaches* would include government-funded building of household latrines, the implementation of policies to support the eradication of open defecation through latrine construction and changes in societal norms.

Sources: Coffey et al. (2014); Gertler et al., (2015); Patwa and Pandit (2018).

UPSTREAM AND DOWNSTREAM APPROACHES

In health promotion we often use the analogy of a river or stream to describe different approaches to promoting health. This originates from a seminal idea from McKinlay (1979) who tells a story as follows:

There I am standing by the shore of a swiftly flowing river and I hear the cry of a drowning man. So I jump into the river, put my arms around him, pull him to shore and apply artificial respiration. Just when he begins to breathe, there is another cry for help. So I jump into the river, reach him, pull him to shore, apply artificial respiration, and then just as he begins to breathe, another cry for help. So back in the river again, without end, goes the sequence. You know, I am so busy jumping in, pulling them to shore, applying artificial respiration, that I have no time to see who the hell is upstream pushing them all in.

The story is a simple analogy about health promotion being concerned with going upstream to find out why people are falling in the river in the first place, or why people are becoming unhealthy, hence the term *upstream* approach. The upstream idea is very important in health promotion. Focusing upstream leads us to consider the wider, social determinants of health – the sets of circumstances and conditions that people live in that influence health outcomes and health experience. In contrast, *downstream* approaches are concerned with action, treatment and cure once people are already sick or afflicted. For example, with reference to the global public health issue of obesity, it is easy to identify a number of downstream approaches or interventions that might be put in place for an individual who has already put on weight such as restricting dietary intake or increasing physical activity (changing 'obesogenic behaviours' – Lakerfeld and Mackenbach, 2017: 216). Upstream approaches, on the other hand, would be concerned with changing obesogenic environments or tackling the social determinants of obesity (Lakerfeld and Mackenbach, 2017). This would mean a critical examination of the environments in which obesity flourishes. Lakerfeld and Mackenbach (2017) categorise four different types of obesogenic environment as follows:

- physical (infrastructure, modes of transport, land use);
- socio-cultural (attitudes and beliefs);
- economic (cost of healthier foods or taking exercise);
- political (consumer regulation and protection).

Of course, obesity like many other public health concerns, is caused by a complex interplay of upstream and downstream factors which calls for multiple ways of addressing the issue.

TOP-DOWN AND BOTTOM-UP APPROACHES

In health promotion we also distinguish between two further types of approach that are polar-opposite in nature: these are referred to as *top-down* and *bottom-up* approaches. We can broadly define all health promotion activity as being either top-down or bottom-up. By top-down we mean that the agenda is led by experts or professionals. This might be through advising someone how to eat more healthily or through policy directives that tell us what to do or aim to shape our behaviour in some way, such as seat-belt laws or speeding limits. In top-down approaches the experts or professionals decide and define what the issue is and how to tackle it. The behaviour change approach and educational approach outlined in Box 3.1 are examples of top-down approaches to promoting health. Bottom-up, on the other hand, starts with the health concerns of individuals or communities as defined and identified by them.

Once these are identified the means for addressing them can be determined. The empowerment approach in Table 3.1 is distinguishable as a bottom-up approach. This way of typifying two different approaches is linked to who has the power to decide what the issue is. In top-down approaches power lies with the experts or professionals; in bottom-up approaches power lies with the individual or community. Considerations of who has power and what they have power over is a crucial part of health promotion, as highlighted in the Ottawa Charter's definition which is centrally concerned with empowering people ('enabling people to take control over their lives and health' – WHO, 1986: 1).

CASE STUDY 3.2: REDUCING TRAFFIC SPEED

Road traffic accidents are a major global public health problem that cause significant injury, disability and death, particularly in low-middle-income countries (Adeloye et al., 2016). *Top-down* approaches to reducing traffic speed include setting speed limits and imposing fines for non-compliant drivers. A *bottom-up* approach would be a community identifying speeding traffic as problematic in their neighbourhood and lobbying for the introduction of pedestrian-only areas, safe spaces for children to play or the introduction of local traffic calming measures such as road humps.

Sources: Adeloye et al. (2016); WHO (2018a)

COMMUNITY DEVELOPMENT APPROACHES

Community development approaches to promoting health can also be described as 'bottom-up'. Such approaches are necessarily linked to community participation and empowerment. As Case Study 3.2 shows they involve communities taking control over issues that concern them and working to address the factors that impact on their health and the health of their community. Community development approaches have a long history and, in some cases, are more likely to be described nowadays as community engagement or community participation but essentially these terms are referring to the same thing (Green et al., 2019). Community development approaches start with the concerns of the community and involve working with communities to identify what their issues are and how to address them. This is typically a longer-term approach underpinned by values that are central to health promotion such as social justice, equality, respect for autonomy and empowerment. Community development necessarily involves the engagement and participation of the community members and advocacy is also an important part of community development approaches (Gottwald and Goodman-Brown, 2012). The central aim of bottom-up or community development approaches is to redress the balance of power enabling the community to take control over what is happening rather than prescribing solutions or imposing top-down strategies on the people concerned. Such approaches can promote a sense of ownership and are more likely to be successful in the longer term (Sykes, 2014). There can be some challenges, however, such as competing interests, lack of short-term gains and differing valued outcomes (Scriven, 2017).

GO FURTHER 3.1

With reference to the health promotion campaigns you found for Reflective Exercise 3.1 consider what specific approaches were used. Were they individual or structural? Upstream or downstream? Top-down or bottom-up? Or was a combination of approaches used? Was there any evidence of community development? Which approaches do you think are likely to be more successful in relation to the public health issue that was being tackled?

MODELS OF HEALTH PROMOTION

Health promotion can be conceptualised in a number of different ways. Here we will look more closely at different *models* of health promotion. Models provide a way of understanding how something works or how different things fit together (or relate to one another) and can represent an aspect of the real world in some way enabling us to make better sense of a phenomenon. Models of health promotion can therefore be useful for describing or explaining what health promotion *is* and *does*, they can inform practice and they can also underpin ways of working (Green et al., 2019; Naidoo and Wills, 2016). There are several models of health promotion in the wider literature but, for the purposes of this chapter, we are going to consider only four different models, each in turn. These are Tannahill's model, Beattie's model, Caplan and Holland's model and, finally, the Red Lotus model.

Tannahill's model (Tannahill, 1985)

Tannahill's model was developed as a useful tool for 'planning and doing health promotion' (Tannahill, 2009: 396).

As you will see from Figure 3.1 the model looks like a Venn diagram. It has three circles which overlap. According to this model, each circle relates to a different type of health promotion activity – health education, prevention and health protection. Health education is concerned with communicating information to people and attempts to try to change attitudes, behaviour, knowledge and beliefs or to develop skills. Prevention is about any activity that is intended to minimise or eliminate risks to health (Warwick-Booth et al., 2021). Health protection includes any activity that is designed to protect population health. As you will see from Figure 3.1 health education and prevention

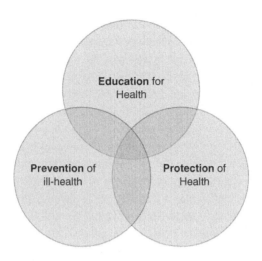

Figure 3.1 Tannahill's model

Source: Tannahill (1985)

overlap, health education and protection overlap, and prevention and health protection overlap. Table 3.2 provides examples of health promotion activities within each part of the model.

Table 3.2 Application of Tannahill's (1985) model of health promotion

Health education	Advising someone about the benefits of doing regular physical activity
Prevention	Vaccination against rubella for young women
Protection	Health and safety in the workplace
Preventative health education	Developing skills in cooking healthier food
Preventative health protection	Legislation to limit alcohol consumption
Education for positive protection	Lobbying for a ban on alcohol advertising

This is the least complex model of health promotion that we are considering in this chapter and, as such, it is open to criticism. It is relatively simplistic (Warwick-Booth et al., 2021) and it is limited to *describing* health promotion activity rather than explaining it (Naidoo and Wills, 2016).

Beattie's Model of Health Promotion (Beattie, 1991)

Beattie's model of health promotion offers a different way of conceptualising health promotion activity. As you will see from Figure 3.2, it is based on the intersection of two axes.

The horizontal axis distinguishes between activities that are either aimed at the individual (or small groups) or aimed at collectives (larger groups or whole populations). The vertical axis distinguishes between activities that are authoritative/expert-led (very similar to the 'top-down' approach discussed earlier) or negotiated/client-led (very similar to the 'bottom-up' approach discussed earlier). Each axis can be viewed as a continuum (Warwick-Booth et al., 2021). The two axes divide the model into four sections. The top two sections are health persuasion and legislative action respectively. Health persuasion is any activity that is authoritative or top-down in nature and is aimed more towards the individual; for example, telling someone to stop smoking. Legislative action is any activity that is authoritative or top-down in nature and is aimed at whole populations; for example, banning smoking in public places. The bottom two sections are personal counselling and community development respectively. Personal counselling is any activity that is aimed more towards the individual but that is negotiated in that the individual has more control over the process and isn't simply being told what to do or not to do; for example, using motivational interviewing to help someone identify whether and how they would like to become healthier. Community development is about activities that involve larger groups of people or whole populations and are more negotiated in that the community has more control or power. Community development approaches were discussed in more detail earlier in this chapter.

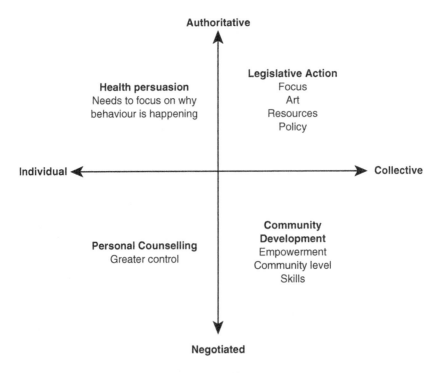

Figure 3.2   Beattie's model of health promotion

Source: Beattie (1991) Reproduced by kind permission of Routledge & CRC Press

GO FURTHER 3.2

Beattie's model of health promotion presents a more nuanced way of examining health promotion activities. Take some time to think about a public health issue that is affecting the city, country or region where you live. What different types of activity could be carried to address that public health issue? Where would they fit on Beattie's model? Do they sit neatly within one of the four quadrants? Alternatively, try to think of one activity for each quadrant that might address the issue you have chosen. In practice a combination of different approaches is often used.

Caplan and Holland's (1990) 'model'

As you will see from Figure 3.3 Caplan and Holland's (1990) 'model' of health promotion looks quite similar, at first glance, to Beattie's model. It has two intersecting axes resulting in four distinct quadrants. However, it offers a more complex way of conceptualising health promotion and the quadrants represent four different political perspectives on health promotion. The horizontal axis represents the nature of knowledge or how knowledge is conceived and created. Objective knowledge, at the one end, is measurable and quantifiable whilst subjective knowledge, at the other end, is not. The vertical axis represents the nature of society, what it is like and whether there is conflict or consensus (Cross, 2010).

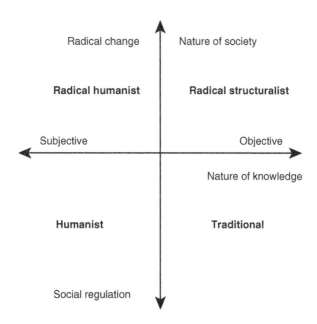

Figure 3.3 Caplan and Holland's four perspectives on health promotion

Source: Capland and Holland (1990)

Each quadrant offers a different perspective on the nature of health and health promotion practice. See Table 3.3 for details – refer to Figure 3.3 whilst you are reading the table to help you understand how the model works.

Table 3.3   Caplan and Holland's (1990) four perspectives on health promotion

Humanist	Health is defined by experts but subjective experience is acknowledged. Interventions would include working with people to enable them to understand what they can do for themselves and equipping them with the skills/knowledge needed to change.
Traditional	Health is objective and related to biomedical knowledge. Interventions are expert-led and would include telling people what to do (education) or doing things to them in order to improve their health (biomedical intervention).
Radical Humanist	Health is subjectively experienced and the individual determines, in dialogue with an 'expert', how they might want to change.
Radical Structuralist	Health is objectively measured but created by socio-economic and environmental factors such as inequalities. The nature of society needs to change in order to improve health.

Source: Adapted from Warwick-Booth et al. (2021)

The Red Lotus Health Promotion Model (Gregg and O'Hara, 2007a)

The Red Lotus Health Promotion Model (Gregg and O'Hara, 2007a) is a more recent conceptualisation of health promotion that draws explicitly on the core values of health promotion (Cross et al., 2021) (see Chapter 6 for a more in-depth exploration of health promotion values). The Red Lotus model is described as a 'new model for holistic, ecological, salutogenic health promotion practice' (Gregg and O'Hara, 2007a: 9).

This model differs from the other models that we have discussed so far in that it is the only one which explicitly draws on the value and principles that underpin health promotion. It considers these in relation to the process of health promotion planning. The name of the model comes from the Red Lotus plant. Gregg and O'Hara (2007a) use the structures of the Red Lotus to represent various aspects of health promotion. For example, the stem represents the principles, the leaves represent sustainability and the pod represents people (see Figure 3.4 for details). The model takes into account the environmental determinants of health, the holistic nature of health, health needs assessment and planning for health promotion. It is necessarily intricate since it is seeking to represent something that is very complex – health promotion. There isn't the space to describe and explain the Red Lotus model in detail here, so see Gregg and O'Hara (2007a) for more information.

A SOCIO-ECOLOGICAL APPROACH TO HEALTH PROMOTION

The final approach to promoting health that we will consider in this chapter is the socio-ecological approach. A wide range of different contextual factors influence our health at

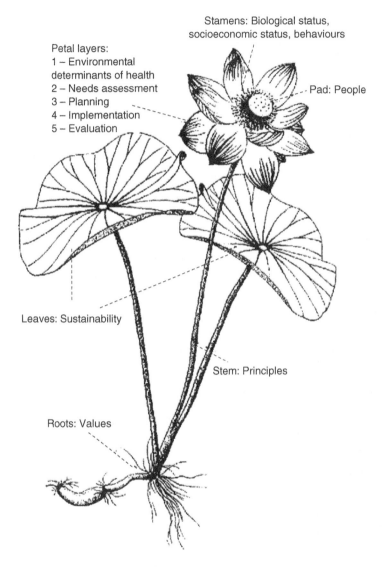

Stamens: Biological status, socioeconomic status, behaviours

Petal layers:
1 – Environmental determinants of health
2 – Needs assessment
3 – Planning
4 – Implementation
5 – Evaluation

Pad: People

Leaves: Sustainability

Stem: Principles

Roots: Values

Figure 3.4 The Red Lotus Health Promotion Model

Source: Gregg, O'Hara – Australian Health Promotion Association (2007) reproduced by kind permission of John Wiley & Sons

the individual level. We have previously signposted these as the wider, social determinants of health (see Chapter 1). Socio-ecological approaches recognise the interactions between people and their environments acknowledging that individual choices and behaviour do not occur within a vacuum but are influenced by the environment(s) that we live in (Golden and Earp, 2012). These include our physical environment, social environment, political environment, global environment and virtual environment. Townsend and Foster (2011: 1101) note that there are two key features to socio-ecological approaches – firstly, that 'behaviour affects and is affected by multiple levels of influence' and, secondly, 'individual behaviour shapes and is shaped by' our environment ('reciprocal causation'). There are a number of different socio-ecological models in the wider literature and each illustrate different layers of influence and interaction describing the multiple factors that impact on health highlighting opportunities for action or intervention to improve health (Harper et al., 2018). For example, McLeroy et al.'s (1988) model has five hierarchical layers starting with the individual (intrapersonal), then the interpersonal, the organisational, community and, finally, public policy. See Table 3.4 for an application of this model to promoting physical activity in young children.

Table 3.4 **McLeroy et al.'s (1988) model applied to physical activity in young children**

Level	Influence/Intervention
Intrapersonal	Age and ability of the child (motor skills, levels of fitness, self-efficacy). Intervention - teaching and enabling play (physical activity)
Interpersonal	Primary groups including family and peers. Intervention - parent and teacher involvement and encouragement in physical activity.
Organisational (or institutional)	Home, school, neighbourhood Intervention - structured play time at school, safe neighbourhood spaces and equipment to play
Community	Social networks, norms, culture, social traditions Intervention - child-friendly local services
Public Policy	Local and national regulation and laws Intervention - child-friendly policies, i.e. around accommodating children in public spaces

Sources: Harper et al. (2018); Mehtälä et al. (2014); Robinson (2008)

As Table 3.4 shows multilevel interventions are most often needed to tackle public health issues in a comprehensive and more successful way. Whilst an intervention at one level, say at the interpersonal, might have *some* effect it is more likely that a greater effect will occur if multilevel approaches are used simultaneously (Harper et al., 2018). Furthermore, using multilevel approaches will help to mitigate against neglecting the environment(s) in which behaviours occur and are shaped (Robinson, 2008) as well as enabling us to tackle the wider, social determinants of health. The socio-ecological model provides the conceptual basis for the settings approach (Townsend and Foster, 2011) which is discussed in more detail in Section 5 of this book.

REFLECTIVE EXERCISE 3.2

Choose another public health issue that is affecting the city, country or region where you live. How might McLeroy's socio-ecological model be applied to that issue? What kinds of health promotion intervention might be put in place at each of the five levels?

SUMMARY

This chapter has discussed different approaches to promoting health including individual and structural approaches to promoting health, upstream and downstream approaches, and top-down versus bottom-up approaches. Each approach has been discussed with reference to relevant examples relating to health promotion, and in terms of the advantages and disadvantages of using such approaches. In addition, a number of theoretical models of health promotion have been introduced and explained including Tannahill's model, Beattie's model, Caplan and Holland's model and the Red Lotus model. Finally, the chapter has provided an overview of the socio-ecological view of health promotion and related this to health promotion practice.

SUGGESTED READING

Gregg, J. and O'Hara, L. (2007) The Red Lotus Health Promotion Model: a new model for holistic, ecological, salutogenic health promotion practice. *Health Promotion Journal of Australia*, 18 (1), 9–12.

Naidoo, J. and Wills, J. (2016) Models and approaches to health promotion. In *Foundations for Health Promotion*. 4th edn. London, Elsevier. pp. 75–92.

Warwick-Booth, L., Cross, R. and Lowcock, D. (2021) Health promotion. In *Contemporary Health Studies: An Introduction*. 2nd edn. Cambridge, Polity Press. pp. 142–161.

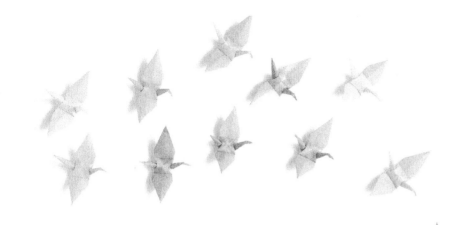

SECTION 2

WHY HEALTH PROMOTION?

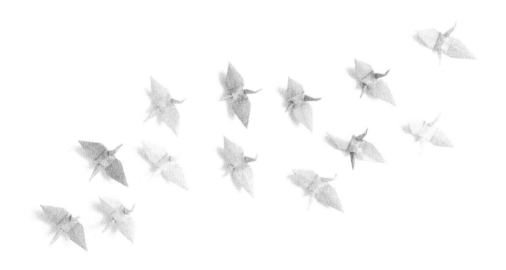

THE ROLE OF HEALTH PROMOTION IN TACKLING CONTEMPORARY HEALTH CHALLENGES

4

INTRODUCTION

Health promotion is a relatively young discipline as outlined in Chapter 2. Since the inception of health promotion in the mid-1980s much has changed in the world that could not have been foreseen. Despite such rapid change, health promotion offers a great deal for addressing significant health challenges and threats in contemporary society. In very recent times, we have seen the devastating impact of new and contemporary challenges not only mortality and morbidity, but also on economic prosperity and our ability to interact at work and in our personal lives. This chapter outlines a series of health issues and threats demonstrating the potential for adverse impacts. The chapter offers indication as to the value and utility of health promotion in addressing these.

CONTEMPORARY HEALTH CHALLENGES

Contemporary society has been described as VUCA – an acronym that suggests we live in times characterised by: *v*olatility, *u*ncertainty, *c*omplexity and *a*mbiguity (Worley and Jules, 2020). This results in fast-paced, dynamic contexts that are difficult to predict or plan for. These challenges emerge in all aspects of society, such as economics, but especially in the health sector. History suggests that health challenges can be specific to a period in time and that many of the health challenges identified as priorities have now been eradicated (small pox, for example). As a recent example, smoking and tobacco use was a major public health priority, but now in many countries smoking prevalence rates are declining rapidly due to concerted efforts to shift policy and practice. In more contemporary society, the impact of pandemics (e.g. COVID-19) has had a devastating impact on the health of individuals and communities and, of course, the economies of almost every global nation.

Although there are national and localised views in relation to the threats that impact on individuals and communities, there is a broad consensus in relation to some of the current global challenges. The WHO (2019a) identify ten challenges, these being:

1. Air pollution and climate change
2. Non-communicable diseases
3. Global influenza pandemic
4. Fragile and vulnerable settings
5. Antimicrobial resistance
6. Ebola and other high-threat pathogens
7. Weak primary healthcare
8. Vaccine hesitancy
9. Dengue
10. HIV

Other commentators have offered a variation on the major global health challenges. Warwick-Booth and Cross (2018b), for example, have suggested, in addition to the WHO, issues concerning population growth and competition for resources linked to the ageing population in many countries. They also highlight the health implications of war and terrorism as well as the social and economic damage caused by these. Surprisingly the WHO did not acknowledge mental health as a contemporary threat or challenge and yet there is evidence that shows that people's mental health experiences are becoming ever more negative (Warwick-Booth and Cross, 2018b). Warwick-Booth and Cross (2018b) also suggest that poverty and inequality are global challenges because this underpins many disease patterns – with poorer communities and individuals facing greater health challenges.

GO FURTHER 4.1

Thinking about your own country of origin, which of the identified health challenges is a 'real' concern and which are not? In addition, try to identify other contemporary challenges that your country faces that have not been mentioned.

Given the scope, spectrum and complexity of issues, it would be foolish to suggest that health promotion can effectively contribute to addressing all of these issues. Indeed, in some cases it may not be appropriate. That said, some have suggested that health promotion is more relevant today than ever in addressing public health problems (Kumar and Preetha, 2012). The remainder of the chapter will focus on those issues that may be effectively tackled using health promotion principles and strategies.

CLIMATE CHANGE

The data on climate change seems undeniable, with a broad consensus that climate change is causing huge damage to human health and well-being. The impact is not evenly distributed, as evidence suggests that there will be certain groups and populations who will be more adversely affected than others – Aboriginal communities, Pacific Island countries, the elderly and people with low income are just some examples (McMichael et al., 2003).

REFLECTIVE EXERCISE 4.1

List the reasons why climate change has implications for the health and individuals and communities (think about social and environmental determinants of health - clean air, safe drinking water, sufficient food and secure shelter). What arguments would you use to convince climate change deniers that climate change is a health issue?

Several commentators in health promotion have been clear in suggesting that climate change should be part of the agenda in the discipline (Catford, 2008), with some arguing that 'health promotion practitioners have a set of competencies that are highly transferable to action on climate change' (Patrick et al., 2011: 484). Indeed, the issue of climate change and addressing its effects fits coherently with the values and principles of health promotion – particularly because the Ottawa Charter demanded that individuals and communities should have access to clean air and water, sufficient food and adequate shelter (Patrick et al., 2011). Some have argued that the planet should be considered a key setting for health promotion with action taken to ensure that sufficient care is taken of the planet to mitigate climate change effects (Hancock et al., 2017). This would be operationalised through principles of 'one planet living' (see Box 4.1).

BOX 4.1 ONE PLANET PRINCIPLES

HEALTH AND HAPPINESS

Encourage active, social, meaningful lives to promote good health and well-being.

EQUITY AND LOCAL ECONOMY

Create safe, equitable places to live and work, which support local prosperity and international fair trade.

(Continued)

CULTURE AND COMMUNITY

Nurture local identity and heritage, empowering communities and promoting a culture of sustainable living.

LAND AND NATURE

Protect and restore land for the benefit of people and wildlife.

SUSTAINABLE WATER

Use water efficiently, protecting local water resources and reducing flooding and drought.

LOCAL AND SUSTAINABLE FOOD

Promote sustainable humane farming and healthy diets high in local, seasonal organic food and vegetable protein.

TRAVEL AND TRANSPORT

Reduce the need to travel and encourage walking, cycling, and low carbon transport.

MATERIALS AND PRODUCTS

Use materials from sustainable sources and promote products and services that help people reduce consumption.

ZERO WASTE

Reduce consumption, and reuse and recycle to achieve zero waste and zero pollution.

ZERO CARBON ENERGY

Make buildings and manufacturing energy efficient and supply all energy with renewables.

Source: Hancock et al. (2017)

Despite the coherent fit between health promotion and the climate change agenda, there remains some ambiguity in how best health promotion can address this issue. Clearly, one of the main strengths of health promotion is the ability to work across multiple sectors and with partners (see Chapter 12). It is abundantly clear that in order to address climate change, this will require multiple agencies and partners coming together to take collective action. Moreover, the ability for practitioners to work both in bottom-up and in top-down approaches seems crucial for both encouraging grass-roots activism and in addressing stakeholders and decision-makers at global levels.

WAR AND TERRORISM

In recent times, there has been an unprecedented focus in relation to the impact of war and terrorism on communities and societies. War and collective violence cause more deaths globally than disease or illness (Sidel and Levy, 2008). War can clearly cause mortality and morbidity and profound human suffering is undeniable (Warwick-Booth and Cross, 2018b), including:

- disruption to families, communities and sometimes entire cultures, including forcing people to leave their homes and become displaced;
- the diversion of resources away from the promotion and protection of health, medical care and other health and social services;
- the degradation of the physical environment of countries.

(Sidel and Levy, 2008)

CASE STUDY 4.1: ARMED CONFLICT IN COLOMBIA

Research by Ricaurte et al. (2019) assessed the relation between exposure to the armed conflict and violence with mental health disorders in Colombia. Their analysis showed that 3 per cent of the population in Colombia had been victims of a violent crime and 13 per cent victims of the armed conflict. Victims of the armed conflict had 1.74 times higher odds of suffering mental health disorders compared to non-victims.

Evidence also shows a rise in the number of far-right extremism incidents and associated deaths in parts of Western Europe and North America (Tremblay, 2019). These devastating incidents have had irreversible damage on communities and have highlighted deep divisions in society, based on religion, politics and ideology. Extreme violence – designed to cause maximum disruption and shock – has created huge consequences for health systems. Moreover, the fear of terrorism is also not inconsequential – simply the fear and disruption that this can cause to people is, in itself, detrimental to mental health and well-being. Terrorism is designed to induce fear and moreover can create situations where people are frightened to do their normal activities.

Given the scale of the impact of war and terrorism, it may seem unusual to anticipate that health promotion can provide meaningful support. Nevertheless, some believe that health promotion offers several answers, including: (1) surveillance and documentation; (2) education and awareness-raising; (3) advocacy for sound policies and programmes;

(4) implementation of programmes aimed at both prevention and the provision of acute and long-term care (Sidel and Levy, 2008).

FRAGILE AND VULNERABLE SETTINGS

While quite ambiguous in the title proposed by WHO (2019a), fragile and vulnerable settings refer to countries where challenges such as drought, famine, conflict and population displacement, coupled with weak health services, leave them without access to basic care. There are several countries which could be described as 'fragile' and, indeed, such categorisations can be seen as unfair or even inaccurate. Dixey (2013) has argued cogently that health promotion in Africa has considerable scope for development. Indeed, others have argued that health promotion is a Eurocentric idea (MacDonald, 1998) which has progressed at a faster rate than in other continents. In relation to the Ottawa Charter, one overwhelming critique has been that it was, in effect, exclusionary in its approach with its focus on the Western, industrialised nations (Nutbeam, 2008), excluding other communities around the world: 'the discourse informing the development of the Ottawa Charter masked underpinning power imbalances and Western-centric worldviews, while also silencing non-Western voices' (McPhail-Bell et al., 2013: 27).

Loss of trained health workers in sub-Saharan Africa, due to migration, death and other issues, threatens the sustainability of health systems in many African states. The crisis facing healthcare systems raises a larger and more fundamental question of whether healthcare workforce planning based on 'Western' models are sustainable (Dixey, 2013). Despite these considerable challenges, which are significant, several countries in the African continent have a clear commitment to health promotion and preventive models – Ghana, as an example, has an explicit health promotion department with dedicated resource and budget. That said, Amuyunzu-Nyamongo et al. (2009) point to six areas which require attention if health promotion is to develop in Africa. These are:

1. to invest in health;
2. to develop more robust health systems;
3. to build capacity in health promotion;
4. to work within traditional and new settings;
5. to cultivate political will;
6. to generate evidence of health promotion effectiveness.

We are suggesting that health promotion offers some, not all, of the answers to the contemporary challenges in fragile settings. If the African continent is to take forward the health promotion agenda, the infrastructure of research and training requires strengthening. Outside South Africa, the academic infrastructure for health promotion is under-developed, and where health promotion is offered, it tends to be as part of a medically dominated university public health department (Dixey, 2013).

EBOLA AND OTHER HIGH-THREAT PATHOGENS

Globalisation has created considerable benefits to health, but also significant challenges. The spread of disease and viruses are now, arguably, far more likely given the ability for people to travel across borders. The coronavirus, for example, in 2020 spread quickly from Wuhan in China soon after Chinese New Year celebrations and the numbers of people travelling to celebrate with friends and family. The traditional public health response to control the spread of viruses and other disease is relatively well rehearsed – with surveillance of disease and quarantine procedures well understood in most parts of the world. Health promotion, with its social model of health and distinct value-set, also has a role to play in disease emergencies (see Box 4.2).

BOX 4.2 COVID-19 AND THE ROLE OF HEALTH PROMOTERS AND EDUCATORS

The global health challenges that have been posed by COVID-19 have been far-reaching, devastating and tragic. Arguably, the response of health promoters was slow in reacting to COVID-19, but evidence has shown that health promoters play a critical role in pandemics (Laverack and Manoncourt, 2016). Elsewhere, it has been argued that a settings approach in health promotion, the fostering of critical health literacy and 'salutogenesis' may be worthy of further debate and discussion in health promotion's response (Woodall, 2020a). These are briefly described below:

- A settings approach in health promotion – a settings approach has been viewed as a plausible way to strengthen public health responses to COVID-19. Any effective activity is ensured when settings 'join up' and work mutually to ensure holistic and integrated activities. This pandemic has perhaps amplified frailties in settings working together – how health messages from schools to homes are communicated, for example, or how health activities are managed and co-ordinated in environments where people live in close-proximity (prisons, care homes, etc.). Settings are discussed in more detail in Chapters 13, 14 and 15.
- Critical health literacy – scholars have noted the importance of health communication during COVID-19 and the importance of critical health literacy (Abel and McQueen, 2020). There are several examples where untrustworthy sources have caught the public imagination and have provided illegitimate concerns, including xenophobia (Shimizu, 2020). In many cases this is perpetuated by social media (through statements such as #ChineseDon'tComeToJapan) that can circulate stories quickly, highlighting the need not only for critical health literacy but also digital health literacy for individuals in responding appropriately. One essential role for

(Continued)

> health educators is to translate this information into credible sources to promote public understanding and provide accurate and timely information in culturally specific ways.
> • Salutogenesis - there is no doubt that a focus on pathogenesis is absolutely fundamental during COVID-19 and the role of disease prevention central. However, it may also be important not to lose sight of the question, 'What makes people healthy?' Data is continually emphasising that COVID-19 impacts disproportionately on certain groups in our communities. How the health promotion and education community supports these groups now and when the recovery post-COVID commences is fundamental to ensure that these groups are not further marginalised.

Community participation is a backbone of health promotion (Green et al., 2019) and can be a hugely effective strategy in addressing high-threat pathogens. Laverack (2017) has suggested how the bottom-up philosophy, which forms a central part of health promotion practice, has a key role in disease emergencies and outbreaks. It is suggested that in relation to these threats, health promotion can play a crucial role in:

• Rapid data collection
• Communication
• Community engagement
• Rumour management
• Conflict resolution
• Promotion of vaccination
• Education leading to behaviour change and empowerment
• Building support mechanisms.

The outbreak of the Ebola virus in West Africa, particularly in Guinea, Liberia and Sierra Leone, between 2014 and 2016, demonstrated the value of community engagement and participation in efforts to control the virus transmission. There was a view that during the crises there was a tendency to adopt 'pre-packaged and top-down approaches' which may have potentially worsened the effects. However, observers commented that community engagement offered an added value through the self-management of quarantines, control of cross-border movement, safe and dignified burials, and the siting of community care centres (Laverack and Manoncourt, 2016).

WEAK PRIMARY HEALTHCARE

The WHO (2019a) have identified weak primary healthcare as a contemporary health challenge. This is particularly identified in low- and middle-income countries, but also the demand placed on primary healthcare in all parts of the world is unsustainable. Health promotion has had a long-standing relationship with primary care (Green et al., 2019), often seen as aligning coherently with the prevention agenda.

The situation in primary care services – where service demand often outstrips supply – has been seen as a 'wicked' health problem and difficult to solve (Southby and Gamsu, 2018). With increasing demands placed on primary healthcare, there have been calls to encourage more self-care, but also calls for the voluntary and community sector to support patients who may not require medical intervention – this has been described as 'social prescribing'. Social prescribing schemes are very new, but have become more popular in recent times (Pescheny et al., 2018). Social prescribing services and programmes have grown quickly as a result of the growing voluntary and community sector's role in health and intense pressure on primary care services to manage patients presenting conditions that can be addressed without medical intervention (South et al., 2008). Such schemes provide GPs with non-clinical choices that can be delivered alongside existing primary care services to improve individuals' health and well-being (Bickerdike et al., 2017). Frequently patients are referred to befriending services, nature-based activities, volunteering opportunities, debt advice, bereavement groups or prescribed hobbies (Kilgarriff-Foster and O'Cathain, 2015; Pescheny et al., 2018; South et al., 2008). Social prescribing resonates with health promotion ideas as it has been defined as: 'harness[ing] assets within the voluntary and community sectors to improve and encourage self-care and facilitate health-creating communities' (Moffatt et al., 2017: 1). Social prescribing is often delivered using link workers or social prescribers who are trained to act as the broker between primary care services and organisations in the voluntary and community sector (Kilgarriff-Foster and O'Cathain, 2015; South et al., 2008). The link workers' ability to understand a social and holistic view of health is critical to the success of the schemes and moreover their interpersonal qualities are essential in the execution of social prescribing schemes and patients' satisfaction of the service – a finding reiterated throughout the literature (Bertotti et al., 2018; Moffatt et al., 2017; South et al., 2008).

CASE STUDY 4.2: SOCIAL PRESCRIBING

A social prescribing service in the UK used 'wellbeing coordinators' to support patients and divert them away from primary care services. The service showed improvements in participants' well-being, and perceived levels of health and social connectedness as well as reductions in anxiety as a result of the services. In many cases, the social prescribing service had enabled individuals to have a more positive and optimistic view of their life often through offering opportunities to engage in a range of hobbies and activities in the local community. Some of the processes which increased the likelihood of success on the social prescribing scheme included the sustained and flexible relationship between the service user and the 'wellbeing coordinator' and a strong and vibrant voluntary and community sector (Woodall, Trigwell et al., 2018).

NON-COMMUNICABLE DISEASES

Non-communicable diseases account for 70 per cent of all worldwide deaths, some of which accounts for people dying prematurely (WHO, 2019a). The rise of non-communicable diseases is attributed to five issues: tobacco use; physical inactivity; the harmful use of alcohol; unhealthy diets; and air pollution. Non-communicable diseases have traditionally been seen as a Westernised problem, but many nations in Africa and Asia are seeing challenges such as obesity, diabetes and cardiovascular disease (Lunyera et al., 2018).

Health promotion has historically addressed 'lifestyle issues' through using a range of approaches, but most prominently behaviour change approaches. These have been outlined in the previous chapter. The recognition that non-communicable disease can be addressed through behaviour change alone is short-sighted and moreover some of the more effective approaches to such issues cannot be addressed only by changing individual behaviour. The obesity challenge, which is commonly associated with a rise in non-communicable diseases, has been most effectively addressed through 'whole systems' approaches which recognise that obesity is caused through a range of factors. Bagnall et al. (2019) identified several factors which supported a whole systems approach to tackling obesity and other public health challenges:

1. Strong leadership and full engagement of partners
2. Engaging the local community in activities and interventions
3. Ensuring time to build relationships, trust and community capacity
4. Good governance and shared values
5. Appropriate partnerships to allow environmental changes
6. Consistency in language used across organisations delivering interventions to avoid confusion
7. Evaluating ongoing progress
8. Financial support and resources.

Health promotion is well positioned to help address non-communicable disease, not through addressing lifestyle issues necessarily (though important) but highlighting and addressing the social and economic circumstances which cause lifestyles. This is important as focusing on behaviour alone will be ineffective, say to tackle obesity, unless the social context is broadly supportive.

MENTAL HEALTH

There has been a growing recognition of the importance of mental health – some may suggest that this falls significantly short of the efforts still placed on physical health dimensions (Warwick-Booth and Cross, 2018b). According to WHO (2019b) poor mental health leads to premature death, human rights violations and global and national economic loss.

There are now global efforts to address mental health, which are primarily based on the recognition that:

- There can be no health or sustainable development without mental health.
- Depression and anxiety disorders cost the global economy US$1 trillion per year.
- There are 800,000 deaths from suicide, which is a leading cause of death in young people.
- People with mental health conditions often experience severe human rights violations, discrimination and stigma (WHO, 2019b).

In relation to the contribution of health promotion, there has been a tradition to focus on mental health promotion and more positive conceptualisations of mental health. In this regard, there has been increasing attention on mental health promotion for young people – in response to the modern challenges that social media can play in young people's health and well-being. However, this has been seen far less in low- and middle-income countries. Interventions that promote positive mental health in young people can provide them with the necessary life skills, supports and resources to fulfil their potential and overcome adversity (Barry et al., 2013). Much health promotion in this area has focused on settings where young people engage (see Chapter 14) and systematic review evidence has demonstrated the utility of schools for promoting mental health. There is particularly robust evidence to suggest that school-based interventions in low- and middle-income countries can have significant positive effects on students' emotional and behavioural well-being, including reduced depression and anxiety and improved coping skills (Barry et al., 2013).

Workplaces are also often used to promote mental health, given that contemporary pressures and a '24-7' culture has led to greater incidences of stress in the workplace. Evidence shows that burnout in workplaces is becoming more common – burnout is 'a prolonged response to long-term emotional and interpersonal stressors on the job. The key dimensions of this response are overwhelming exhaustion, feelings of cynicism and detachment from the job, a sense of ineffectiveness and a lack of accomplishment' (Bagnall et al., 2016). As will be shown in Chapters 13 and 14, a holistic approach to tackling these issues in settings is often seen as being more effective. This means that individual and organisational level approaches combined often produce better health outcomes for people (Bagnall et al., 2016).

REFLECTIVE EXERCISE 4.2

What interventions and activities do you think would be helpful in supporting mental health in workplace settings? Taking into consideration that all workplaces are different, how may the suggested approaches differ between small and medium sized workplaces and multinational companies? Why may some workplaces be reluctant to embed health promotion activities in their organisation?

AGEING POPULATIONS

Population increases in many countries has created significant pressures on the health sector and in providing quality care services. The fact that more and more people will reach their 100th birthday is becoming a reality in many parts of the world. In addition, there is little indication of this shift slowing down – even in developing countries, life expectancy is lengthening at a considerable rate (Christensen et al., 2009). As populations age, so do the incidences of disease and ill health and a greater likelihood of years of illness and disability. One area of growing concern is dementia and the implications this has for health and social care (see Box 4.3).

BOX 4.3 DEMENTIA AS A GLOBAL HEALTH ISSUE

- 50 million people worldwide were living with dementia in 2018. This number will more than triple to 152 million by 2050 (WHO, 2017b).
- Globally over 46 million people are estimated to live with dementia; around 7 per cent of the population over 60 years old (Prince et al., 2013).
- The number of people living with dementia worldwide is estimated at 47.5 million and is projected to increase to 75.6 million by 2030 (WHO, 2017b).
- Rates of dementia are increasing worldwide, with the largest growth in numbers expected amongst those living in low- and middle-income countries (LMICs).
- In 2010, 58 per cent of people with dementia resided in LMICs and this is set to rise to 63 per cent by 2030, and 71 per cent by 2050 (Prince et al., 2013).
- In 2005, the number of people with dementia in Malaysia, a middle-income country, was estimated at 63,000 with 20,100 incident cases per annum. This is projected to be 126,800, with 39,000 annual cases by 2020 (Akter et al., 2012), although this is likely underestimated (Cheong et al., 2018).

Health promotion has a clear research, practice and policy agenda in relation to healthy ageing (see Box 4.4). Indeed, with health promotion's clear prevention focus there is little doubt that such interventions could counter the costs associated with ageing populations in many countries.

BOX 4.4 HEALTHY AGEING

Healthy ageing may be considered as the promotion of healthy living and the prevention and management of illness and disability associated with ageing. Ageing can be thought of as an accumulation of changes over the life course that increases frailty. If we can design and execute effective interventions to prevent or delay the onset of chronic disease and increase healthy life expectancy, there will be social, economic and health dividends for us all.

Source: Age UK, n.d.: 6

A systematic review of evidence (Cattan et al., 2002) showed the value of health promotion in alleviating and addressing social isolation in older people. What proved particularly effective were group activities involving some form of educational or training input and social activities that targeted specific groups of people (i.e. women, care-givers, the widowed, the physically inactive, or people with serious mental health problems). Encouraging volunteer activities has also been shown to be effective in approaches to supporting healthy ageing (Age UK, n.d.), especially for older people acting in volunteer roles who often gain a sense of purpose and improve their own self-confidence and self-esteem.

SUMMARY

This chapter has identified a series of significant health threats and challenges that many countries now face. Perhaps the most acute example of this has been the impact of the recent pandemic, which has devastated national security, economic prosperity and, of course, individual and community life chances and health. The challenges threaten life expectancy and have implications for health systems in almost all parts of the world. This chapter argues that health promotion can play a major role in addressing these challenges and argues that health promotion can be a powerful discipline to foster change and to address challenges differently. As shown later in the book, health promotion has distinct values (see Chapter 6) that can empower and support individuals and communities. Moreover, the breadth of health promotion approaches – crudely characterised as bottom-up and top-down – provides a menu of options for tackling extremely complex issues.

SUGGESTED READING

Laverack, G. (2017) *Health promotion in disease outbreaks and health emergencies*. London, CRC Press.

Warwick-Booth, L. and Cross, R. (2018) *Global health studies: a social determinants perspective*. Cambridge, Polity.

Woodall, J. (2020) COVID-19 and the role of health promoters and educators. Emerald Open Research 2.

INEQUALITIES IN HEALTH

5

INTRODUCTION

A commitment to addressing inequalities in health has been a key concern for health promotion and is a common strand running through this book. This chapter, however, will specifically show how health inequalities exist between individuals and communities, examining this from a global and national perspective. The chapter explores why communities have different health experiences and why, ultimately, some people die sooner than others – not based on their genetic profile necessarily, but on their living and working conditions or, by virtue of where they were born and raised. Explanations for these inequalities are provided using sociology and psychology to provide theoretical insight. The chapter will suggest that one of the key reasons for health promotion practice is to reduce health inequalities in society, but why, in some cases, inequalities in health have widened rather than reduced.

WHAT ARE INEQUALITIES?

Inequalities relate to differences in people's health as a result of a range of social or economic factors. Differences in people's health could relate to how long they live (their life expectancy) or the likelihood of facing a particular condition (e.g. cancer or obesity). Differences in health based on social and economic factors are avoidable and unfair, but manifest consistently in many ways – physical health, mental health, social connectiveness and, of course, many others. Recognising that health inequalities exist suggest we need to reallocate resources not equally but equitably to balance up this unfairness. Some people may argue that in most societies we treat everyone with equal worth and are equitable with resources so that everyone can lead a full and healthy life, but this cannot be the case. Children would not be dying in the 'developing' world due to preventable diseases such as diarrhoea, respiratory infections or measles, whilst others live in some luxury if we readdressed health inequalities (Dixey, Cross, Foster and Woodall, 2013).

There are several ways in which health inequalities have been described and explained. Health inequalities have been documented between population groups across at least four dimensions:

- socio-economic status and deprivation: e.g. unemployed, low income, people living in deprived areas (e.g. poor housing, poor education and/or unemployment);
- protected characteristics: e.g. age, sex, race, sexual orientation, disability;
- vulnerable groups of society, or 'inclusion health' groups: e.g. migrants, Gypsy, Roma and Traveller communities, rough sleepers and homeless people and sex workers;
- geography: e.g. urban, rural.

This is perhaps summed up most effectively by Graham (2007) who suggests three meanings of health inequalities:

1. health differences between individuals;
2. health differences between population groups;
3. health differences between different groups based on the social position they occupy.

Health inequalities are evident between population groups at a global level as well as within countries and within communities. As an example, average global life expectancy at birth in 2016 was 72.0 years ranging from 61.2 years in the WHO African Region to 77.5 years in the WHO European Region (WHO, 2020b). Data on inequalities in health is abundant, whether this is within rich countries such as the UK, between richer countries, such as the USA and Japan, or in poorer countries of the global South (Cross, Rowlands and Foster, 2021). Within countries differences exist yet further – as an example in England's most deprived areas, life expectancy was 74.0 years in the years 2015 to 2017, whereas it was 83.3 years in the least deprived, a gap of 9.3 years. Women in the least deprived areas of England were expected to live 78.7 years in 2015–17, while those in the most affluent were expected to live 86.2 years, a gap of 7.5 years (Iacobucci, 2019). Some differences in life expectancy can literally be seen between two communities in very close proximity, but, as shown, health inequalities manifest also at global and national levels for a range of health indicators and outcomes.

REFLECTIVE EXERCISE 5.1

A version of the London Underground map has been produced to show how life expectancy varies from station to station. Travelling east on the Tube from Westminster, every two Tube stops represented more than a year of life expectancy lost. For example, if you travel eastbound between Lancaster Gate and Mile End - 20 minutes on the Central line - life expectancy decreases by 12 years (Cheshire, 2012). What explanations do you propose cause this inequality in life expectancy? What factors may be at play in creating these differences in life expectancy?

BOX 5.1 INFANT MORTALITY AS AN INDICATOR OF HEALTH INEQUALITIES

Using the example of infant mortality as a crude indicator of health we can map clear health inequalities at local, regional and global levels. If we start with Leeds, which is where the authors are based, we can see differences within the city itself:

- In 2016 in Leeds there were 4.8 infant deaths for every 1000 live births compared with 3.9 for the rest of the country. The most deprived parts of the city had a higher rate (above 5) and the least deprived had a lower rate (below 4).

Moving to the regional level, we can see differences between Yorkshire and Humber (the region where Leeds is located) and the rest of England:

- In 2014-2016, the average infant mortality rate for the whole of England was 3.9 deaths per 1000 live births and 4.1 deaths per 1000 for Yorkshire and Humber. Within the Yorkshire and Humber region, there were variations from 2 (East Riding) to 5.7 (City of Bradford).

There are differences between England and the rest of Europe:

- In 2014-2016, the average infant mortality rate was 3.9 in England per 1000 live births. Compare this with, for example, the highest rates - 6.7 in Malta and Romania - and the lowest - 1.3 in Cyprus or 2 in Finland - whilst the average in Europe in 2017 was 3.6 deaths per 1000 live births.

There are differences between Europe and the rest of the world:

- In 2018, the average infant mortality rate in the countries comprising Latin America and the Caribbean was 14 per 1000 live births compared with the average infant mortality rate in the countries of the European Union, which was 3 per 1000 live births. There is a clear difference here between 'developed' and 'developing' countries.

There are also differences within continents:

- Within the continent of Asia for example, in 2018, the infant mortality rate was 48 per 1000 live births in Afghanistan, compared with 2 per 1000 live births in Japan in the same year. In Africa for the same year South Sudan's IMR was 62 whilst South Africa's was 29.

Source: adapted from Cross, Rowlands and Foster (2021)

SOCIAL CLASS AND HEALTH INEQUALITIES

People's social class has been consistently used by researchers, politicians and health practitioners as a way to examine health differences across groups in society (see Box 5.2). In short, people in the 'higher' socio-economic groups do better on many health indicators compared to people in poorer circumstances working in routine and manual occupations.

Social class is a way of producing a classification or hierarchy of people (Sayani, 2019). Social class can be determined by several factors, but often relates to economic, social and cultural capital – or, in other words, how much wealth, networks and knowledge someone has. Identifying and measuring social class is very difficult and there have been several attempts throughout history to do this. Reports on inequalities in health in the United Kingdom make heavy use of the concept of social class and a five-point social-class classification was the principal classification of socio-economic status used in the UK when it first appeared in the Registrar General's Annual Report for 1911. Analysis using this classification has consistently shown social gradients for a wide range of health indicators, with social classes IV and V having a disproportionate amount of ill health (Hubley et al., 2021). The Registrar General's class schema was one example of how social class was defined – it classified people based on their job role:

    I. Professional
   II. Intermediate
IIIN. Skilled non-manual
IIIM. Skilled manual
  IV. Semi-skilled manual
   V. Unskilled manual

While this classification was, and remains, popular, it has faced some strong critique. It is based, fundamentally, on employment relations and therefore is quite narrow in its focus – social class is made up of far more than occupation (Savage et al., 2013). More recently, researchers have developed a more sophisticated way of approaching class, looking at cultural, social and economic capitals (using different measures of economic capital, including household income, but also savings and the value of owner-occupied housing) which provides seven classes (Savage et al., 2013):

1. Elite (e.g. barristers and judges)
2. Established middle class (e.g. police officers)
3. Technical middle class (e.g. pharmacists)
4. New affluent workers (e.g. sales and retail assistants)
5. Traditional working class (e.g. electrical and electronic technicians)
6. Emergent service workers (e.g. chefs)
7. Precariat (e.g. cleaners).

BOX 5.2 BLACK REPORT TO THE MARMOT REVIEW

Social class has been used throughout as a variable to see how disease patterns vary based on these classifications. The Black Report of 1980 was the first major report in the UK to highlight how health is systematically related to social class (Cross, Warwick-Booth and Foster, 2021). Later work has continued to look closely at health inequalities – perhaps the most significant being the Marmot review of the social determinants of health that highlights the role of psychosocial factors in explaining the differences in health between social groups. Professor Sir Michael Marmot in his report *Fair Society, Healthy Lives* (Marmot, 2010) emphasised the link between health and social groups, showing that the lower a person's social position, the worse his or her health. Marmot argues that a reduction in health inequalities requires the following action:

- Give every child the best start in life;
- Enable all children, young people and adults to maximise their capabilities and have control over their lives;
- Create fair employment and good work for all;
- Ensure a healthy standard of living for all;
- Create and develop healthy and sustainable places and communities;
- Strengthen the role and impact of ill health prevention.

Health Equity in England: The Marmot Review 10 Years On (Marmot et al., 2020) examined the decade that had passed since the publication of the original Marmot Review in 2010 (Marmot, 2010). Despite the set of recommendations that were made to government in the original review there has been a slowing in improvements in life expectancy, and in some areas it even went down (Marmot et al., 2020).

As noted, social class impacts on health. You are more likely to die sooner if you are in a lower social class position (Green et al., 2019). People of lower socio-economic status are more likely to experience mental health problems – those who are unemployed or economically inactive have higher rates of common mental health problems than those who are employed (Mental Health Foundation, 2020). Moreover, obesity is linked to social class and socio-economic status; however, these differ according to whether they are measured in lower- or higher-income countries. In higher-income countries, levels of obesity are greater in the lower social classes, and this is associated with a poorer diet (Warwick-Booth and Cross, 2018b). Box 5.4 in the chapter shows some of the explanations for why health inequalities occur. In relation to social class, there is little doubt that a materialist or structuralist explanation is very persuasive. Being materially deprived in terms of income and employment can reduce people's access to important health resources – as an example people on lower social class groups may not have a car and may be more likely to not attend important cancer-screening programmes (Sayani, 2019). There may also be implications for accessing fresh produce and food for those on lower incomes. This can result in people feeling a lack of control over their health and their social circumstance which can be highly stressful which in turn affects biological pathways that impact negatively on health (known as a psycho-social impact) (Warwick-Booth et al., 2012).

REFLECTIVE EXERCISE 5.2

Could a consensus be formed whereby we *accept* that some people will predictably have healthier lives than others and live longer and happier? Similarly, people will also experience differences based on whether they are in a highly industrialised economy or from developing nations? Put simply, isn't inequality a natural by-product of the economically prosperous lives that most of us wish to lead?

As a health promoter, why would you argue against this statement? How would you potentially challenge this view of inequalities? What counter-arguments would you develop and how would you articulate or communicate the necessity for more equal societies? Can you hold capitalist viewpoints and also be committed to reductions in health inequalities and improvements in health equity?

ETHNICITY AND HEALTH INEQUALITIES

Ethnicity is a term defined by some as: 'a form of collective identity that draws on notions of shared ancestry, cultural commonality, geographical origins and shared biological features' (Salway et al., 2014: 4–5). The data is unequivocal in demonstrating that people, based on their ethnicity, face disproportionate health challenges. These relate to several outcomes; for example, experiences of discrimination and exclusion (including the fear of such negative incidents) have been shown to impact on health (Toleikyte and Salway, 2018). To equate poor health with differences based on biology is therefore incorrect (Bartley, 2017).

There are some challenges to recording people's ethnicity. Terminology does vary (see Box 5.3) and, in many countries, data is collected via a national census where individuals can self-declare their ethnicity (Bartley, 2017). Often when analyses are done on data based on ethnicity, the categorisation can be extremely broad. So, for example, 'Black African' or 'White British' is a very broad classification and somewhat unhelpful for understanding the data or in designing appropriate and culturally tailored interventions, programmes and policy.

BOX 5.3 TERMINOLOGY

Terminology relating to ethnicity varies. Terms such as: 'ethnic group' and 'minority ethnic' are seen in the literature. Other common terms used in English health publications include 'Black, Asian and minority ethnic' (BAME), 'Black and minority ethnic' (BME) and 'ethnic minority groups'.

While it is not possible to report all health outcomes for all ethnicities, a brief list of some of the health inequalities faced by some groups includes:

- Individuals identifying as Gypsy or Irish Traveller, and to a lesser extent those identifying as Bangladeshi, Pakistani or Irish, stand out as having poor health across a range of indicators.
- Black men have higher reported rates of psychotic disorder than men in other ethnic groups.
- Prostate cancer makes up over 40 per cent of Black men's cancer compared with around 15 per cent among Chinese men and 25 per cent among all men.
- The National Child Measurement Programme in England indicates that among children most minority ethnic groups have higher levels of overweight or obesity at age 10–11 than the White majority. Those in Black groups have the highest levels.

(Data from Toleikyte and Salway, 2018)

Inequalities in health as a result of ethnicity reflects other inequalities in terms of socioeconomic position and social class. Therefore, it is a complicated and complex web of interacting factors and issues. A recent example of this was COVID-19 and how people's living conditions could have a detrimental impact (see Box 5.4).

BOX 5.4 COVID-19 SHOWS HEALTH INEQUALITIES IN SOCIETY

COVID-19 has exposed deep inequalities in society. Data has shown that deaths and people experiencing COVID-19 were disproportionately Black or from another minority ethnic background. People from Black, Asian and minority ethnic communities are more likely to live in densely populated urban areas and are often overly represented in high-risk key worker jobs (The Health Foundation, 2020).

There is also evidence that shows how people from some ethnicities are less likely to seek healthcare services or advice. The lack of accessible information, language barriers, poorer knowledge about services, inadequate surgery premises and longer waits for appointments all contribute to difficulties in terms of healthcare access (Evandrou et al., 2016). Imagine walking into primary care services and feeling that they in no way reflect your background, cultural identification, language or rituals? This can have significant consequences in terms of delayed treatment and management of conditions (Marlow et al., 2015).

CASE STUDY 5.1: BARRIERS TO CERVICAL CANCER SCREENING AMONG ETHNIC MINORITY WOMEN: A QUALITATIVE STUDY

Background Ethnic minority women are less likely to attend cervical screening.

Aim To explore self-perceived barriers to cervical screening attendance among ethnic minority women compared to white British women.

Design Qualitative interview study.

Setting Community groups in ethnically diverse London boroughs.

Methods Interviews were carried out with 43 women from a range of ethnic minority backgrounds (Indian, Pakistani, Bangladeshi, Caribbean, African, Black British, Black other, White other) and 11 White British women. Interviews were recorded, transcribed verbatim and analysed using Framework analysis.

Results Fifteen women had delayed screening/had never been screened. Ethnic minority women felt that there was a lack of awareness about cervical cancer in their community, and several did not recognise the terms 'cervical screening' or 'smear test'. Barriers to cervical screening raised by all women were emotional (fear, embarrassment, shame), practical (lack of time) and cognitive (low perceived risk, absence of symptoms). Emotional barriers seemed to be more prominent among Asian women. Low perceived risk of cervical cancer was influenced by beliefs about having sex outside of marriage and some women felt a diagnosis of cervical cancer might be considered shameful. Negative experiences were well remembered by all women and could be a barrier to repeat attendance.

Conclusions Emotional barriers (fear, embarrassment and anticipated shame) and low perceived risk might contribute to explaining lower cervical screening coverage for some ethnic groups. Interventions to improve knowledge and understanding of cervical cancer are needed in ethnic minority communities, and investment in training for health professionals may improve experiences and encourage repeat attendance for all women.

Source: Marlow et al. (2015)

GENDER AND HEALTH INEQUALITIES

Data shows that women live longer than men, but spend fewer years in good health (EuroHealthNet, n.d.). Like other sections in this book, the relationship is complex but we know that social structures do not, and continue to not, favour women. That could relate to progression in workplaces; pay and salary; expectations for childcare and family responsibility; sexism and many, many others. Patriarchy – a social system where men hold power and political authority – is a major obstacle to women achieving their full potential and it remains difficult to maintain issues in the political spotlight, such as: gender-based violence, traditions harmful to women (such as genital cutting), sexual harassment and forced marriage (Cross, Warwick-Booth and Foster, 2021). Patriarchy is apparent in many situations and contexts – in Zambia, for example, men hold the power over money within most family contexts (Warwick-Booth et al., 2012).

CASE STUDY 5.2: THE STATE OF WOMEN'S HEALTH IN LEEDS

- Twice as many women as men are recorded as having a common mental health disorder. Black women, asylum seekers, refugees, and Gypsy and Traveller women have higher rates of common mental health issues and are less likely to receive mental health treatment.
- Women are more likely than men to become addicted to smoking, alcohol and drugs and find it harder to stop.
- 30% of women accessing support for drug/alcohol treatment have a mental health condition, compared to 21% of men.
- Problem gambling – predominately seen in men – is now increasing for women.
- More women than men are diagnosed as underweight.
- Women over 65 years have twice as many emergency admissions due to a fall as men.

Source: Thomas and Warwick-Booth (2019)

REFLECTIVE EXERCISE 5.3

Take one of the statements presented in the case study above and try to explain why there is a difference in the health issues between men and women. Discuss why these inequalities are happening in a large city in the UK with good access to healthcare services?

MARGINALISED POPULATIONS AND HEALTH INEQUALITIES

Data on many sources of inequalities go uncollected, particularly certain populations – information on the health of refugees, asylum seekers, prisoners, the homeless, and a range of other marginalised groups is not available (Cross, Rowlands and Foster, 2021). In many cases, albeit, not all, many marginalised populations face complex challenges. It is difficult to ascertain the number of people faced with severe and multiple disadvantage (Rankin and Regan, 2004), although the estimated figures are not inconsequential. Over 250,000 people in England have contact with at least two out of three of the homelessness, substance misuse and/or criminal justice systems and at least 58,000 people have contact with all three (Bramley et al., 2015). Evidence suggests that severe and multiple disadvantage results from myriad factors including structural, systemic, family and personal influences (Bramley et al., 2015) – resonating strongly with ecological views of health promotion which seek to intervene at macro, meso and micro levels (McLeroy et al., 1988). The lack of affordable, available or suitable accommodation is a tangible illustration of a structural factor that impedes intervention with people with multiple and complex need (Macias Balda, 2016). Other systemic challenges include poor management sharing and a lack of collective recording processes across agencies working toward supporting those with severe and multiple disadvantage (CLES, 2016). This can mean that individuals 'fall through the gaps' of service provision (Bringewatt and Gershoff, 2010, Warwick-Booth and Cross, 2018a). Finally, unsupportive interpersonal relationships, irregular contact with care services and fractured family dynamics may also characterise the experiences of people facing severe and multiple disadvantage (Social Exclusion Unit, 2002).

We will focus briefly on inequalities facing people in prison specifically. People in prison undoubtedly face significant health challenges to a greater extent to those in the wider community. This relates to almost all health outcomes, but particularly in regard to mental health. De Viggiani (2006) has argued that both 'deprivation' and 'importation factors' are significant health determinants within prison. This suggests that there are factors caused by imprisonment that contribute to ill health and those which are a result of circumstances which pre-dated someone's prison sentence. For example, deprivation factors are based on the premise that imprisonment deprives individuals and renders them powerless. Prison from this perspective is viewed as being counterproductive and harmful to prisoners' health. In contrast, importation factors focus on prisoners' past experiences, biographies and demographic characteristics that influence their negotiation of prison life (Gover et al., 2000).

Prisons are settings in which the health needs of those from marginalised and disempowered groups can be addressed (Woodall, 2020). This has the potential to improve individual health outcomes and lessen health inequalities and improve health equity. There have been some promising signs of individual countries developing their own approaches to delivering a healthy settings approach in prison – England and Wales (Department of Health, 2002) and Scotland (Scottish Prison Service, 2002), for example, have led the way by adopting clear strategies for health promotion in prison. In other countries there has been far less activity – in Norway and in Ireland, for instance, there are no dedicated policies for health promotion in prison (MacNamara and Mannix-McNamara, 2014; Santora et al., 2014) and in several Eastern European regions there is no resource for health promotion in prison (MacDonald et al., 2013). In extreme cases, some countries in sub-Saharan Africa are reported to run prisons that are unjust, unhealthy and sites of human rights abuses (Dixey et al., 2015). These differences often relate to resource allocation and, in some instances, ideological views on who is deserving or not in regard to health intervention.

WHY DO HEALTH INEQUALITIES EXIST?

There are several theories concerning why health inequalities exist in societies. We have grouped these in Box 5.5.

BOX 5.5 EXPLAINING HEALTH INEQUALITIES

ARTEFACT EXPLANATION

This position suggests that the differences seen in health (life expectancy, illness, etc.) between groups is a result of the way variables, like social class, are measured and due to challenges in gathering accurate data. The relationship between class and health is not real, but is instead artificial or statistical anomaly. Overwhelmingly, however, this explanation has been discounted as a way of understanding and explaining health inequalities as evidence clearly shows differences between social class and health. Some groups still argue that this is not the case.

SOCIAL SELECTION

This theory suggest that people with better health tend to occupy higher social class positions. Health therefore has consequences for social life and success or failure in the labour market and class structure. Good health provides upward social mobility, whereas poor health has a downward impact on social mobility.

CULTURAL/BEHAVIOURAL EXPLANATION

This theory suggests that health behaviours are associated with cultural influences and therefore causes increases in disease. In short certain social groups 'choose' an unhealthy lifestyle because of either fatalism, recklessness of ignorance and therefore at higher risk of poor health. Lower social classes experience poorer health because they choose to smoke more, drink more, eat sugary foods, etc. This position, however, has been viewed as victim blaming and having an overly individualistic view on how health and disease patterns occur in society - failing to fully consider wider social influences.

MATERIALIST OR STRUCTURALIST EXPLANATION

The inequalities that are presented in society are due to material differences in people's lives such as unemployment or poor living conditions. This can lead to chronic stress and impact negatively on health. This, for many, is the most plausible theory for health inequalities.

WHY ARE HEALTH INEQUALITIES WIDENING?

There have been significant interventions to try to rebalance health inequalities operating at individual and state (government) levels (see Chapters 10 and 11). In many cases, there has been an expectation that in many countries life expectancy and quality of life will increase for us all. There is a long-held assumption that your generation will live longer than the previous generation as a result of improved healthcare and eradication of diseases and conditions through prevention activities. Throughout the twentieth century, the UK saw significant increases in life expectancy. Of people born in 1905, only 62 per cent lived to 60 compared with 89 per cent of those born in 1955. For people born today, 96 per cent can be expected to live to 60 (Marshall et al., 2019).

This improving historical picture is not now the case: 'The UK has been seen as a world leader in identifying and addressing health inequalities but something dramatic is happening' (Marmot et al., 2020: 5).

GO FURTHER 5.1

Advances in public health and healthcare in the last century drove big improvements in life expectancy: the eradication of many infectious diseases in the 1950s and 1960s, reductions in smoking rates from the mid-1970s, advances in treatment of heart disease in the 1990s and, more recently, better diagnosis and treatment of cancer (Marshall et al., 2019).

Societies have already made significant gains in life expectancy, so is it becoming increasingly difficult to achieve further big improvements? Discuss this statement and try to consider how life expectancy and quality of life can continue to improve further. Where or what would you prioritise to achieve these gains?

We have seen a stalling in life expectancy as a result of a wide range of factors which broadly relate to social and economic determinants (see Box 5.5). Some of these have been political decisions by governments not to invest substantially in improving people's living and social conditions. This is indeed an ideological position and relates back to whose responsibility poor health is and whether health inequalities are in themselves seen as a statistical artefact or a matter of individual choice.

BOX 5.6 STALLING LIFE EXPECTANCY IN ENGLAND

The evidence we compile in this 'ten years on' report, commissioned by the Health Foundation, explores what has happened since the Marmot Review of 2010. Austerity has taken its toll in all the domains set out in the Marmot Review.

> From rising child poverty and the closure of children's centres, to declines in education funding, an increase in precarious work and zero hours contracts, to a housing affordability crisis and a rise in homelessness, to people with insufficient money to lead a healthy life and resorting to foodbanks in large numbers, to ignored communities with poor conditions and little reason for hope. And these outcomes, on the whole, are even worse for minority ethnic population groups and people with disabilities. We cannot say with certainty which of these adverse trends might be responsible for the worsening health picture in England. Some, such as the increase in child poverty, will mostly show their effects in the long term. We can say, though, that austerity has adversely affected the social determinants that impact on health in the short, medium and long term. Austerity will cast a long shadow over the lives of the children born and growing up under its effects.
>
> (Marmot et al., 2020: 5)

Health promoters, whose remit leans heavily on reducing inequalities, should be concerned by the current picture of widening health inequalities. Epidemiological data showing the life expectancy of the poorest and wealthiest widening is troubling. This is happening in many countries across the world. Indeed, it may be time for an increased focus on 'big picture health promotion' (Cross, Warwick-Booth and Foster, 2021) which looks at important, but complex, factors concerning our health and well-being. Yet, even the most optimistic health promoter will be aware that such a call to action is difficult and such rhetoric for 'big picture health promotion' has been around for many decades now (St Leger, 1997). Climate change and globalisation are just two examples where health promoters can work towards making change through activism, lobbying and raising health consciousness. Developing countries are ill-equipped to cope with the forces of globalisation and furthermore have seen a decline in their independent policy-making capacity, whilst having to accept the policies made by outside agencies (Cross, Warwick-Booth and Foster, 2021). The fact that Coca-Cola can be purchased in even the most remote parts of the world suggests the forces of globalised marketing. Health promotion, as a global profession, needs to question whether as a community we are doing enough to challenge this.

SUMMARY

Health inequalities are differences in outcomes – like how long we live and the chances of becoming unwell – as a result of a range of social and environmental factors. While this chapter has only just touched upon some of the main issues, it is clear that factors such as someone's gender, their ethnicity and their social position have significant impacts on their health. There are several explanations for why this happens, but most commonly material disadvantage plays a huge role. The role of health promotion is to undoubtedly tackle health inequalities and yet there are indications that current efforts are not enough. Life expectancy is not continuing to rise as it once was and the health gap between the wealthiest and poorest in many countries is widening. The impact of forces such as climate change and globalisation cannot be underplayed here and requires health promoters to adopt new ways of working to reverse the trend of growing health inequalities in society.

SUGGESTED READING

Bartley, M. (2017) *Health inequality: an introduction to concepts, theories and methods.* Cambridge, Polity Press.

Marmot, M., Allen, J., Boyce, T., Goldblatt, P. and Morrison, J. (2020) *Health equity in England: the Marmot Review 10 years on.* London, Institute of Health Equity.

Warwick-Booth, L. and Cross, R. (2018) *Global health studies: a social determinants perspective.* Cambridge, Polity Press.

THE IMPORTANCE OF HEALTH PROMOTION VALUES

6

INTRODUCTION

In continuing this section on *why* health promotion is important, we turn to the importance of values and how they provide a coherent backdrop to health promotion endeavours and more practically guidance for action. We suggest in this chapter that values provide the discipline of health promotion with a unique edge which positions it apart from other approaches to health improvement and protection. There are several values synonymous in health promotion; some of these are not unique to health promotion (such as equality and social justice), but collectively these demarcate health promotion from other disciplines such as health education and public health. The chapter presents values based on both desired outcomes (i.e. what health promoters should view as end goals, like health equity or social justice) and processes or ways of achieving these goals (i.e. autonomy of individuals and participation).

We are not uncritical of values in health promotion and challenge the notion of values in health promotion arguing that the practice and policy of health promotion is often inconsistent. The chapter outlines some of the tensions between values, practice and evidence.

WHAT ARE VALUES?

We all operate by a set of values. These often guide the way we live our life and the decisions we take. Some of these have been passed to us via family traditions or social norms and others may be personally defined through our moral or political beliefs. Our values help shape the people we are and influence the way we communicate, the way we conduct ourselves and interact with others and how we approach life issues. Nevertheless, few of us will not have thought fully about what our own core values are. People may be consciously aware of the values they hold, but, in some cases, people can hold subconscious values that they are not fully aware of. Some of us, for example, may hold 'kindness' and 'honesty' as a core value (though we may not have thought about it as a value, rather an intuitive thing to do) and our behaviours become consistent with this.

According to the literature, values are end states or behaviours that we hold as important and that we take with us across the various domains of our life (in work, in relationships, etc.) (Schwartz and Bilsky, 1987). According to some of the key theorists on values (see Rokeach (1973)), humans hold relatively few values – indeed as you are reading this, you may be struggling to really articulate or think through what values you hold. Most of us will not have an extensive list of values but would hold three or four that are important to us. Often people rank these and identify which hold more importance than others (Schwartz and Bilsky, 1987). There is also a great deal of overlap in the values that people have, but these may be held to a greater or lesser extent – as an example, some may hold politeness as a value, but some would value this more than others. In addition, our values are shaped by the society that we live in – religious beliefs and cultural traditions can influence our personal value base.

REFLECTIVE EXERCISE 6.1

Think about the values that you adopt in your daily life. Try to list all of the values and try to rank them into an order of importance. If you feel able to, share these with someone else and compare the two lists. Where are there commonalities and differences? What values concern 'end goals' and which are about general principles of behaving and interacting?

AN OVERVIEW OF VALUES IN HEALTH PROMOTION

Many professions and disciplines have explicit values. Nursing, for instance, holds altruism, autonomy, human dignity, integrity and social justice as key influences on professional practice (Shaw and Degazon, 2008). Health promotion is no different in being driven by values. However, there is not an agreed 'set' which can be referred to, with different professional organisations, bodies and institutions in health promotion subscribing to different and nuanced positions (see Box 6.1). This is arguably quite surprising given that health promotion is a relatively small professional discipline with less than a handful of major global bodies. Perhaps this is because many health promotion professionals hold tacit assumptions about practice and yet this is not always helpful as it can promote inconsistencies and a lack of clarity.

BOX 6.1 PROFESSIONAL VALUES

The International Union for Health Promotion and Education (IUHPE) are committed to a series of values which they believe will enable professionals to ensure that everyone achieves optimum health and well-being. These values include:

- Respect - for the innate dignity of all people; for cultural identity; for cultural diversity; and for natural resources and the environment;
- Inclusion and involvement of people in making the decisions that shape their lives and impact upon their health and well-being;
- Equity in health, social and economic outcomes for all people;
- Accountability and transparency - within governments, organisations and communities;
- Sustainability;
- Social justice for all people; and
- Compassion and empowerment.

Source: IUHPE (2018)

However, in contrast, the Galway consensus (Barry et al., 2009), which outlines global competencies for health promoters, sees the core values of the discipline slightly differently. For example, these include:

- A social-ecologic model of health that takes into account the cultural, economic and social determinants of health;
- A commitment to equity, civil society and social justice; a respect for cultural diversity and sensitivity.

A dedication to sustainable development; and a participatory approach to engaging the population in identifying needs, setting priorities, and planning, implementing and evaluating the practical and feasible health promotion solutions to address needs.

As already noted, values are culturally shaped and structured and the same is true in the values espoused in health promotion. Take, as an example, the Health Promotion Forum of New Zealand – their values position is heavily influenced by Te Tiriti o Waitangi, a document that is central within the history and political constitution of the state of New Zealand, and the concept of hauora (well-being). Clearly these values are culturally contextualised and resonate with practice in that part of the world. Taken from the Health Promotion Forum of New Zealand (2012: 9), the values encompass:

- **Te Tiriti o Waitangi** – Respect for, and commitment to, and protection of Te Tiriti o Waitangi, including the application of Te Tiriti o Waitangi to the actions and everyday practice of health promotion
- **human rights** – Respect for and commitment to hauora as everyone's right based on the mana and dignity of people, communities and individuals; everyone being able to realise their human rights; and respect for and commitment to rangatiratanga, manaaki, tapu and noa
- **equity** – Commitment to improving health equity and the fair distribution of the determinants of health and well-being, taonga tuku iho, tinana, wairua, hinengaro and mana

- **determinants** – Commitment to improving the social and environmental determinants of health which include social justice, equity, participation – whakamana tāngata, whai oranga, whai wāhi, taiao me nga mea katoa e whakapiki ake i te hauora
- **interdependence** – Recognition of the interdependence of individuals, families, communities and the broader environment. This includes recognition of te ao turoa, whakawhānaungatanga, whānau, whānau ora, kotahitanga and whatumanawa
- **aroha** – Respect for peoples' rights to aroha, awhi and hauoratanga
- **integrity** – Commitment to acting honestly, ethically and with integrity – he mahinga i runga i te mahi tika me te mana tāngata me he ngakau tapatahi.

GO FURTHER 6.1

Examine the values of global and national health promotion organisations (perhaps using the examples above). Where is there commonality in the values base and where are there differences? Why may these differences exist and, if you were drawing up a set of values for health promotion, which would you include and why?

Values are important as they shape not only the methods and approaches used in health promotion, but also the outcomes that are valued. Whether you value free will and individual choice might, for instance, shape the way you may deliver interventions to tackle health issues in obesity. The impact of these values is therefore critical to decisions about what health promotion approaches and methods are appropriate (see Chapter 3). However, values in health promotion have a secondary function in distinguishing the discipline from other approaches to health improvement and protection, such as health education or public health (Green, 2004a). Health promotion and public health, for example, clearly have overlapping values and intentions, but health promotion has a stronger value-set around involvement, participation and autonomy contributing to empowerment (Tilford et al., 2003). Public health in contrast emphasises more firmly values relating to paternalism; positivist research; and protection (Green, 2004a) – these values became very clear during the recent COVID-19 pandemic when they were highly evident in communication from public health experts. Values play out and manifest both in practice and in the approach to tackling health issues, but also in professional training competencies, education and training.

Based on discussions at international conferences and events, it is clear that there is some shared understanding of certain values in health promotion. In Chapter 2, which tracks the development of health promotion, it is clear that certain values have been a salient feature of international conferences and declarations. Some of these were values identified in the mid-1980s and still remain prominent today (Gregg and O'Hara, 2007b). One striking issue has been the lack of empirical research on the values associated with health promotion and this continues to be an overlooked research gap. As previously mentioned, it is likely that values are implicit or tacit between health promotion professionals but teasing out a common framework for understanding, through research, would seem highly beneficial.

One study attempted to define the values in health promotion (Tilford et al., 2003) and reported a list of 'terminal' (i.e. the desired goals) and 'instrumental' values (i.e. the process and activities to achieving the 'terminal' values) based on responses from UK health promotion specialists and academics. The approach used postal questionnaires and gained 25 responses. The questionnaire asked a series of questions, but specifically sought views on the core values in health promotion. Analysis drew out a series of values and these can be seen in Box 6.2. Careful examination between Boxes 6.1 and 6.2 will reveal considerable overlap and some slight nuances between international statements on health promotion values and the empirical literature.

BOX 6.2 TERMINAL AND INSTRUMENTAL VALUES IN HEALTH PROMOTION

Terminal values: Equity, Equality, Social justice, Empowerment, Autonomy, Participation.

Instrumental values (activities): Addressing health inequalities, Tackling determinants of health, Holistic, Community development, Non-positivist.

Instrumental values (processes): Partnerships, Voluntarism, Beneficence/non-maleficence, Sustainability, Participation, Advocacy, Respect, Inclusiveness.

Source: Tilford et al. (2003)

So why does this actually matter? Well, as already noted, values guide the way that practice and policy in health promotion is delivered. They shape practice and give health promotion a distinctive 'voice'. Without these values, it is likely that health promotion will lose its unique contribution – this could lead to health promotion being consumed or confused with other disciplines, such as public health; our position is that health promotion should be regarded very differently (see Chapter 1) and that values are one way of making this case.

Take as a practical example reductions in depression; this is an outcome that a health promoter and a general practitioner would unanimously subscribe to. However, it is less likely for a general practitioner to be guided by values such as empowerment, participation or autonomy. In fact, the approach taken from a general practitioner perspective may be completely at odds with these values. Health promoters may be more inclined to recognise lay perspectives and embrace a social view of health, whereas a general practitioner may privilege scientific and biomedical explanations of the condition. This has been noted by others: 'When people are working on matters relevant to health, following a health promotion approach obligates them to encourage openness and participation, strive for the empowerment and autonomy of others, and hold equity and justice as the highest of principles' (Mittelmark et al., 2001: 3).

VALUES IN ACTION

This section of the chapter now describes some of the core values in health promotion in some detail. It is not exclusive in its reporting of these, but nonetheless some of the values which frequently and consistently are mentioned in the literature are outlined and discussed.

Equity and equality

Equity and equality are often values that are used interchangeably, but they in fact have quite different meanings. They are both prominent ideas in health promotion and have underpinned efforts to promote the health of individuals and communities. Equality relates to things being equal so that regardless of background, gender, social status or any other factor, people receive an equal distribution of services or resources. Equity, on the other hand, relates to fairness and is a judgement on who is more or less deserving of support based on their social circumstances or conditions of living (see Box 6.3).

Equality aims to promote fairness, but it can only work if everyone has a similar starting point in life. We know that in many countries, particularly in the Western world, some people live in poverty and others in excessive wealth; this is not equality. Efforts to achieve equity in health are therefore aimed at creating opportunities and removing barriers to achieving the health potential of all people. This means the fair distribution of resources needed for health, fair access to the opportunities available and fairness in the support offered to people when ill. This is no easy task as it involves rebalancing the distribution of power and tackling inequities along the lines of class, education, gender, age, ethnicity, disability and geography (Dixey, Cross, Foster and Woodall, 2013). At first glance, the idea of equity seems grossly unfair but it is a value which seeks to 'level the playing field' so that people have the chance to reach their health potential and health goals.

BOX 6.3 EQUALITY OR EQUITY IN PRISON HEALTH

Many progressive countries are committed to providing 'equal' healthcare and health promotion to people in prison compared to the general population. The premise is that individuals detained in prison must have the benefit of care equivalent of that available to the general public (Niveau, 2007).

Though government policy for prison health is saturated with references to equivalence, this does not reflect the complexity and reality of delivering services in the setting (Birmingham et al., 2006). Critics have deconstructed the notion of equivalence in prison health services and have argued that an equivalent health service is an 'insufficient public health response' (Lines, 2006: 276). These commentators argue that the inputs needed to generate equivalence of health outcomes in prisoners must be greater than those expected at a community level as research demonstrates that prisoners have poorer health than the general community (Levy, 2007). This suggests that the idea of health equity may be better than equality. Supporting this, Niveau (2007) suggests that prison health services cannot be taken in a manner equivalent to those in the general population. He suggests that they must be directed in a more intense and precise approach and never fall short of community standards. Indeed, Lines (2006) proposes that prison health services should move beyond the notion of equivalence and endorse standards that achieve equivalent objectives instead.

Social justice

Social justice is a value in health promotion, linked closely to equity and views around fairness. If it is accepted that health inequalities exist by virtue of social and economic conditions (see Chapter 5), then social justice is about working towards un-doing socially created differences in conditions of living which impact on health outcomes for people (Calderwood, 2003). Why, for example, is it fair or acceptable for a child to be born today in one part of the world, say Japan, and expect to live well into their 80s and in another country, say Sierra Leone, this may only be their 50s. Broadly speaking then, social justice is about re-balancing power and fighting oppression. It is closely linked to empowerment which is often regarded as the 'tool' to reconfigure social injustice and structural divisions in society.

Social justice issues can be wide-ranging, covering gender, ethnicity, social background and geography. It is an ideologically contested idea, but follows what Seedhouse (1997) calls 'social health promotion' where health and justice are entwined – health promoters with this value base would view that it is unjust that people suffer deprivation in a plentiful world. Ideas around social justice are largely associated with the political left. For example, this perspective in health promotion would see disadvantaged groups having limited power and choice in affecting the determinants that influence their health. A left-wing view would advocate for collective solutions and interventions aimed at social justice to reduce inequalities in health (Davison and Davey Smith, 1995). Moreover, it would support a systems or structural approach to health promotion, grounded predominantly in macro-level or environmental interventions which draws its focus towards the social, economic, political, institutional, cultural, legislative, industrial and physical environments of societies in order to modify behaviour change (Green and Raeburn, 1988). Nettleton and Bunton (1995: 44) summarise: 'Essentially the structural critique argues that attempts to prevent illness and to promote health have failed to take into account the material disadvantages of people's lives. This works at three levels: the political environment, the social environment and the physical environment.' The structural approach avoids focusing on the individual and instead intervenes at a political or systems level (Stokols et al., 2003).

Social justice has been a prominent feature of debate and discussion concerning health. Recent discussions have seen debates on access issues, especially in Western societies, in relation to healthcare professionals, services or treatment. Much of this has been coined the 'postcode lottery', effectively arguing that health outcomes and experiences of the health sector can differ simply based on where you live. Some have suggested that health promotion forms part of 'a professional community for social justice' (Mittelmark, 2008: 5). Indeed in order to achieve social justice, it is necessary for health promoters to work across boundaries and professional lines. This could include, for instance, working alongside different groups and organisations and adopting a partnership approach (see Chapter 12).

Autonomy

The idea that people have autonomy in their decisions is a fundamental concept in health promotion, but at the same time it has been a profoundly contentious principle. In theory, autonomy works at its best when people have the information to hand and choose how to behave based on this information. Underlying this, however, is a view that there is a 'right' and 'wrong' decision and that, provided with the right information in a meaningful way, people will make choices that *they* believe to be 'healthy'. Much health promotion has assumed that if you tell people what is best for them to do, they will do it! This is quite misguided.

One of the criticisms of health promotion has been that it has a streak of 'moral superiority' in knowing what is best for others. It has been accused of prescribing ways of living and in demonising unhealthy choices. Autonomy is therefore an issue which has been divisive in health promotion circles.

Values are often politically and ideologically underpinned and none more so in the case of autonomy and in its manifestation, 'choice'. Those with a more right-wing view of health promotion may subscribe to the free availability of epidemiological risk information and total liberty of autonomy and choice (Davison and Davey Smith, 1995). The strength of the right-wing critique of health promotion lies in its defiance of intrusion into other people's personal life or choice (Fitzpatrick, 2001; Kelly and Charlton, 1995). This perspective argues that health choices are decisions which individuals make, not governments or other organisations, and that individuals have the autonomy and fundamental human rights to choose their own health-related behaviours (Jochelson, 2006; Minkler, 1999). Those challenging this outlook suggest that this perspective oversimplifies disease causation and fails to address the influences on people's autonomy – particularly the social determinants of health, such as poverty, unemployment and poor housing (Davison and Davey Smith, 1995; Naidoo, 1986). However, on this point, and extending the value of autonomy to its logical end, health promoters should be prepared and accept that people have the fundamental right to choose to be 'unhealthy':

> It is arrogant to assume that people consume alcohol, chocolate, or cream cakes because they are irrational or are simply behaving thoughtlessly or stupidly. Human actors are profoundly knowledgeable about their own behaviour, they can account for it in meaningful ways which not only make sense to them, but if we take the trouble to hear those accounts, the rationality within them is clear.
>
> (Kelly and Barker, 2016: 112)

Any attempt to block people's choices can be regarded as a form of paternalism or health fascism which is often levelled at health promoters (Downie et al., 1996). There may be some exceptions to this, though; for example, where the autonomous decisions of individuals impacts on the health of others (e.g. the impact of passive smoking).

Our view is that people have the right to choose how they lead their life. However, the concept of 'free choice' on being healthy can be somewhat 'illusory' as the environment plays a major role in whether people are in a position to choose a healthy way of life (Green, 2004b: 2; Tones, 1998). The notion that health promotion should 'make the healthy choice the easy choice' is a simplistic but useful idea. Few of us have unfettered freedom to do as we please as we are constrained by other factors. Structural conditions, for example, perform an important role in an individual's ability to exercise free choice. Material, environmental, social, political and cultural determinants can all influence people's capacity to take action (McKee and Raine, 2005). This has been illustrated in Chapter 5.

REFLECTIVE EXERCISE 6.2

Examine the quotation below and consider the extent to which you agree or disagree with this statement. To what extent do you feel that people 'choose' their lifestyle decisions?

Can individuals act healthily in a wholly voluntary manner, or do the social structures in which they live or social norms and values limit what is possible or likely? To what extent do people choose unhealthy habits, and to what extent are they imposed upon them?

(Blaxter, 2004: 86)

Participation and empowerment

The values of social justice, participation and empowerment are very closely interlinked and difficult to separate. Empowerment has become a flagship value for health promotion and is seen as 'the holy grail' of the discipline (Rissel, 1994). It has become one of the key ideas in health promotion because empowerment concerns combating oppression and injustice and is a process by which people participate collectively to increase the control they have over events that influence their lives and health (Fisher and Gosselink, 2008; Laverack, 2006). To this extent, it resonates particularly well with the Ottawa Charter and a whole host of WHO declarations and Charters indicating the requirement for individuals and communities to 'take control' of the determinants influencing their lives.

Importantly, empowerment cannot be given to people, but comes from individuals and communities empowering themselves. Health promoters may create a situation where empowerment may be more likely, through facilitation and support, but only when groups of people gain their own momentum, acquire skills and advocate for their own change will empowerment have been fully realised (Wallerstein, 2006). Wise (1995) believes that the underlying philosophy of empowerment involves enabling people to collectively understand how structural processes (e.g. gender inequality, social inequalities) impact upon them and through this realisation mobilise people to take community action (Baum, 2003).

Participation is an important feature of empowerment. Individuals have a better chance of achieving their health goals if they can share these matters with other people who are faced with similar problems. Through participation, individuals are likely to experience some degree of control as they are better able to define and analyse their concerns and together they are capable of finding joint solutions to act on their issues (Laverack, 2005). However, while participation forms 'the backbone of empowering strategies' (Wallerstein, 2006: 9) participation alone does not guarantee empowerment as it can often be manipulative, tokenistic and passive, rather than truly engaging.

Individual empowerment (also referred to as psychological empowerment) relates to a number of attributes which are needed for people's personal capacity to be realised. This may include building people's confidence or self-worth, boosting their self-esteem, developing their coping mechanisms or enhancing their personal skills in order for them to make health related choices. Individual empowerment basically means people feeling and actually having a sense of control over their lives (Woodall et al., 2010). Whilst individual empowerment is fundamental to people gaining increased control over their lives, it is limited because it does not consider the wider environmental influences on people's health, such as poverty and employment.

Community empowerment concerns power relations and intervention strategies which ultimately focus on collective participation in challenging social injustice through political and social processes (Wallerstein, 2006). The overall aim is to allow people to take control of the decisions that influence their lives and health. As a process (see Figure 6.1), community empowerment can be regarded as a series of actions which progressively contribute to more organised community and social action (Laverack, 2004). Starting with an individual's concerns about a given issue, the process of community empowerment starts with the development of small mutual groups, then community organisations, partnerships and ultimately to groups of people taking political and social action to create social change through the redistribution of resources and power (Laverack, 2006; Wallerstein, 2002).

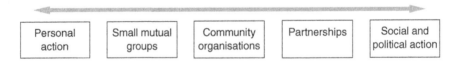

| Personal action | Small mutual groups | Community organisations | Partnerships | Social and political action |

Figure 6.1 Community empowerment as a continuum

Source: Laverack (2004)

GO FURTHER 6.2

Empowerment is a word used very frequently in health promotion. We have argued that at best the term 'empowerment' has been diluted and at worst lost within health promotion. This, we would suggest, has happened as a result of broader shifts in health promotion which has moved more towards individuals (focused largely on behaviour change), rather than a discipline that focuses on addressing social justice and wider power structures through social and structural change (Woodall et al., 2012). What do you understand by empowerment? What does it mean to you? Can you provide your own definition of empowerment, encompassing individual and community aspects?

THE CHALLENGE OF VALUES IN HEALTH PROMOTION

Critics have suggested that there are tensions between practitioners *understanding* values in health promotion and *enacting* them in practice (Gregg and O'Hara, 2007a). Practitioners may hold values in relation to empowerment, but adopt ways of working that may neglect listening to people or by adopting very individualistic interventions that fail to recognise broader social factors.

There is further controversy in relation to 'values' and 'evidence'. On this point, we see the tension, but don't necessarily subscribe to the position. The lack of evidence in relation to empowerment approaches in promoting health is an example perhaps of where a values position has overtaken an evidence-based position (Woodall et al., 2010). This brings a further dimension into the identification of values in health promotion which is moral position – what we feel is the 'right' or 'wrong' thing to do.

Seedhouse (1997) has provided a very detailed book which throughout critiques the application of values in health promotion. His view is that values inherently create prejudice and that this should be fully acknowledged by health promotion practitioners. Indeed, his argument is extended much further in that Seedhouse suggests that values overrides evidence in health promotion, with alternative views to this being 'blinkered' to reality. Whether health promotion is indeed 'blinkered' by its values is a debating point; however, what this stresses is perhaps the requirement for an agreed set of values that can be subscribed to and made transparent.

GO FURTHER 6.3

The values outlined in Box 6.2 were derived from a specific group of specialists working in a specific part of the world. The extent to which these values are shared across different continents and countries is unknown. There may be some divergent perspectives on the values underpinning health promotion linked to how people conceptualise health promotion itself. What values would you identify as being critical to health promotion? If you were trying to gauge what health promoters perceived were the core values of health promotion how would you go about doing this? What methods would you choose and why?

Some of the values identified as being important in health promotion may be contradictory in themselves (Duncan, 2004); the value of autonomy and the 'right to choose', for example, and the value to tackling health inequalities which may use state intervention as a way to improve health equity and deny personal choice. Personal choice is favoured so long as it does not impact on others: 'the principle of voluntarism urges freedom of choice unless good reason can be provided for coercive measures on the basis of utilitarianism, paternalism or "social justice"' (Green et al., 2019: 42). Linked very closely to this is how values in health promotion are undermined by some approaches and methods to facilitate improvements to individual and community health. Several approaches to health promotion may actively contradict some of the values espoused. Focusing on lifestyle behaviours, for instance, at the exclusion of addressing wider social and environmental determinants may not align with values such as empowerment or social justice.

SUMMARY

This chapter has outlined the core values in health promotion and has discussed why values are important in distinguishing disciplinary boundaries. The chapter has outlined a series of values which are salient in health promotion and are broadly subscribed to. We argue that these values provide the 'backbone' of professional practice and shape the way that health promotion is delivered and operationalised. We are not uncritical of values in health promotion and have outlined some of the main challenges associated with adopting a values position in practice.

SUGGESTED READING

Downie, R.S., Tannahill, C. and Tannahill, A. (1996) *Health promotion: models and values.* Oxford, Oxford University Press.

Gregg, J. and O'Hara, L. (2007) Values and principles evident in current health promotion practice. *Health Promotion Journal of Australia*, 18: 7–11.

Tilford, S., Green, J. and Tones, K. (2003) Values, health promotion and public health. Leeds, Centre for Health Promotion Research, Leeds Metropolitan University.

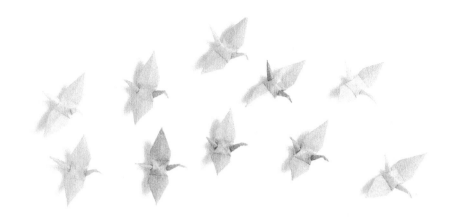

SECTION 3

WHEN IS HEALTH PROMOTION RELEVANT?

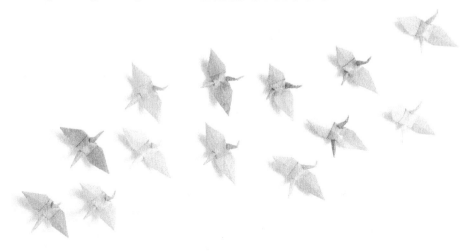

ASSESSING HEALTH NEEDS

7

PRINCIPLES AND PRACTICE

INTRODUCTION

Assessing health needs is a crucial part of planning health promotion activities and there is growing recognition of the importance of determining health need so that finite resources in health promotion can be used effectively. This chapter discusses various interpretations of health need and the different implications of these. It considers assessing health needs in the light of positive and negative concepts of health and, for example, whether or not a professional or lay perspective on health is prioritised. This chapter describes and explores what type of data can be used to assess health need and how routine information can enable health needs to be better understood. Finally, different approaches to health needs assessment are considered including participatory methods, rapid appraisal and asset-based approaches.

DEFINING 'NEED'

Before we go any further we suggest you undertake the first Reflective Exercise for this chapter (7.1).

REFLECTIVE EXERCISE 7.1

Take some time to think about what you need on a day-to-day basis. What do you need to live? What do you need to be healthy? What do you need to feel fulfilled? What do you need to live your best life? Write a list. Can you distinguish between the things that you actually *need* rather than the things you might *want* but are not really essential for survival?

The concept of need is an interesting one. Often when we talk about needing something we are actually expressing a want or desire as you will have appreciated from undertaking Reflective Exercise 7.1. In relation to health therefore Naidoo and Wills (2016: 269) define need as 'something which is required or essential rather than merely desired or wanted'. However, there is no agreed definition of what a health need actually *is* (Green et al., 2019). Some people suggest that needs should be defined according to whether or not they can actually be met and NHS Scotland (2019) suggests that a useful definition of need is 'the capacity to benefit from services' which reflects a similar understanding.

THEORIES ABOUT NEED

Maslow's hierarchy of needs

In 1943 a humanist psychologist called Abraham Maslow proposed a 'hierarchy of needs' in a paper he wrote entitled 'A Theory of Human Motivation' (cited in Cherry, 2019). This theory of motivation proposes that our behaviour is motivated by a variety of needs. Whilst Maslow's hierarchy of needs was originally developed as a theory of motivation it still has considerable influence today. It also provides an understanding of the concept of need. As you will see from Figure 7.1 the hierarchy is presented as a pyramid with a wide base and a narrow top. In this pyramid there are five different levels which represent various types of need. Starting from the lowest level there are basic physical needs. These are what we need to survive as human beings from day to day; for example, food, water and shelter. These can be defined as 'physiological' needs and are conceptualised by Maslow as being the most necessary (Hopper, 2019). The next level is concerned with 'safety' or

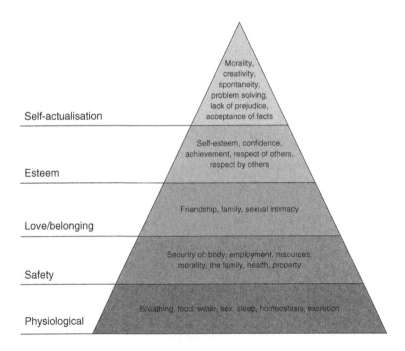

Figure 7.1   Maslow's hierarchy of needs

'security' needs and relates to the need for a safe and secure environment. The needs at the middle level are defined as 'social' needs; for example, having a sense of belonging and feeling connected to other people which is sometimes referred to as 'love and belonging' (Hopper, 2019). The fourth level is need to do with esteem factors – feeling good about ourselves and feeling valued by others. The final level at the top of the pyramid Maslow termed 'self-actualisation' by which he meant needs related to fulfilling our individual potential, achieving what we want to or, essentially, 'being all we can be' (Green et al., 2019: 16). Maslow theorised that each level of the pyramid cannot be reached unless the level below it has been achieved. Therefore, Maslow saw basic needs as the foundation for everything else. Without these being met nothing further up the hierarchy of needs can be attained. All of Maslow's human needs can actually be understood as 'health' needs (Naidoo and Wills, 2016). Indeed, the different levels of the pyramid reflect the prerequisites for health outlined by the Ottawa Charter (World Health Organization, 1986), namely shelter, food, peace, sustainable resources, income, education, social justice, equity and a stable ecosystem.

Bradshaw's (1972) taxonomy of need

Bradshaw (1972) identified four different types of need that still have currency today – see Table 7.1 for details.

Table 7.1 Bradshaw's taxonomy of need

Type of Need	Described as...	Defined by...	For example
1. Normative need	When someone is identified as needing something on the basis of a desirable standard, criterion or benchmark	Experts or professionals	A healthcare professional decides that a person needs some kind of intervention
2. Felt need	When someone feels that they need something (equates with 'wants')	Lay people	An individual feels that they need some kind of resource or intervention
3. Expressed need	When a felt need becomes a demand	Lay people	An individual requests some kind of resource or intervention. Expressed need can also be 'inferred' from people's demands (Morgan, 2006).
4. Comparative need	When a group of people or an area lacks something in comparison to another group of people or area	Experts or professionals *or* lay people	One community has access to safe green space and another does not

Source: Adapted from Naidoo and Wills (2016) and Green et al. (2019)

Issel (2014: 120) offers a fictitious account depicting Bradshaw's four different types of need which is adapted here:

A group of health practitioners identify a community as having a need for a primary healthcare centre based on the fact that the members of the community frequent a local emergency department to meet their health needs (*normative need*). A nearby community has a primary healthcare centre and the members of that community attend the local emergency department a lot less frequently (*comparative need*). When the community was informed that a new primary healthcare centre was going to be built they asked if the money could be used to build a swimming pool instead (*expressed need*). The community felt (*felt* need) that they needed somewhere for leisure and recreation as an alternative to 'the gang activities that were contributing to the shootings' in the neighbourhood which were impacting on everyone's quality of life and feelings of well-being.

This example and Bradshaw's taxonomy of need illustrates how need can be defined in different ways by different groups of people. It is important to consider this since perspectives on need can be very different. For example, from a professional perspective an expert might decide that a community without adequate sanitation needs money to sink boreholes for fresh water and to build latrines (*normative* need) particularly when compared to a nearby community who has access to both (*comparative* need). However, as in the example above, the community themselves may think they have other needs (*felt* need) and may state that they want the money spent on something else (*expressed* need).

WHAT IS A 'HEALTH' NEED?

In this chapter we are paying particular attention to *health* needs. However, as stated previously, there is no agreed definition of what a health need actually *is* (Green et al., 2019). As part of Reflective Exercise 7.1 you were asked to write down what you thought you needed to be healthy. Perhaps you put things like eating well, taking regular exercise and not drinking too much alcohol. On the other hand you may have considered factors which lie outside of your immediate control such as access to healthcare services or a supportive environment. Similarly, Hubley et al. (2021) differentiate between two elements of health promotion need – 'health service-determined needs' and 'community-determined needs or wants' (see Box 7.1 for details).

BOX 7.1 TWO ELEMENTS OF HEALTH PROMOTION NEED

HEALTH SERVICE-DETERMINED NEEDS

These are determined by health or other services, relate to the allocation of resources and are based on the distribution of indicators of health and disease. As per Bradshaw's taxonomy of needs this includes normative and comparative judgements about need.

COMMUNITY-DETERMINED NEEDS OR WANTS

These are determined by the community itself. As per Bradshaw's taxonomy of needs this includes felt need and expressed need.

Source: Hubley et al. (2021)

Health service-determined needs and community-determined needs may overlap to some extent but there will be differences in what is defined as a need depending on who is defining it – health professionals or the individual/community concerned (Hubley et al., 2013). Alongside the concept of need it is also important to consider 'supply' and 'demand'. Need generates demand which requires a supply in order for the need to be met (Morgan, 2006). In a world where resources are finite not all needs can be met. The simple fact is that it is impossible to meet everyone's health needs – demand (need) is always bigger than supply (resources). For that reason we need to prioritise how resources are used and where they are allocated. This is where health needs assessment comes in.

WHY IS IT NECESSARY TO ASSESS HEALTH NEEDS?

It is recognised that the concept of needs assessment is not straightforward and therefore some prefer to use terms like 'situation analysis' that are more 'neutral' (Hubley et al., 2013: 30); however, for ease here, we will use the terms 'health needs' and 'health needs assessment'. There are a number of different reasons why we need to assess health needs. Here we outline six key reasons. First and foremost, health needs assessment is an integral part of the health promotion planning process (for more on health promotion planning see Chapter 18). In order to design effective health promotion interventions and policies we have to identify the public health concerns we are trying to tackle (Cavanagh and Chadwick, 2005). Secondly, health needs assessment is necessary in order to assist with planning and commissioning services (NHS Scotland, 2019). Thirdly, health needs assessment is necessary in order to prioritise areas of action and to make decisions about what issues should be addressed. Fourthly, health needs assessment is essential in order to help understand the needs of individuals or groups of people and how best to address them. Fifthly, health needs assessment is key to appreciating what type of intervention and/or resources will make the most difference. Lastly, health needs assessment is absolutely crucial in reducing or tackling health inequalities; thus, for example, community health needs assessment provides a way of tackling the social determinants of health (Caffrey et al., 2018).

Health needs assessment has been defined as 'a systematic process of identifying priority health issues, targeting the populations with most need and taking action in the most cost-effective and efficient way' (Morgan, 2006: 21). Note that this definition implies some sort of structured, organised procedure and that it focuses on people who have the greatest needs as well as suggesting that what might be done to tackle that need should be worthwhile, effective and achievable. Before you read any further we recommend you undertake Reflective Exercise 7.2.

Given what has been discussed so far how do you think health needs could be determined? What would you want to find out? How would you do that? What types of information would you need? Where would you get it from and how? What types of methods could you use? Who would you need to talk to? Use the internet to help you answer these questions if you want to.

APPROACHES TO HEALTH NEEDS ASSESSMENT

Health needs assessment can be carried out at different levels – at the individual level, group level, community level or organisational level. As Morgan (2006: 22) argues, 'the purpose of needs assessment is to determine health priorities and unmet health and social need, the desired outcome should be action to address the needs identified to ensure improvements in health are made'. According to Naidoo and Wills (2016: 278) the following questions should guide health needs assessment:

• What information is needed?
• How am I going to find out this information?
• What am I going to do with the information?
• What scope is there to act on the information?

Scriven (2017) offers a similar set of questions as follows:

• What type of need is it?
• Who decided that there is a need?
• What are the grounds for deciding that there is a need?
• What are the aims and the appropriate response to the need?

NHS Scotland (2019) suggest that there are some common steps to health needs assessment as follows:

1. Identify the issue – why are you doing the needs assessment and what do you want to understand?
2. Identify the population – is it everyone within a geographical area, or people with a particular characteristic or health condition?
3. Identify the sources of data you can use – these may include community profiles, local and national statistics, existing evidence about what works and stakeholder views
4. Identify the gap between need and supply

Clearly there are some similarities in the different frameworks available. We have considered three here as offered by Naidoo and Wills (2016), NHS Scotland (2019) and Scriven

(2017). In short, the key steps or questions necessary to carry out a health needs assessment can be summarised as follows:

- What is the need?
- Who says so?
- What (if anything) can be done about it?

It is important to have some sense of what you are trying to achieve at the outset which is why it is useful to have a set of questions or some sort of strategy in mind for identifying need or carrying out a health needs assessment.

GO FURTHER 7.1

Look back at what you discovered when you undertook Reflective Exercise 7.2. Consider the list you came up with. Can you group or categorise your findings in any way? Reflect on and refer to this as you engage with the next section of this chapter.

USING DIFFERENT TYPES OF INFORMATION

Information can be gathered using a variety of approaches and these are underpinned by different perspectives on health. Think back to the ground we covered in Chapter 1, 'What Is "Health"?' How we define health has implications for how we might assess health needs. We can carry out assessments of health need using *negative* definitions of health, i.e. focusing on patterns of ill health, disease and death, or we can carry out assessments of health needs using *positive* definitions of health, i.e. focusing on indicators of happiness or well-being. Health needs assessment can be done using professional or *expert* concepts of health, or *lay* concepts of health, or utilising both in tandem.

Health needs can be determined by using epidemiological approaches which help identify population health status. Epidemiological approaches are concerned with the 'distribution and determinants of disease' (Scriven, 2017: 90) and are discussed in more detail in Chapter 9, 'Understanding Epidemiology and Health Profiling'. Other types of data are also very useful in determining health needs. For example, data on lifestyles, socio-economic data, professional views and lay perspectives (Scriven, 2017). Issel (2014) offers a comparison of five different perspectives on health needs assessment which is presented in Table 7.2. The table presents each perspective alongside what types of data sources would be used, examples of such data sources and the types of needs that would be assessed.

Health needs assessment can take different forms, entail different methods and involve different stakeholders. There is no prescribed way of carrying out a health needs assessment. It will vary according to the context, the issue and the resources available. Case Study 7.1 illustrates this with two examples of health needs assessment that both used a combination of different approaches.

Table 7.2 Health needs assessment: five perspectives

	Data Sources	Examples	Types of needs assessed
Epidemiological Assesses whole populations	Quantitative, numerical data such as statistics	Data sets, i.e. disease and death rates	Normative, Comparative
Public Health Assesses communities or local regions	Existing data including epidemiological data	Surveys, data sets	Normative, comparative
Social Assesses populations or groups therein	Social data such as education, income levels as well as social norms and connections	Surveys	Normative
Asset Assesses communities or neighbourhoods	The community themselves including assets and competencies	Focus groups, transect walks, asset mapping	Felt, expressed
Rapid Assess communities or neighbourhoods	Various but a quick superficial appraisal rather than an in-depth analysis	Use of existing data, interviews, focus groups	Normative, felt

Source: Adapted from Issel (2014)

CASE STUDY 7.1: SOURCES OF DATA IN HEALTH NEEDS ASSESSMENT

INJECTING DRUG USE IN PUBLIC PLACES IN GLASGOW, SCOTLAND

Injecting drug use is a significant public health problem in many cities. A health needs assessment was carried out in Glasgow, Scotland for people who inject drugs in public places. A 'tripartite' health needs assessment framework was employed that comprised three different types of approaches - epidemiological, comparative and corporate. The methods included an analysis of local and national secondary data sources on drug use, rapid literature reviews, and an engagement exercise (using interviews and focus group discussions) with people who were injecting drugs in public places, people in recovery from injecting drug use, and staff from relevant health and social care services. The aims were to investigate the characteristics and health needs of people who inject drugs in public and to examine the factors relevant to the implementation of safer injecting facilities and heroin-assisted treatment.

Source: Adapted from Tweed et al. (2018)

MENTAL HEALTH SUPPORT FOR WOMEN WHO HAVE BEEN RAPED IN THE WESTERN CAPE, SOUTH AFRICA

Rape and sexual assault are significant public health issues in many different contexts however, the mental health support to survivors available varies widely despite the severe impact on mental health. Qualitative methods were used in a rapid appraisal of mental health services for rape survivors in an attempt to better understand service provision. The methods included semi-structured interviews with rape survivors, service providers from post-rape sexual assault services and observations of survivor sessions with counsellors, nurses and doctors.

Source: Adapted from Abrahams and Gevers (2017)

Another health needs assessment carried out in Iran by Khami et al. (2018) sought to determine women's sexual and reproductive healthcare needs. Khami et al. used a specific questionnaire to gather information – the Sexual and Reproductive Health Needs Assessment Questionnaire (designed by the United Nations Population Fund). The women who could not self-administer the questionnaire (due to not being able to read or write) were interviewed by midwives who they knew and trusted. The women had health needs in six areas: safe motherhood, family planning, sexual history and activity, sexually transmitted infections, HIV/AIDS and violence.

PARTICIPATION AND HEALTH NEEDS ASSESSMENT

As discussed in Chapter 1, 'What Is "Health"?', health promotion emphasises lay perspectives on health. In order to hear people's voices and understand what concerns them they must be involved in the health needs assessment process. This is why participation is an underlying principle of health promotion. Participation implies taking part and also recognising that what people say should be listened to and acted upon (Lowcock and Cross, 2011). Participation in health needs assessment is vital because it is essential that the people whose needs are being assessed are involved in the process (NHS Scotland, 2019). 'People have to be at the centre of health promotion action and decision-making processes for them to be effective' (WHO, 1997: n.p.). In order to appreciate what a community needs it is important to understand the perspective of its members or the 'lay perspective' (this is discussed in more detail in Chapter 8, 'Valuing Lay Perspectives'). As Green et al. (2019) point out, people are much more likely to engage with an intervention if they have been involved in the process of identifying the issue and solution than if an expert comes along and decides what the problem is and how to address it without involving them – see Case Study 7.2, 'Community-led Total Sanitation' by way of example.

CASE STUDY 7.2: COMMUNITY-LED TOTAL SANITATION

As established in Case Study 3.1, open defecation (OD) is a major problem for a significant proportion of the world's population (Zeleke et al., 2019) adding to the burden of disease in the communities where this is an issue. From a health expert perspective the need to address open defecation is clear (*normative* and *comparative*) - it causes disease and death. However, many communities have not, historically, identified (*felt*) the 'need' to address this practice given that it has been going on for decades if not centuries. The principles underpinning the CLTS approach include working with communities to identify what the problem is and finding local solutions (*assets*) to address it supported by the programme staff (Gebremariam et al., 2018). The methods used commonly include 'OD mapping' and 'transect walks' intended to identify where OD takes place within the community setting (Sigler et al., 2014).

Participation is, of course, linked to empowerment which is another key principle of health promotion (Green et al., 2019). Participation in health needs assessment can increase a sense of ownership of the problem as well as enable potential solutions (Issel, 2014). Including people in the process creates buy-in (Berkley-Patton et al., 2018). Working in this way recognises that people are autonomous and possess the skills, knowledge and power to take part and make decisions about things that affect them (Warwick-Booth et al., 2021). There are many examples in the wider literature of community-based health needs assessment. For instance, Berkley-Patton et al. (2018) reported on a faith-based community health needs assessment that took place in African American churches involving church leaders and members. Clearly working in collaboration with communities provides a crucial source of data when carrying out health needs assessment (Shah, 2018). In order to gain a better perspective on people's lived experiences and to 'understand the reality of the impact of social determinants on health experiences and outcomes' qualitative research methods are often the most appropriate, as advocated by Ndomoto et al. (2018: 43) who carried out a health needs assessment in deprived communities in Kenya and the United Kingdom using key informant interviews, focus groups and participant observation. Despite the different contexts there were several common health issues affecting the health of the communities in both countries. These included access to healthcare, poverty, sanitation and hygiene, infectious disease, gender inequality and nutrition (Ndomoto et al., 2018). Participatory approaches to health needs assessment are especially important when working with marginalised communities and can serve as means to build community and nurture social development, as illustrated by Al-Qdah and Lacroix (2017) who carried out a participatory needs assessment with Syrian refugees in Jordan.

CITIZENS' JURIES

We have already established the importance of community participation in the needs assessment process. Community participation is discussed in greater depth in Chapter 8, 'Valuing Lay Perspectives'; however, the concept of 'citizens' juries' is worth mentioning here whilst we are considering participation in health needs assessment. Citizens' juries are a specific means of ensuring community involvement in health needs assessment and decision-making (Laverack, 2014a). They are a method for engaging people and involve small groups of people coming together to debate or deliberate certain issue/s which concern them. Questions such as 'What would improve the health and well-being of your community?' can be used in order to enable the jury to discuss local issues and reach a verdict about what can be done about them (Green et al., 2019). See Box 7.2 for an example of the use of citizens' juries.

BOX 7.2 CONNECTED HEALTH CITIES

The Connected Health Cities project has used citizens' juries to explore a number of issues with groups of ordinary people. In January 2018 a jury of 17 people were asked to consider how people's personal data is used in healthcare settings. They were given a fictional scenario to talk about that involved a patient called Anita. Anita first visits her GP with an eye problem. The jury then 'followed' Anita through her healthcare journey and were given ten different scenarios to consider. At each salient point, the jury were asked whether or not Anita would have reasonably expected privacy or sharing of her personal data and the views of the jury subsequently shaped how personal data is being used.

Source: Adapted from www.connectedhealthcities.org – visit website for more information about the use of citizens' juries

RAPID APPROACHES TO HEALTH NEEDS ASSESSMENT

Rapid approaches to health needs assessment cover a range of strategies which might also be referred to as 'rapid appraisal', 'participatory appraisal' or 'participatory needs assessment' (Green et al., 2019: 257). Essentially such approaches are participatory in nature and involve the members of the community (or key stakeholders) in the process of collecting and analysing information/data. The aim of these approaches is to appropriately and accurately inform intervention planning for health improvement. The term 'rapid' implies that this is a quick process resulting in a quick outcome that seeks to address this question – 'What are the most immediate and pressing needs that can be addressed with readily available resources?' (Issel, 2014: 125). A number of different methods can be used – see Box 7.3 for further details.

BOX 7.3 COMMON TECHNIQUES FOR RAPID APPROACHES

- Mapping
- Transects (transect walks)
- Social mapping
- Body mapping
- Timelines and trends, including seasonal trends
- Historical transects
- Photography
- Ranking and scoring exercises
- Sequence matrices
- Causal and flow diagramming
- Chapatti (Venn) diagramming
- Case histories
- Life histories
- Diaries
- Focus groups
- Observations

Source: Green et al. (2019)

Rapid appraisal can be applied in many different contexts to examine any number of public health concerns. For example, in the Republic of Georgia, Murphy et al. (2018) undertook a rapid appraisal which investigated why displaced persons with mental health disorders were not accessing mental health services. The methods used included a review of existing policy documents and other published data, and interviews with key informants including patients, psychiatrists and senior health officials. The authors found a number of factors affecting service provision for people with mental health problems including inadequate insurance coverage, case identification and referral to treatment, underfunding, inadequate human resources, poor information systems, patient out-of-pocket payments, and stigmatization (Murphy et al., 2018). Identifying what the issues are in this way can lead to the design of effective interventions. Once the issues are known, they can be tackled with the resources available.

ASSET-BASED APPROACHES TO HEALTH NEEDS ASSESSMENT

The concept of need can be quite a negative one implying some kind of deficit or deficiency or that something is lacking. More recently there is greater recognition of the notion of 'assets' in health needs assessment (Green et al., 2019). In short this means paying attention to the positive things that are already in existence in a situation or community that might help address the health problem. Assets might include, for example, community knowledge, expertise and existing resources as well as the strengths and abilities that are available and accessible (Issel, 2014). Community asset mapping has therefore been defined as 'an inventory of the strengths (assets) of the people who make up a community; the interconnections of these assets and how to access them' (Morgan, 2006: 21). Asset-based approaches to health needs assessment looks for resolutions to health issues in the capabilities and capacities of the community itself (Issel, 2014).

SUMMARY

This chapter has highlighted the importance of assessing health needs which is a vital component in the health promotion planning process. It has considered the concept of need drawing on different understandings of this. We have looked at several different aspects of health needs assessment including the different approaches that are used which, in turn, reflect alternative perspectives. This has included participatory needs assessment, rapid appraisal and asset-based approaches to health needs assessment. Throughout the chapter the importance of the lay perspective has been a key theme; however, this is now discussed in more detail in the next chapter.

SUGGESTED READING

Hubley, J., Copeman, J. and Woodall, J. (2013) Part 1: Health promotion needs assessment. In *Practical health promotion*. 2nd edn. Cambridge, Polity. pp. 5–103.

Lavender, M. (2013) Doing a health needs assessment. In J. Harvey and V. Taylor (eds), *Measuring health and wellbeing*. London, Sage. pp. 42–68.

Scriven, A. (2017) Identifying health promotion needs and priorities. In *Ewles and Simnett's promoting health: a practical guide*. 7th edn. London, Elsevier. pp. 85–98.

VALUING LAY PERSPECTIVES

8

INTRODUCTION

Understanding the value of lay perspectives of health and well-being has long been recognised. The importance of subjective experiences in understanding health and disease is often overlooked; however, knowledge and beliefs about health and illness causation by 'non-experts' can shed interesting light which may ultimately be more effective in tackling inequalities in health. This chapter considers lay perspectives on health and well-being. It begins by discussing what we mean by 'lay perspectives'. This leads into a debate about the contested nature of knowledge and issues of power. Different influences on lay perspectives are then discussed before we consider why lay perspectives are so crucial to health promotion. Finally, we turn to community participation as an essential means of taking lay perspectives into account and we consider ways that the lay perspective can be heard and included.

WHAT ARE LAY PERSPECTIVES?

Green et al. (2019: 126) argue that since 'health is essentially a subjective experience, the lay perspective is particularly relevant'. By 'subjective' we mean *personal* or *individual* and by 'lay' perspective we mean *non-expert*. Before we go any further we suggest that you undertake Reflective Exercise 8.1.

REFLECTIVE EXERCISE 8.1

Think back to Chapter 1 where you were asked to reflect on what you understand health to be. What informs or influences your understanding of what health is? What do you do when you are sick? How do you interpret different symptoms? What (or who) influences the decisions you make and the actions you take? Where do you seek help or who from? Why?

As you will have appreciated from doing Reflective Exercise 8.1, what people *think* or *believe* can influence what they *do* so people's ideas about health will have an impact on their health-related behaviour. Green et al. (2019) argue that understanding subjective health experience is of central importance to health promotion. The lay perspective provides insight into how individuals experience, understand and manage their health (and their ill health) (Moon and Gould, 2000) and acknowledges that everyone is the expert of their own experience. Therefore, lay perspectives (or understandings) of health should be given attention and priority. This is important since, as Cross, Rowlands and Foster (2021) rightly point out, not everyone who engages in 'unhealthy' behaviours gets ill, and, conversely, some people who 'do the right things' get sick.

As Shaw (2002) argued, lay understandings of health and illness often encompass medical understandings, and this is particularly the case in more wealthy industrialised contexts where the medical model of health dominates (Western countries). This is inevitable because we constantly interact with the world around us and our opinions and beliefs are influenced by many different things including our interactions with healthcare professionals and the information that is available to us. For instance, Green et al. (2019) note how germ theory has been subsumed into most Western lay concepts of illness.

The term 'lay epidemiology' is also used in the wider literature. Allmark and Tod (2006: 460) define lay epidemiology as 'the processes through which health risks are understood and interpreted by lay people' and suggest that this has two elements: firstly, 'empirical *beliefs* about the nature of illness'; and, secondly, '*values* about the place of health and risks to health in a good life' (our emphasis). For example, a study in Northern England and Scotland explored lay epidemiology in relation to how people who drink alcohol made sense of public health guidance about levels of consumption (Lovatt et al., 2015). The authors found that the participants interpreted the guidelines in different ways including having the opinion that the guidelines were irrelevant (specifically by those who mostly drank heavily at the weekend), and that they weren't realistic for people who drank to get drunk. They also didn't measure alcohol intake by units but by the number of drinks. Where participants said they drank less it wasn't because they were worried about their health but because they were more concerned about the impact on being able to work or to fulfil commitments to their families. The authors therefore concluded that the participants moderated their own alcohol intake according to their own understandings or frames of reference and not with regards to official guidance. Findings like these have major relevance for how health promotion and public health interventions are developed and implemented.

Lay perspectives are informed by many different things aside from medical and scientific knowledge. History (personal and collective), other people, the internet, mass media and our own personal experience all have a bearing. In addition, social media has increasing influence on lay perspectives of health and illness (Baker and Rojeck, 2019). The anthropology of health and illness can give us a lot of insight into lay perspectives.

Anthropology is the study of all aspects of society from a cross-cultural perspective whilst the anthropology of health and illness explores the social and cultural dimensions of health, ill health and medicine, and is concerned with the 'experience and practices of health, illness, and healing in different social and cultural contexts' (Warwick-Booth et al., 2021: 104). Psychology and sociology have also become more concerned with lay beliefs alongside increasing recognition that understanding why people do what they do is important for improving health experience (Cross, Rowlands and Foster, 2021).

THE NATURE OF (VALUED) KNOWLEDGE

'Understandings of health are constructed by interactions between people in the real world' (Dixey, 2013: 40). Expert models of knowledge (those that rely on scientific interpretations of the world) tend to ignore people's everyday experiences and reality (Cross et al., 2017). In addition, 'lay perspectives are often regarded as irrational and trivial in contrast to the rational [...] view of the so-called experts' (Green et al., 2019: 91). The problem is that, if people's experiences and knowledge are not taken into account, there is a risk that the experts can get it wrong; that is, there will not be enough understanding of an issue for it to be dealt with in the most successful way. Lay understandings about health and illness causation can be very different to expert, medical and scientific understandings. For example, medical expertise states that strokes are caused by a number of risk factors such as high blood pressure, being overweight and physical inactivity; however, Moorley et al.'s (2016) study on African-Caribbean women's lay beliefs about the causes of stroke revealed alternative explanations related to witchcraft and curses. Historically, as noted by Green et al. (2019) earlier, lay understandings of health and illness have been devalued and dismissed with more importance being given to medical expertise; however, this is changing. After all, we all have the best knowledge of our own lived experiences and the circumstances of our personal lives. In the study mentioned previously the authors concluded that 'lay beliefs such as witchcraft can co-exist amicably alongside modern medicine, as long as they do not hinder access to medication, treatment or risk factor management of stroke' (Moorley et al., 2016: 403).

HOW DO LAY PERSPECTIVES DIFFER?

Lay perspectives on health are 'complex and multidimensional' (Green et al., 2019: 11). There are many different influences on lay perspectives and beliefs about health. These include gender, social class, socio-economic status, culture, geography (location), age, time, personal experience of health, illness, disease and disability, and ethnicity. Socio-economic status leads to different health behaviours and experience because it impacts on how people think and feel (Manstead, 2018). What may be viewed as a part of normal human experience in one culture may be seen as abnormal in another culture (Geeraert, 2018). This is particularly the case with mental (ill) health since, for example, emotional expression varies according to culture and social norms (Hechanova and Waelde, 2017). Rosser (2019) notes how more people are reporting anxiety disorders and mental distress than ever before and puts this down to an increasing culture of uncertainty in contemporary life resulting in people feeling less able to cope and being more fearful of the future. At the time of writing this chapter the coronavirus pandemic is causing an increased burden of mental ill health on a global scale. Ornell et al. (2020) note how, in such situations, the number of people whose mental health is affected (for example by increased fear, anxiety, stress or worsening of existing psychological conditions) often significantly outweighs the number of people who experience infection.

Lay perspectives can encompass many different explanations for the origins (or causes) of ill health such as evil spirits or curses. For example, Tedeschi (2017) described different perspectives between a Western medical doctor and a Hmong immigrant in the United States of America – the doctor diagnosed a cancerous tumour and the patient believed their discomfort was being caused by an evil spirit. This illustrates the contrast between explanations of ill health in physiological terms versus mystical terms. Good and Hannah (2015) argue that culture influences a number of things including the way that people present with symptoms and consequently how they might be diagnosed, the way that health professionals and patients interact, the way an individual experiences illness, and the way the individual might perceive and communicate their symptoms. It is important to appreciate such different perspectives in order to tackle certain diseases in some communities. By way of example, breastfeeding is less common in Western culture than it used to be for many complex reasons and in lower-income countries there is also a belief that formula feed is better for infants than breast milk despite scientific evidence to the contrary (Thorley, 2019). Radzyminski and Callister (2016) point out that many factors affect the decision about whether or not a mother will breastfeed including level of education, age, culture, marital status and self-confidence. There are probably more factors too because, as Scriven (2017: 5) argues, 'people assess their own health subjectively, according to their own norms and expectations'. This results in rich, varied and complex ideas about health which need to be taken into account for health promotion efforts to be effective (Cross et al., 2021). Lay people's ideas about health and ill health are situated within different contexts such as cultural context, social context and temporal context. Case Study 8.1 illustrates this with reference to smoking.

CASE STUDY 8.1: SMOKING

Smoking is a good example of a behaviour which has changed over time in response to changing medical and scientific knowledge that has been subsumed in lay perspectives. Burns (2014) noted that dramatic changes in both smoking behaviours *and* attitudes to smoking have occurred since the 1960s, particularly in the wealthier parts of the world. These have occurred for a number of complex and interrelated reasons. Whilst it is commonly less easy now to smoke due to restrictions laid down by governments and ruling states social attitudes have also changed. 'Race, ethnicity, income, sex, education, occupation, and other individual characteristics lead to different life experience with smoking and different resultant smoking behaviours, attitudes, and norms' (Burns, 2014: n.p.). In addition, where people live makes a difference – within and between countries. Over the past two decades smoking has been on the decline in some parts of the world accompanying (or as a result of) a shift in culture and social attitudes which are more anti-smoking than they were previously (Schudson and Baykurt, 2016). Taking up smoking is a behaviour that has typically been associated with youth yet anti-smoking attitudes have also increased among young people (McKelvey and Halpren-Felsher, 2016). However, smoking is on the increase in some parts of the world such as the Eastern Mediterranean and Africa (WHO, 2019c). When asked why they continued to smoke despite being chronically ill people suffering with chronic obstructive pulmonary disease gave a number of different responses including that cigarettes were their friends and that it wasn't worth stopping having been diagnosed with a chronic disease (Wilson et al., 2011). Doctors, medical students and nurses in some European countries have a surprisingly high rate of smoking given their profession. Some research has found that healthcare professionals who smoke were less likely to view smoking as harmful compared to their non-smoking colleagues (Cattaruzza and West, 2013). A study in New Zealand exploring why Māori women continue to smoke in pregnancy found a number of reasons such as habit, stress, addiction, feeling more calm/relaxed, satisfaction, liking smoking, social benefit, boredom/something to do, time out and depression (Glover and Kira, 2011).

As Case Study 8.1 illustrates, people make sense of their health and illness experience within a frame of reference that takes into account social and cultural norms. Responses to different symptoms vary across different cultures, as does the perception of whether or not a sensation or experience is viewed as a 'symptom' in the first place. In traditional Chinese medicine disease is viewed as a result of an imbalance between yin and yang whilst the traditional Indian healing system of Ayurveda positions ill health as a product of karma (Gopalkrishnan, 2018). Garthwaite and Bambra (2017) carried out a study in the North East of England that explored lay perspectives on the causes of health inequalities. They compared and contrasted the views of people living in two different areas – one more affluent than the other. As expected there were some similar views on causation such as notions of fatalism, lack of control and choice, and fear of the future. However, there were also differences between the two groups in terms of inequitable access to healthcare services, and in terms of experiences of stigma related to where people lived. Garthwaite and Bambra (2017) concluded that the experiences of communities should be listened to, understood and prioritised in order to address health inequalities.

HEALTHWORLDS

Germond and Cochrane (2010) talk about 'healthworlds', a concept that has direct relevance here. Healthworlds relate to 'people's conceptions of health, to their health-seeking behaviour and to their conditions of health. Individual's healthworlds are shaped by, and simultaneously affect, their social shared healthworld constituted by the collective search for health and well-being' (Germond and Cochrane, 2010: 309). Healthworlds are not static and consistent, however; they change as people (and communities) change. With reference to the acceptability of pharmaceutical intervention in the United States, Adams et al. (2019) noted how minority ethnic groups, particularly those who are less acculturated to Western culture (and therefore western medicine), were more sceptical about using prescription drugs. Their healthworlds were not as narrowly focused on Western medicine as a treatment option as the majority of the population's were. Also using the concept of healthworlds, Fried et al. (2015) undertook research in South Africa into the acceptability of health services in relation to tuberculosis treatment and antiretroviral therapy. They concluded that the patients' healthworlds need to be acknowledged and incorporated into patient–provider interactions and that the importance of this was underestimated which had significant implications for policy and practice.

THE IMPORTANCE OF LAY PERSPECTIVES

As emphasised in Chapter 1, 'What Is "Health"?', health promotion gives more weight to the social model of health which, in turn, is concerned with valuing lay perspectives. As Williams (2014) points out, increased attention has been paid to lay knowledge and expertise particularly in relation to health and illness experience. It is important to acknowledge lay perspectives because they inform people's capacity for self-care and manage their own (ill) health which can reduce the strain on healthcare services. When people's own experiences and understandings are not taken into account expert opinion is likely to be inaccurate or incomplete which can then result in mismanagement of a situation (Cross, 2020). Cross, Rowlands and Foster (2021) argue that understanding the relationship between what people think and how they interpret health messages is crucial for health promotion, particularly that which is focused on trying to encourage people to change their behaviour in some way. Lay perspectives should inform health needs assessment which, in turn, promotes effective health promotion practice.

Exploring the lay perspective is also vital for developing understanding about how to address the social determinants of health (Cross et al., 2017). Popay (2008) argues that the theoretical and conceptual insights offered by work on lay knowledge and lay people must be incorporated into public health research and practice if contemporary health problems are to be tackled in more effective ways. Case Study 8.2 illustrates the importance of local knowledge and insights, and how these need to be fused with professional knowledge for maximum success.

CASE STUDY 8.2: LAY BELIEFS AND ELEPHANTIASIS

Elephantiasis is a complication of lymphatic filariasis which was identified as a neglected tropical disease in 2011 by the World Health Organization (Deribe et al., 2018) yet continues to be a major public health threat in certain parts of the world. Elephantiasis is a mosquito-borne tropical disease. It is caused by the filarial worm which is transmitted via mosquitos into the human lymphatic systems when they bite (Mandal, 2019). The disease leads to gross swelling of the limbs and other parts of the body, hence the name elephantiasis. It has a significant social and economic impact on the communities it affects and commonly results in stigma related to disfigurement (Abdulmalik et al., 2018). Studies have shown that communities believe this condition is caused by several different things including supernatural forces and there is, in some communities, a lack of awareness that it can actually be successfully treated with medication (Babu et al., 2004).

Qualitative research carried out with communities in Sierra Leone who are affected by this condition reveal very interesting findings about lay beliefs of causation. The members of the communities did not believe themselves to be in control of whether or not they contracted the disease. They cited several reasons how they might become infected such as stepping on a nail and walking on the same soil as an infected person. Mostly, however, they believed that 'divine will' caused the spread of the disease and that, therefore, only divine intervention could cure them of it. Consequently, they relied on praying as the means of preventing and treating the disease and did not engage with health promotion or healthcare activities designed to educate them about how to prevent and treat it. This case clearly illustrates the importance of involving communities in the planning and implementation of disease control measures and the design of health communication messages.

With acknowledgements to Mustapha Sonnie - unpublished Master of Science dissertation (2013) 'Exploring Traditional Beliefs Affecting Elephantiasis (Lymphatic Filariasis) Prevention in Sell Limba Chiefdom, Bombali District, Sierra Leone'.

COMMUNITY PARTICIPATION

In Chapter 7, 'Assessing Health Needs: Principles and Practice', we outlined a number of different important aspects of health needs assessment; however, one of the most important is the role and contribution of the community itself. This is where community participation comes in although it should be acknowledged that the concept is not unproblematic. Naidoo and Wills (2016: 69) define community participation as 'the active involvement of people in formal or informal activities to bring about a planned change or improvements in community life, services and/or resources'. There are a number of different frameworks that try to determine different levels of participation. One of the oldest is Arnstein's (1969) ladder of participation. Arnstein uses a ladder to depict different 'levels' of participation illustrating how communities might be truly participating (at the top of the ladder) whilst simply being manipulated at the bottom end. The rungs in between the two ends of the ladder represent different levels of participation between these two extremes (see Figure 8.1 for more detail). Clearly the aim (and ideal) of health promotion should be to operate at the top end of the ladder where communities are completely in control of what is happening to them although this is not always possible in practice for various reasons (Hubley et al., 2021).

Community participation might also be referred to as community engagement or involvement (Naidoo and Wills, 2016) but essentially these are the same thing. Participation is closely linked to empowerment since it is concerned with the amounts of power and control people have in making decisions about the things that affect them (Green et al., 2019). Taylor (2007) offers four different approaches to promoting lay contributions to public health (see Box 8.1 for details).

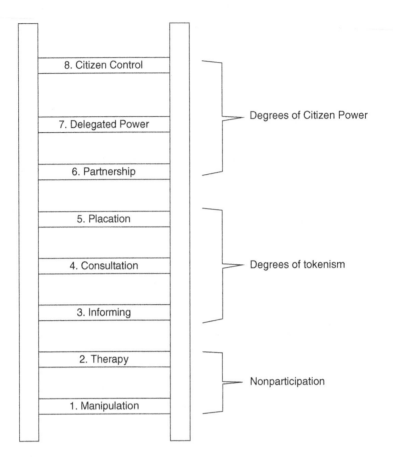

Figure 8.1 Arnstein's ladder of participation. Reproduced by kind permission of Taylor and Francis

BOX 8.1 FOUR APPROACHES TO PROMOTING LAY CONTRIBUTIONS TO PUBLIC HEALTH (TAYLOR, 2007)

Consumerist approach: lay people are consulted as consumers of services.

Representative approach: lay people sit on committees as representatives for the public.

Interest group approach: lay people form interest groups on a specific cause.

Network approach: health professionals find out about the lived experiences of communities through networking with them.

Participation is very much linked to empowerment. In order to participate in something a person has to feel (or be) empowered to do so. Green et al. (2019) map out the relationship between participation and empowerment in their gradient as shown in Figure 8.2.

The gradient clearly shows that the more empowered person, group or community is, the more control they will have and the more 'true' participation is likely to be happening. Conversely, people who are less empowered are more likely to be excluded or coerced than to really participate in terms of making a difference to their lived experience.

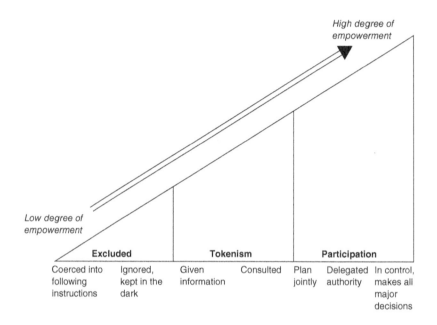

Figure 8.2   Participation and the empowerment gradient

Source: Green et al. (2019)

GO FURTHER 8.1

Using the internet or other appropriate sources find an example of where a community has been involved in tackling an issue at a local level. Using the frameworks presented here (Arnstein, 1969; Green et al., 2019; Taylor, 2007) try to establish the extent that the community was involved. Was it merely consultation and tokenism or was there true participation and community control? You could also reflect on an intervention that has taken place in the community in which you live, or another one that you are familiar with. Again, use the three frameworks to reflect on the extent to which the community was participating (or not).

In order to determine what people think and believe we need to talk to them or engage them in some way. Qualitative methods of research lend themselves to finding out about people's experiences and opinions on all kinds of things and are particularly suited to investigating lay perspectives on health (Cross et al., 2017). Qualitative methods of research are discussed in more detail in Chapter 19, 'Health Promotion Research', and were introduced in Chapter 7 with reference to assessing health promotion needs. As you will appreciate, there are many different methods that can be used under the umbrella of 'qualitative' research that lend themselves to finding out about the world from the people concerned, exploring their subjectivities.

SUMMARY

This chapter has explored the importance of lay perspectives for health promotion. As illustrated the lay perspective has a great deal to offer in terms of our understanding of health and illness and experience. Not only can lay perspectives contribute to, and inform, efforts to improve health, they can also help to tackle health inequalities which is a major pursuit of health promotion. This chapter has also considered participation as the key mechanism to include lay perspectives. The next chapter will look at different ways of exploring health and illness through the discipline of epidemiology.

SUGGESTED READING

Blaxter, M. (2010) *Health*. 2nd edn. Cambridge, Polity.

Lupton, D. (2012) *Medicine as culture: illness, disease and the body*. 3rd edn. London, Sage.

Warwick-Booth, L., Cross, R. and Lowcock, D. (2021) Social anthropology and health. In *Contemporary Health Studies: An Introduction*. 2nd edn. Cambridge, Polity. pp. 105–122.

UNDERSTANDING EPIDEMIOLOGY AND HEALTH PROFILING

9

INTRODUCTION

The previous chapter considered lay epidemiology and the importance of lay perspectives for promoting health. In this chapter we will consider epidemiology more broadly. Epidemiology is a key discipline in health promotion. This chapter presents key concepts in epidemiology such as risk as well as introducing descriptive and analytical epidemiology. The final part of the chapter looks at positive health concepts such as well-being and happiness and how patterns of health, rather than disease, are gaining more attention.

KEY CONCEPTS IN EPIDEMIOLOGY

Scriven (2017: 90) defines epidemiology as the 'study of the distribution and determinants of disease in populations'. Essentially epidemiology is the study of patterns of disease and illness in populations (Naidoo and Wills, 2016) and of the factors that affect patterns of disease and illness (Crichton and Mulhall, 2015). Epidemiological data is typically quantitative, numerical and statistical. By using such data we can establish things like how many people within a given community are affected by a health issue, how many people have died from a certain illness and who is most at risk of certain illnesses by identifying the conditions ('risk factors') that might make it more likely for certain people to become sick (Crichton and Mulhall, 2015). Scriven (2017: 90) summarises this as follows: 'epidemiological data provide essential information on the health of the population [and] the causes and risk factors related to ill-health'. As the discussion in Chapter 7, 'Assessing Health Needs: Principles and Practice', outlined, using data is an important part of the health needs assessment process and therefore for designing health promotion interventions. In addition it can help to direct and prioritise healthcare delivery which is very important in resource-finite contexts.

REFLECTIVE EXERCISE 9.1

Take some time to find out about one of the following diseases/conditions:

- Heart disease
- Depression
- Breast cancer
- Malaria

Or choose something else that interests you. Who does the condition affect? Where do the people that it affects live? What are the 'risk factors' for the condition; i.e. who is most likely to be affected by it and why? Note where you found the information from and consider how reliable your sources might be.

Naidoo and Wills (2016) offer a number of key questions in health promotion that can be answered by using epidemiological approaches to the distribution and determinants of disease as outlined in Box 9.1. Undertaking Reflective Exercise 9.1 will have enabled you to appreciate some of these already.

BOX 9.1 KEY QUESTIONS FOR EPIDEMIOLOGY

GENERAL QUESTIONS:

- *Who* is becoming sick, or is most likely to experience a disease or condition?
- *Why* do certain people become sick (and not others)?
- *When* are people most likely to be affected?
- How effective are the available treatments and prevention strategies?

QUESTIONS CONCERNING *DISTRIBUTION* OF DISEASE:

- How many are there?
- How often are they occurring? (frequency)
- Where are they occurring? (places)
- When are they occurring and how do they change over time?
- Who has them and who does not? (which populations are at higher risk?)

QUESTIONS CONCERNING *DETERMINANTS* OF DISEASE:

- Why do diseases happen?
- What causes ill health?

> - What works to reduce the burden or risk of disease? Is there a relationship between the disease and the factors surrounding people's lives? Which factors are associated with a higher risk of getting the disease? How much higher is the risk associated with these factors?
> - What kind of factors (e.g. genetic or lifestyle) determine which populations are most at risk?
>
> Sources: Adapted from Naidoo and Wills (2016: 41) and
> Crichton and Mulhall (2015: 79)

We can differentiate between two types of epidemiology – descriptive and analytic. *Descriptive* epidemiology is concerned with the question *'what* is happening?' whilst *analytic* epidemiology is concerned with the question *'why* is it happening?'. Each type will now be considered in some detail.

DESCRIPTIVE EPIDEMIOLOGY

One of the most common ways of establishing the health of a population is to look at how many people die (*mortality* rates) and how many people are sick (*morbidity* rates). Using such data are a means of *describing* the state of a population in terms of the 'occurrence of disease according to people, place and time' (Hubley et al., 2013: 36), hence the term 'descriptive epidemiology'. Mortality and morbidity rates give us a sense of what is going on (how many people are dying and how many people are sick) but they don't tell us *why* this is happening. Now let's consider each in turn.

Mortality rates

Mortality rates are death rates, i.e. the number of people who die in a given population. A death rate is a very basic indicator of the health of a community or population. Death rates can be expressed in different ways as follows:

- *Crude mortality rate* = the number of deaths per 1000 people per year.
- *Standardised mortality ratio* (SMR) = (see later explanation).
- *Infant mortality rate* (IMR) = the number of infants who die in the first year of life per 1000 live births that year.

Crude mortality rates give us limited information about a population's health since they will be affected by how old people are within that population. Clearly the older the population the higher average number of deaths there will be over any period of time as the risk of dying increases with age. Standardised mortality rates (SMR) adjust for differences in ages. So, the SMR is 'the number of deaths experienced within a population or group compared to what would be expected for that group if national averages were applied, taking age differences into account' (Naidoo and Wills, 2016: 42). As Hubley et al. (2013: 39) explain, 'an SMR of 100 indicates that the death rate adjusted for age differences is the same as the national or regional average so, SMRs greater or lower than 100 indicate that the age-adjusted death rates are higher or lower than the national or regional average'.

Infant mortality rates are a good indicator of the health of a population because they reflect a number of factors that impact on health such as the health of the mother (also measured as maternal mortality rates), access to healthcare and social services and, at very basic level, access to adequate nutrition. IMRs are therefore often used to compare health between and within countries (see Case Study 9.1).

CASE STUDY 9.1: INFANT MORTALITY

According to data from the World Bank in 2017 Central African Republic had the highest infant mortality rate (IMR) in 2017 - 88. In contrast several countries had an IMR of 2. These were Sweden, Slovenia, Singapore, San Marino, Norway, Estonia, Finland, Iceland, Japan and Luxembourg. The IMR for the United Kingdom (where the authors live) was 4. In terms of regions the European Union averaged an IMR of 3 whilst the least developed countries averaged 47. High-income countries averaged an IMR of 5 whilst low-income countries had an average IMR of 49. Whilst IMR has fallen globally by more than half over the past few decades (from an estimated 65 deaths per 1000 live births in 1990 to 29 deaths per 1000 births in 2017 - World Health Organization, 2019d), data such as these show stark and enduring global health inequalities. It should be noted that there were a number of countries on the list for 2017 that had no information for IMR which illustrates how data is not always complete or reliable.

Source: World Bank (https://data.worldbank.org)

The accuracy of mortality rates varies between countries. Some countries have rigorous methods in place to collect these types of statistics such as death registers however, this is not always the case and therefore access to such information may be more difficult in some contexts.

Morbidity rates

Morbidity rates are concerned with trying to measure rates of illness and disease within communities or populations. This type of information may be found in a number of different places; for example, health services data, census data and household survey data. It should be noted that the data collected often only represents a small proportion of the illness experienced in a population since many sick people do not report as such and the vast majority of incidences are therefore not recorded formally anywhere. This is sometimes referred to as the 'tip of the iceberg', 'the ears of the hippopotamus' or 'the nose of the crocodile' (Green et al., 2019; Schneider and Lilienfeld, 2015). Basically the majority of the disease burden is not seen or reported, it is submerged under water.

Both mortality and morbidity rates are useful but they have limitations. Neither are able to account for people who are experiencing some kind of life-limiting condition that impacts on their health in some way but is not captured by these formal ways of recording information. Hence a number of other measures are also used in order to determine the burden of disease and quality of life of groups or populations – see Box 9.2 for some examples.

BOX 9.2 MEASURES OF POPULATION HEALTH

HALE – health-adjusted life expectancy: 'the average number of years that a person can expect to live in "full health" taking into account years lived in less than full health due to disease and/or injury' (World Health Organization, 2013).

DALYs – disability adjusted life years: 'one lost year of "healthy" life'. Calculated as the sum of the years of life lost (YLL) due to premature mortality in the population and the years lost due to disability (YLD) for people living with a health condition or its consequences as follows:

DALY = YLL +YLD

YLL is calculated by multiplying the number of deaths by the standard life expectancy at age of death in years. YLD is calculated by multiplying the number of incident cases by the disability weight by the average duration of the case until remission or death (years).

QALYs – quality-adjusted life years is life expectancy combined with a measure of the quality of life years remaining. Perfect health for one year equals one QALY.

Sources: www.who.int, www.eufic.org and www.nice.org.uk

RISK IN EPIDEMIOLOGY

Risk is a key term in epidemiology and refers to the likelihood that one thing will lead to another. *Relative risk* is measured in different ways but put simply is an indicator of how likely it is that a person will develop a condition when exposed to something that someone else has not been exposed to. Relative risk therefore provides a measure of the strength of a causal relationship – a *cause* refers to 'any factor that can directly lead to disease e.g. chemicals, radiation, micro-organisms, environment, lifestyle/behaviour' (Hubley et al., 2013: 47). For example, smoking (exposure to harmful chemicals via tobacco smoke) increases the relative risk of developing lung cancer when we compare someone who smokes to a non-smoker. *Attributable risk* basically examines how much disease can be prevented if any causal factors are removed. It is the proportion of disease in people who have been exposed to something that can be attributed to that exposure (Bonita et al., 2006). So, in simple terms, if more deaths occur in people who climb trees as compared to people who do not it would be assumed that climbing trees increases the risk of dying (the deaths would be attributable to the tree-climbing).

A *risk* factor is 'something which can increase the likelihood of disease but on its own is insufficient to cause disease e.g. age, sex, family history, low income' (Hubley et al., 2013: 47) however, if that something does have an impact it will result in negative health outcomes. A *protective* factor, in contrast, decreases the likelihood of disease and leads to positive health outcomes (Carneiro and Howard, 2011). For example, we know that a sedentary lifestyle is a risk factor for a number of chronic diseases whilst partaking in regular physical activity is a protective factor against the same. However, lay understandings of risk often differ to medical or scientific understandings (Crichton and Mulhall, 2015) so what is defined as a risk factor or a protective factor by 'non-expert' people may not chime with what the experts think. This has important implications for how health promotion messages and interventions are designed and delivered.

Epidemiological data can be analysed in a number of different ways and this is sometimes referred to as 'people', 'place' and 'time' (Hubley et al., 2013). *People* is about the nature of who is affected by a certain disease or condition; for example, how old they are, what gender and ethnicity, and their socio-economic circumstances. *Place* refers to which communities are affected and where they are located (geography) – this could be at a local, regional, national or global level. *Time* is about when a disease or condition occurs.

Epidemiological data derives from a number of main sources that are categorised as either 'descriptive' or 'analytical' (Carneiro and Howard, 2011). In each category there are several means of gathering data and information about population health. These are now outlined in turn.

DESCRIPTIVE DATA

Routine monitoring (or routine data sources) is epidemiological information that is gathered routinely or for other reasons such as a population census or household survey. For example, the Community Life Survey in the United Kingdom which is carried out by the government at a household level to find out about people's views on a range of issues but which also asks questions about health, social well-being and lifestyle. Birth and death registers are also examples of routine data. *Descriptive studies* simply describe the existence of a certain condition within a specified population and do not attempt to examine any causal factors/relationships or to find out why the condition may or may not exist in that group of people at that point in time.

REFLECTIVE EXERCISE 9.2

Using the internet and other appropriate sources see what you can find out about the health of the people who live in your neighbourhood, country or region. You could look at the Global Burden of Disease, for example. You could pick an age group, e.g. children aged five years or younger. What are the major diseases being experienced in that age group?

What are those people dying most from? Chronic diseases or infectious diseases or other causes? Most of the information you are likely to come across will give you a good picture of what is happening in that population group; however, it is unlikely to tell you *why* it is happening or what is *causing* it. This is where 'analytical epidemiology' comes in.

ANALYTICAL EPIDEMIOLOGY

In contrast to descriptive studies, *analytical epidemiology* is concerned with 'determining the causes and risk factors for health and disease' (Hubley et al., 2013: 36) and aims to investigate what influences the development (or not) of a condition or disease (Carneiro and Howard, 2011). There are two broad groups of study design in analytical epidemiology. Group 1 comprises 'observation studies' such as ecological studies, cross-sectional studies, cohort studies and case control studies.

Ecological studies are observational studies where populations or groups of people are the units of analysis rather than individuals (Carneiro and Howard, 2011); they are sometimes also referred to as correlational studies (Bonita et al., 2006). Such studies can compare disease patterns in two different regions or countries at the same time, for example. *Prevalence* is an epidemiological term that refers to the disease-status of a given population at a point in time (Crichton and Mulhall, 2015) or 'all cases either at a point in time (point prevalence) or over a defined period in time (period prevalence)' (Green et al., 2019: 72). Prevalence (or *cross-sectional*) studies will therefore give a picture of what is happening in a group of people at a specific time or over a specified period of time – see Box 9.3 for two examples of cross-sectional studies. *Incidence* refers to 'the number of new cases within a particular time period' (Green et al., 2019: 72) and therefore indicates the rate at which a condition is increasing or decreasing in a group of people.

BOX 9.3 CROSS-SECTIONAL STUDIES

Bird et al. (2017) The effects of household income distribution on stroke prevalence and its risk factors of high blood pressure and smoking cross sectional study in Saskatchewan, Canada.

Stroke is a major chronic disease and a common cause of adult disability and mortality. Although there are many known risk factors for stroke, lower income is not one that is often discussed. This study aimed to determine the association between income distribution on the prevalence of stroke in Saskatchewan, Canada. Information was collected from the Canadian Community Health Survey conducted by Statistics for Canada for 2000-2008. The study found that income distribution was strongly associated with

(Continued)

stroke and high blood pressure (which is a risk factor for stroke). That is, having a low household income (defined as below CAD $30,000 per year) increased the likelihood of experiencing a stroke by times seven.

Hobbs et al. (2018) Associations between the combined physical activity environment, socioeconomic status, and obesity: a cross-sectional study.

This study aimed to investigate associations between the combined physical activity environment and obesity and to explore any sub-group effects by individual-level socio-economic status. Drawing on data from a large cohort (n = 22,889) from the Yorkshire Health Study (Yorkshire, United Kingdom), the study found that individuals within favourable physical activity environments were less likely to be obese.

Cohort studies are also sometimes called 'longitudinal' or 'prospective' studies (Crichton and Mulhall, 2015: 101). Such studies usually take place over a longer period of time following the same group of people over several years or even decades. In contrast to case control studies where the development of conditions are examined retrospectively, cohort studies look at how conditions develop over time. An example is the Born in Bradford project. Born in Bradford started in 2007 and is a large cohort study of 13,500 children born at the Bradford Royal Infirmary in Bradford, England during a period of three years. The children are being tracked through childhood into adulthood with researchers collecting medical, educational and social data at different points during their individual lives' trajectories. 'The Born in Bradford cohort study was established to examine how genetic, nutritional, environmental, behavioural and social factors impact in health and development during childhood, and subsequently adult life in a deprived multi-ethnic population' (Wright et al., 2013: 978). For further information see the Born in Bradford website available at https://borninbradford.nhs.uk.

Case control studies are a comparison between two otherwise similar groups of people – one group that has a condition (the cases) and one group that does not have the condition (the controls) (Crichton and Mulhall, 2015). The cases are then investigated for historical factors that might have influenced their developing the condition so the cases are considered in hindsight.

Group 2 are intervention studies. An intervention study is when one group receives an intervention and the outcomes of this are compared with another group that does not receive the intervention in order to determine whether or not the intervention has had an effect. One example of an intervention study is the *randomised control trial* (RCT) which is often referred to as the 'gold standard' in clinical trials as the evidence that they provide about cause and effect relationships is viewed as being more reliable than other sorts of studies (Crichton and Mulhall, 2015). In an RCT the researcher is in complete control of who does and does not receive an intervention and therefore the effectiveness of the intervention can be more easily determined; i.e. does it work? The 'random-ness' of an RCT is in the random allocation of people into either the control group (the group who is not receiving the intervention) and the experimental or intervention (the group that is receiving it). RCTs are often used in clinical settings, i.e. to test a new drug, but can also be used in community settings to determine the effectiveness of an intervention (Gordis, 2013).

BOX 9.4 RANDOMISED CONTROL TRIALS

Kyoko et al. (2019) Effectiveness of an educational program for mid-level Japanese public health nurses to improve program planning competencies: A preliminary randomized control trial.

This study aimed to establish the effect of an education programme for mid-level Japanese public health nurses to improve their competencies in programme planning and therefore better fulfil community health needs. The nurses were randomly allocated to either the control group (not receiving the intervention) or the intervention group. After the intervention the total knowledge and skills scores significantly improved in the intervention group as compared with the control group.

Huybregts et al. (2017) The impact of integrated prevention and treatment on child malnutrition and health: the PROMIS project, a randomized control trial in Burkina Faso and Mali.

The aim of this study was to assess the feasibility, quality of implementation, effectiveness and cost-effectiveness of an integrated child malnutrition prevention and treatment intervention package implemented through a community-based platform in Mali and a facility-based platform in Burkina Faso. The package included behaviour change communication on essential nutrition and hygiene for caregivers of children alongside monthly preventative doses of nutrient supplements for children aged 6–23.9 months. This randomised control trial assesses the effectiveness of this model which combines both prevention and treatment.

GO FURTHER 9.1

Take some time to think about what types of study would be most appropriate if you were trying to achieve the following:

1. investigating the effect of air pollutants on children's asthma;
2. establishing the effectiveness of a new anti-malarial vaccine;
3. investigating the relationship between having a high-fibre diet and developing bowel cancer;
4. establishing the incidence of mental illness in adolescents aged 12 to 19 years.

See the end of the chapter for the answers.

HEALTH PROFILING

Health profiling is the 'technique of describing health using a range of measures' (Hill et al., 2010: 253). In the UK and Ireland health profiling is led by public health observatories (PHOs). This is a relatively recent development and the second health profile for

England was only published in September 2018 (Public Health England, 2018). This health profile brings together data, knowledge and information from different sources in order to present a broad picture of the health of people in England in 2018. It draws on several different types of data for example absolute and relative measures of inequality, breastfeeding at 6–8 weeks, dental decay in children, excess weight in children, the Global Burden of Disease Study (as mentioned earlier in this chapter), healthy life expectancy, serious mental illness and smoking prevalence to name a few. The report covers the following:

- population change and trends in life expectancy;
- trends in mortality;
- trends in morbidity and risk;
- health of children in the early years;
- inequalities in health;
- wider determinants of health;
- current and emerging health protection issues; and
- methods, data and definitions.

The report concluded that 'as a society, people are living longer but often in poorer health and stubborn inequalities persist. Good health is about much more than good healthcare – a high-quality education, a warm home, and a good job are just as important to a healthy standard of living' (Public Health England, 2018: n.p.)

MEASURING POSITIVE CONCEPTS OF HEALTH

So far in this chapter, we have focused much more on patterns of ill health and disease than on *health* itself which reflects a more (bio)medical approach to understanding health and illness on which the discipline of epidemiology is predominantly based. However, there is a growing body of research and literature that is more concerned with how we measure and establish positive indicators of human experience such as well-being and happiness. These attempt to appreciate the complexities of health that were explored in Chapter 1, 'What Is "Health"?' A number of different scales have been devised that are used to measure subjective understandings and experiences of health. See Box 9.5 for details.

BOX 9.5 MEASURING SUBJECTIVE EXPERIENCES OF HEALTH

SF-36 (WARE AND SHERBURN, 1992)

This is a multi-item survey that is widely used to measure health which assesses a number of areas including physical health, mental health, emotional health and experiences of pain.

For further information on this survey tool use an internet search engine using the search term 'SF 36'.

GENERAL HEALTH QUESTIONNAIRE (GOLDBERG AND HILLIER, 1997)

This questionnaire measures psychological well-being and assesses a number of areas including feelings such as depression and unhappiness, sleep disruption and enjoyment of everyday activities.

WARWICK–EDINBURGH MENTAL WELL-BEING SCALE

This scale measures well-being and focuses on mental health including psychological functioning.

Due to the rather narrow way that epidemiology conceptualises 'health' Crichton and Mulhall (2015: 80) argue that a broader definition is needed that takes into the complexities of health experience that traditional epidemiology does not account for – 'a social epidemiology focuses not just on biomedical causes [of disease and illness] but also on socioeconomic factors'. As demonstrated elsewhere in this book (see Chapter 1, 'What Is "Health"?') health is socially determined and is not just about our physical state of being. As discussed, poverty and inequality. As well as focusing on the links between socio-economic factors and (ill) health, social epidemiology looks at why and how this is the case in order to address health inequalities (Crichton and Mulhall, 2015). As Chapter 8, 'Valuing Lay Perspectives', argued, the lay perspective (or 'lay epidemiology') is key to understanding the complexities of health (and illness) experience. This has been demonstrated in a number of different health and illness experiences. See Case Study 9.2 for an example of how lay and expert understandings of health experience can come together to produce more effective measurement tools in relation to mental health recovery.

CASE STUDY 9.2 MEASURING WHAT MATTERS IN MENTAL HEALTH

Accurate clinical outcomes in mental health are important for understanding the burden of ill health and for delivering effective interventions; however, personal recovery – building a valued and socially engaged life – is not typically reflected in such data. There are a number of validated measures of recovery. One example is the 'Hope, Agency and Opportunity' tool (HAO) which was co-produced by people with lived experience of mental ill health and clinicians as a simple means to measure mental health outcomes

(Continued)

in routine clinical care. The tool asks people to rate a number of things on a simple scale (0 = none of the time; 1 = rarely; 2 = some of the time; 3 = often; and 4 = all of the time) as follows:

Over the past few weeks, how much have you experienced a sense of:

1. Hope:

    - Seeing a future for yourself
    - Believing that difficulties in your life will get better
    - Having things that you want to do

Do you believe that you can live well, and pursue your aspirations and goals?

2. Agency (sense of control):

    - Having a choice and information about the support you receive
    - Feeling that you are able to take control of difficulties in your life
    - Knowing how to keep yourself well

Do you have a sense of control over your life?

3. Opportunity:

    - Developing and supporting the things that you are good at
    - Supporting the roles that you already have, e.g. family members, student, job role
    - Having the chance to get involved in your local community

Can you build a full and meaningful life of your choice, with opportunities to be part of a wider society?

4. Working relationships:

    - Being listened to by health and social care professionals and people that support you
    - Working together to build a care plan that fits you
    - Feeling that people supporting you believe in your recovery

Do your relationships with staff foster hope, agency and opportunity for recovery?

Source: Newman-Taylor et al. (2019)

SUMMARY

This chapter has introduced the discipline of epidemiology. It has outlined what epidemiology is and how and why it is a key part of public health and health promotion. Bunton and Macdonald (2004) refer to epidemiology as a 'primary feeder discipline' for health promotion which illustrates the importance of it for developing understanding about what impacts on health experience and, crucially, how we can use epidemiological data and information to inform more effective strategies to improve health experience and health outcomes. Once again, the contribution of the lay perspective and the importance of positive concepts of health have been demonstrated. The next section of this book addresses the question 'Who is responsible for health promotion?' starting with Chapter 10, 'The Role of the Individual'.

SUGGESTED READING

Bonita, R., Beaglehole, R. and Kjellstrm, T. (2006) *Basic epidemiology*. 2nd edn. Geneva, World Health Organization.

Carneiro, I. and Howard, N. (2011) *Introduction to epidemiology*. 2nd edn. Maidenhead, Open University Press.

Gordis, L. (2013) *Epidemiology*. 5th edn. London, Elsevier.

ANSWERS TO GO FURTHER 9.1

1. Ecological study; 2. Randomised control trial; 3. Cohort study; 4. Cross-sectional study.

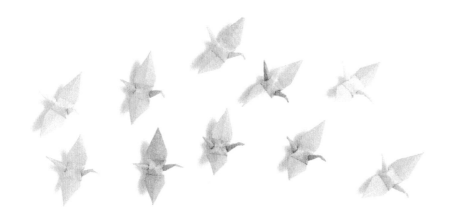

SECTION 4

WHO IS RESPONSIBLE FOR HEALTH PROMOTION?

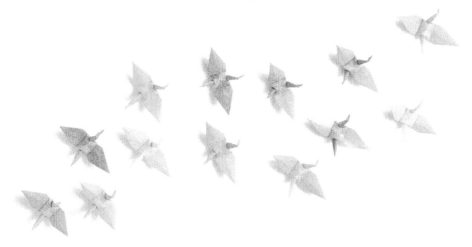

THE ROLE OF
THE INDIVIDUAL 10

INTRODUCTION

The previous chapter explored epidemiology and health profiling. In this section of the book we turn our attention to something quite different and start to consider the question, 'Who is responsible for health promotion?' To this end, Chapter 10 specifically focuses at the micro level; that is, on the role of the individual in the creation and maintenance of health. The chapter presents debates about personal responsibility for health and the notion of the healthy citizen. It introduces, and begins to critique, the neoliberal ideology that underpins these perspectives (a critique that is picked up in more detail in the following chapter – Chapter 11, 'The Role of the State') and describes how it is particularly manifest in recent times through individualised digital health technologies. The role of health education as a method for changing behaviour will also be discussed alongside the value of health communication strategies.

PERSONAL RESPONSIBILITY FOR HEALTH

In Chapter 3, 'Health Promotion Approaches', we introduced the concept of individual approaches to health promotion in the context of contrasting these with structural approaches. As discussed, individual approaches to health promotion operate from the assumption that responsibility for the creation and maintenance of health lies with the individual (Naidoo and Wills, 2016). Health is viewed as something that the individual *can* control and has control *over*. This is a highly individualistic perspective and does not take into account the wider social determinants of health that are discussed elsewhere in this book. There are a number of factors that play a part in our understanding of the role of the individual in health promotion. To begin with we will consider the concepts of risk and lifestyle.

In Chapter 9 we introduced the concept of 'risk' which is also important to this discussion. In this context risk is viewed as a consequence of the lifestyle choices that individuals make which is linked with individual responsibility and self-control (or lack of) (Bell et al., 2011). The concept of 'lifestyle' generally refers to the ways we live our lives and the behaviours that we engage in from day to day which is basically what we do or do not do as a result of the choices that we do or do not make (Korp, 2008). However, it is important to note here that not all of our choices are conscious and that much of our behaviour is also shaped by our environment (physical, social and political). Crucially the focus at the individual level takes very little account of social and structural determinants of health (Cross et al., 2021).

At the individual level people are encouraged to self-police and regulate their own health through a variety of means. This is reinforced by health policy, particularly in more economically wealthy countries. For example, in the United Kingdom, health policy focuses a lot on individual behaviour and the subsequent consequences for personal health which promotes self-regulation and behaviour change. Key public health issues identified for 2019 include smoking, screening, antibiotic use, childhood obesity, and sexual and reproductive health (Brine, 2019). The obligation to look after and monitor our own health is prescribed through the notion of 'healthy lifestyles' which we will now consider alongside the concept of the 'healthy citizen'.

REFLECTIVE EXERCISE 10.1

Consider the term *healthy lifestyle*. What does this mean? Use any information you can find about what it means to live a healthy lifestyle from a range of sources, such as the internet, magazines and social media. What features make up a healthy lifestyle? How does your own life measure up to ideals of a healthy lifestyle? How easy do you think it is to adopt a healthy lifestyle? What barriers stand in your way? What would make it easier?

THE HEALTHY CITIZEN

Neoliberal ideology promotes the idea that individuals have total autonomy over their lives, actions and destiny (Rose, 2000) and it depicts people as having complete control over what they do and the choices that they make – essentially endorsing the idea that they are independent and free agents (Gill and Scharff, 2011). This ideology results in neoliberal policies that shift responsibility onto the individual and away from the collective (government or state). In keeping with this neoliberal ideology is embedded within ideas of how to promote health via notions of personal control and choice, possibility and potential, and self-(re)invention. When health is seen as lying within the control of the individual it stands to reason that they then have a duty and responsibility to ensure and maintain good health, or to strive to achieve as good a state of health as they can. Neoliberal ideas about individual responsibility for health dictate that we should avoid (or at least minimise) behaviours that pose a risk to our health such as smoking, drinking too much alcohol and being sedentary (Robertson and Williams, 2010).

This is reinforced through social and political concerns with healthy lifestyles which result in health-conscious subjects (Ayo, 2012). A health-conscious subject is a person who is aware of their health, the impact that their behavioural choices have on it, and who then makes an effort to improve their health. Being health conscious requires a number of things including self-care and being able to look after oneself, managing one's body appropriately (for example, through undertaking regular physical activity and eating a healthy diet) and the exercise of self-discipline. It is vital to emphasise here that we do, as individuals, have some control over our behaviour but that this is limited for many people in many circumstances. Short and Mollborn (2015: 78) make this point really well when they state that 'at any given point, an individual's health and health behaviours reflect endowments in combination with a cumulated set of experiences and circumstances that have unfolded over time, in distinct and physical contexts'. Nevertheless, a focus on the role of the individual in promoting health is inescapable and we all have a part to play in the promotion of our own health and well-being.

Whilst it might seem quite dated now Peterson and Lupton's (1996) concept of the 'participatory imperative' is still very important. It neatly captures the pressure that is put onto individuals to take an active part in promoting their own health, and in monitoring it. Being a good or valued citizen in society means being a healthy citizen, (or trying to be) and this means engaging in a range of healthier behaviours (Thompson and Kumar, 2011) which includes the idea that we all need to be useful and productive rather than a drain on society's (limited) resources (Patrick, 2012). Being and staying healthy is hard work and it requires time, effort and investment. This links to another neoliberal notion that the body is a project that can be worked on (Rich and Evans, 2008). It is also important to note here that ideas about keeping healthy link to notions of morality and the idea that we all have a duty to take care of/look after ourselves (Gill, 2008). People who exhibit a high level of self-discipline are generally admired and there is a specific set of positive values ascribed to people who appear to be healthy (i.e. slim and toned).

There is also a set of lifestyle behaviours that are held up as being evidence of good citizenship in relation to health – ways in which we should all be behaving. Turn back to Reflective Exercise 10.1 for some examples of these. Good citizenship requires the achievement of health through healthy practice, the pursuit of health and, in turn, self-discipline (Peterson et al., 2010). Being a good citizen means taking good care of one's health (Anderson et al., 2017). Whilst it makes sense at a personal level to try to take care of our own health because of the benefits of doing so, staying well and healthy also reduces our burden on society and associated healthcare costs as pointed out earlier. A book published in 2019 by Carstairs et al. entitled *Be Wise? Be Healthy? Morality and Citizenship in Canadian Public Health Campaigns* highlights how changing our behaviour is no longer a personal choice (if it ever has been). We are increasingly obliged to conform to healthier ways of living and being as part of our social and moral duty as a good (and therefore valued) citizen. A good citizen is therefore a healthy citizen and vice versa. By taking care of our health and our bodies we become perfect neoliberal subjects (Choi, 2019).

REFLECTIVE EXERCISE 10.2

Thinking about health, see if you can create a model of a 'good citizen'. What would they be like? What would they do? How would they behave? What decisions would they make? What activities would they engage in during the course of their lifespan in order to be a good and healthy citizen? You can draw on your work for Reflective Exercise 10.1 to help you here.

A focus at the individual level is important because many behaviours are linked to health experience and health outcomes. 'The evidence for the link between some health behaviours and health outcomes is generally stronger for some health behaviours (e.g. smoking, physical activity) than others (e.g. binge drinking, diet)' (Connor and Norman, 2017: 895). However, research indicates that there are a number of behaviours that increase our risk of developing certain illnesses. For example, up to three-quarters of cancer deaths can be attributed to a person's behaviour (Morrison and Bennett, 2016) and more than 60 medical conditions have alcohol intake as a causal factor (Cameron, 2018). Added to this is the fact that unhealthy behaviours tend to 'cluster' together meaning that they do not tend to occur in isolation or by chance (Rabel et al., 2019). The consequences of this are significant since having two or more unhealthy behaviours (for example smoking, excess alcohol consumption, not taking enough physical activity) increases the risk of mortality (Buck and Frosini, 2012). By way of illustration, research in Australia by Hobbs et al. (2019) showed that the participants with a higher risk of ill health had a range of unhealthy behaviours such as excessive alcohol consumption, excessive sitting time, more fast-food consumption, smoking, more inactivity, and a lack of fruit and vegetables. These participants, however, were also more likely to live in a deprived area which is a very important factor to keep in consideration. Clearly there is a strong link between our environment and the behavioural choices that we have available to us. It is also important to note here that some behaviours can benefit our health and actually protect against illness, such as effective handwashing and eating a healthy diet (Morrison and Bennett, 2016).

INDIVIDUAL FACTORS

Behaviour at an individual level impacts on health in positive and negative ways. We can differentiate between behaviours that have a positive effect on health (health-protective behaviour) and behaviours that have a negative effect on health (health-risk behaviours). Health-protective behaviour are practices that are considered to be beneficial for health. These are also sometimes referred to as behavioural 'immunogens' (Morrison and Bennett, 2016). Such behaviours include regular moderate physical activity, eating a healthy diet, taking part in screening opportunities, being immunised and complying with a treatment regime. Health-risk behaviours are those that are believed to be damaging to our health; these are also sometimes referred to as behavioural 'pathogens' (Morrison and Bennett, 2016). Such behaviours include eating an unhealthy diet, smoking, drinking too much alcohol, illicit drug use, non-compliance with medication or treatment, and unprotected sex.

Behaviour is very complex. There are a number of factors at the individual level that impact on our behaviour. These include our age, personality, motivation, beliefs, perceptions about control and capacity for resilience. As we age our behaviour changes and we adapt as our bodies get older (Rodham, 2019). We are more likely to engage in risky health behaviour whilst we are adolescents, such as binge-drinking and unprotected sex (El Achhab et al., 2016). Our personality type can also influence what we do.

For example, having a Type A personality (being more inclined to competitiveness, hostility and urgency) has been linked to an increased risk of coronary heart disease whilst a sensation-seeking personality will mean that we are more likely to take risks (Morrison and Bennett, 2016). Hardiness appears to offer some protection against ill health, especially experiences of stress. A person with a hardy personality is more likely to be optimistic and open to challenges (Mazzetti et al., 2019). Hardiness is linked to another important notion in health promotion – resilience (see Case Study 10.1 for more detail). Our health beliefs influence on our health behaviours (Dewi et al., 2019) as do our perceptions of personal control (Bennett et al., 2017) whilst motivation is also important. What motivates us (and our levels of motivation) are important drivers in determining health behaviour. Lack of motivation is often a significant factor in why people do not engage in health-enhancing behaviour and motivating people who do not want to change is a challenge (Hardcastle et al., 2015).

CASE STUDY 10.1: RESILIENCE

The concept of resilience has received increasing attention over the past couple of decades (Southwick et al., 2014) and it is perhaps no surprise that this has occurred alongside an increasingly neoliberalised public health context. Resilience is linked to hardiness and our ability to bounce back from adversity (Pooley and Cohen, 2010), cope with the stresses of life and adapt in positive ways to what happens to us (Herrman et al., 2011). As Fletcher and Mustafa (2013: 12) point out, most definitions 'are based around two core concepts: adversity and positive adaptation'. For example, it is defined as 'the capacity to recover from difficulties' (Oxford English Dictionary, n.d.) or 'the ability to be happy, successful, etc. again after something bad or difficult has happened' (Cambridge English Dictionary, n.d.). Essentially the core concept remains the same and can be applied at the individual, community or institutional level. For the purpose of this case study we are focusing on micro-level resilience as linked to the role of the individual in the promotion of health. Resilience is not static; it changes over our life course and in response to our circumstances and relationships with others (Herrman et al., 2011). There is some debate in the literature about whether resilience is innate (a personality trait) or is something that we can acquire but it is acknowledged that resilience is a complex, yet important, concept and is something that is worth enhancing (Southwick et al., 2014). Naturally resilience is closely linked to mental well-being (Barry, 2018) but also to individual health events. However, in a comparison of people who had experienced a single health event during a defined period of time and people who had experienced several health events over the same period resilience was not affected by the number which, it was concluded, is an indication that resilience is generally robust (Morin et al., 2017). The challenge for health promotion, then, is how can we promote and enhance individual resilience?

BOX 10.1 THE ALAMEDA SEVEN

Research suggests that there are seven key behavioural factors associated with health and longevity:

1. Sleeping 7–8 hours per night
2. Not smoking
3. Consuming no more than 1–2 alcoholic drinks per day
4. Getting regular exercise
5. Not eating between meals
6. Eating breakfast
7. Being no more than 10% overweight

(Cited in Morrison and Bennett, 2016: 53)

INDIVIDUALISED DIGITAL HEALTH TECHNOLOGIES

The active, responsible citizen is obliged to participate in various forms of self-governance and self-regulation including those required to maintain good health (Green et al., 2012). Advances in digital technology have resulted in numerous ways that we can monitor and govern our own health; for example, through mobile apps and wearable devices. These can range from a simple pedometer or step-counter on a smart phone to more complex devices that measure and monitor intricate physiological conditions. Lupton (2020) points out that digital health technologies can increase a sense of agency and control over our health enabling people to gain knowledge and better understand their own health and well-being and, in that sense, they can be empowering. The most commonly targeted behaviours are physical activity and healthy eating, the most commonly used technology platform is the mobile phone, whilst goal setting and self-management are the most frequently reported reasons for engagement (Taj et al., 2019).

It is becoming increasingly apparent that digital technology and social media have huge potential to increase population health through different means including individual engagement with these (Allegrante and Auld, 2019). Digital technology can be used to change health behaviour and the amount of research on this has risen significantly in the past two decades as our access to digital technologies has grown (Taj et al., 2019: n.p.). However, Lupton (2020) cautions that there is a potential for personal data to be mined, used and exploited by third parties which people are not always aware of and, as Allegrante and Auld (2019) argue, there are numerous other moral, ethical and legal challenges that have to be taken into account. In addition, this links directly to some of the issues we have raised with the neoliberal ideology embedded in contemporary public health agenda neatly captured in the following quote: 'when a sufficiently large portion of the population starts making positive changes to health-related behaviours, this will lead to lower utilization of healthcare and, eventually, to a significant reduction in healthcare expenditure' (Taj et al., 2019). Nevertheless, such digital technologies can be harnessed to improve people's health in many different ways.

'Wearables' refer to wearable devices that people can use to aid healthier lifestyles through being able to measure, track and record things like physical activity levels and diet (O'Neil, 2019). Deborah Lupton has written extensively on this phenomenon in her work including her book *The Quantified Self: A Sociology of Self-Tracking* (2016). Whilst such devices can result in healthier behaviour it seems that the effects, for various reasons, can be relatively short-lived and that the efficacy of using wearables to change individual behaviour actually decreases over time (Ledger, 2014; Stephenson et al., 2017). Next, we will consider the role that health education has to play at the individual level.

HEALTH EDUCATION AND THE INDIVIDUAL

Health education is defined as 'any combination of learning experiences designed to help individuals and communities improve their health, by increasing their knowledge or influencing their attitudes' (WHO, n.d.). Health education puts the onus on the personal responsibility for health and reinforces what Gustafson (2011) refers to as the civic duty to maintain (individual) health. Attempts to improve health often take the form of health education interventions designed to persuade people to change their behaviours, reduce any risks to their own health and adopt healthier lifestyles (Green et al., 2019). This comes from the simple hypothesis that knowing what is good for you will mean that you will do it. However, the assumption that more knowledge, better education or increased awareness leads to positive behaviour change is problematic because it is never this simple (Thompson and Kumar, 2011). Consider your own behaviour. You may know, for example, that it is important for your health to eat at least five portions of fruit and vegetables per day, or that you should do at least 30 minutes of moderately vigorous exercise a recommended five times per week, but do you manage to do this? Also see Case Study 10.2 for further illustration of this conundrum in relation to knowledge, attitudes and practice.

CASE STUDY 10.2: THE K-A-P FORMULA

The K-A-P formula is a simple way of trying to explain health behaviour (Green et al., 2019). K is for knowledge, A is for attitude(s) and P is for practice (or behaviour). Despite the limitations of this model it is utilised quite frequently in the wider literature to explore different types of health behaviour using self-administered surveys that question people about their knowledge, attitudes and practices in relation to different phenomena. An Iranian study that explored K-A-P relating to hypertension found that knowledge levels about the symptoms and causes of this condition were high but that this did not translate into appropriate avoidance behaviours such as

(Continued)

eating less salt or taking regular exercise (Lookian et al., 2019). Similarly a study on breast self-examination in Ethiopia found that, although the participants had a high level of knowledge and expressed positive attitudes towards it, this did not result in them regularly examining their breasts for any abnormalities (Yosef et al., 2019). Interestingly both studies found that levels of formal education were linked to levels of knowledge which points to the importance of education as a social determinant of health. A final example is that research indicates that university and college students are generally more likely to develop and maintain unhealthy diets than the general population despite knowing what a healthy diet comprises (Lalot et al., 2019). This is likely for a number of complex reasons; however, lack of knowledge does not appear to be a key factor. Some of the reasons cited include lack of time and lack of money which could also be linked to the social determinants of health.

GO FURTHER 10.1

Explore the academic journal literature using your institution's library service or even Google Scholar. See if you can find two or three journal papers which use the K-A-P formula to investigate health behaviours. Was knowledge a good predictor of behaviour? What about attitudes towards the behaviour? Did they serve as a useful indicator about the likelihood that behaviour would result? What conclusions do the author/s draw based on their findings? Do you agree with them? Why, or why not? What are the implications for health education?

Health education aligns with individualistic and top-down approaches to promoting health (see Chapter 3, 'Health Promotion Approaches', for more details). Such approaches operate under the assumption that the expert knows best and that, by imparting expert knowledge to people, change will happen resulting in better health outcomes. The educational approach is one of five different approaches to health promotion outlined in Naidoo and Wills's (2016) typology of approaches which also includes the medical approach, the behaviour change approach, the empowerment approach and the social change approach. For more detail on the other four approaches see Naidoo and Wills (2016). For the purpose of this chapter we are focusing on the educational approach. The aim of the educational approach is 'to ensure that people are well informed and able to make healthier choices' (Naidoo and Wills, 2016: 76) by providing knowledge, information and advice. The purpose of using an educational approach (health education) is not to try to persuade people to change behaviour but to provide the necessary knowledge in order to raise awareness, and the assumption is that a change in knowledge or awareness will ultimately lead to a change in behaviour.

Health education takes many forms for example, leaflets, posters, one-to-one advice and information on websites as well as working in small groups – see Table 10.1 for some examples.

Table 10.1 Health education

Health Topic	Health Education
Physical Exercise	Promotion of benefits of exercise, understanding of the kinds of exercise that will improve health and skills in specific exercise methods.
Tobacco Smoking	Promotion of increased awareness of the risks of smoking, the benefits of quitting and practical skills in resisting peer pressure, refusing cigarettes and different ways of stopping smoking.
Alcohol Abuse	Directed at young people, young adults and other age groups on appropriate alcohol use, self-monitoring of alcohol consumption, resisting peer pressure, etc.
Nutrition - promotion of fruit and vegetable consumption	Using schools and mass media to promote awareness of the health benefits of eating fruit and vegetables.

Source: Hubley et al. (2021) reproduced by kind permission of Polity Press. Ltd.

Health education does have a role to play in the promotion of health and education for skills development is particularly important. For example, a person may know that it is beneficial to eat a healthy diet but not possess the cooking skills needed to prepare healthy foods. It does appear that skills-based health education methods are more likely to be successful than traditional health education methods and can lead to deeper and longer-lasting knowledge (Simbar et al., 2017). However, it is also important to note that health education and educational approaches tend to fail to acknowledge or address the barriers to changing behaviour that exist in people's physical and social environments (Dorling et al., 2018).

In any instance using an educational approach adopts an expert-led model whereby the recipient is deemed to be lacking in some way, usually because they do not know something or are misinformed. This is often referred to as the 'deficit' model (Cross et al., 2017: 7). Consequently, health education rarely takes into account the lay expertise which we have signalled the importance of in Chapter 8, 'Valuing Lay Perspectives'. Nevertheless, educational approaches have an important role to play in the promotion of health and it is arguably difficult to promote behaviour change without some element of education.

VICTIM-BLAMING

Education and behavioural change approaches to health promotion theoretically hold a lot of promise; however, in reality outcomes are limited. In addition such approaches can lead to victim-blaming and stigmatisation (Tengland, 2016) which, from a health promotion perspective, we would seek to avoid because victim-blaming clearly does not sit well with notions of empowerment (Cross et al., 2017). We have to be especially careful of implying that ill health is self-inflicted and that people who are experiencing ill health deserve to as this distracts from addressing structural health inequalities.

'The essence of victim-blaming lies in attempts to persuade individuals to take responsibility for their own health while ignoring the fact that they are victims of social and environmental circumstances' (Green et al., 2019: 20). Victim blaming holds the individual to account for their health behaviour and the choices that they make. Emphasising individual responsibility puts the responsibility onto individuals to avoid behaviours that are damaging or risky to health and to engage in behaviours that promote better health outcomes. We can turn to the issue of overweight and obesity to illustrate this very clearly. Varea and Underwood (2016) carried out a study exploring Australian physical education teachers' constructions of fatness and found that certain bodies were classified as 'decent' and 'normal', and 'indecent' and 'abnormal' depending on their size (no prizes for guessing how people who were judged to be overweight or obese were classified!). Comments in Varea and Underwood's (2016) data such as 'you are just an idiot for not doing any physical activity right now', 'unless they are quite lazy they should all be able to have quite a fit body', and 'I just looked at them and wow! What are you doing? You are 14 and could have a BMI over 35 ... that's huge!' illustrate a victim-blaming mentality. People who carry excess weight are often judged for doing so and labelled as lazy, greedy or lacking in self-control; however, the issue is much more complex than this. Whilst it might be assumed that becoming overweight is simply to do with eating too much there are many other factors at play which should be taken into account in order to avoid blaming people. For example, we need to consider this within the context of an obesogenic environment. An obesogenic environment is 'an environment promoting high energy intake and sedentary behaviour' (Rendina et al., 2019: 562). It is no surprise, then, that neighbourhoods with higher numbers of fast-food outlets, higher volumes of road traffic and less public space amenable to taking part in physical activity have higher rates of obesity nor is it a mere coincidence that, in wealthier countries, less well-off people are more likely to be overweight then their wealthier counterparts (Wilkinson and Pickett, 2009). Clearly the wider, social determinants of health play a significant role in the development of obesity.

HEALTH COMMUNICATION STRATEGIES AND THE INDIVIDUAL

The focus on individual-level behaviour change over recent decades has led to the development of several theories that try to account for how behaviour change takes place (or not). These derive from the discipline of psychology and are collectively referred to as 'social cognitive models'. They include, for example, the Health Belief Model (Janz and Becker, 1984), the Transtheoretical Model (Prochaska and DiClemente, 1982), the Theory of Planned Behaviour (Ajzen, 1988) and the COM-B model (Michie et al., 2011). This is not an exhaustive list and there isn't the space to go into each model in-depth in this chapter so for more information see Connor and Norman (2015). Suffice to say, such models attempt to identify the different factors that influence behaviour change including, for example, beliefs, motivation, self-efficacy and behavioural intention.

Social cognition models are subject to a number of general criticisms. Firstly, they do not take into account the wider social, political and environmental determinants of health that can constrain the choices we are able to make at an individual level (Ayo, 2012). Secondly, they are reductionist and tend to objectify human experience in contrast to the more holistic approach that characterises health promotion (Green et al., 2019). Thirdly, they do not take into account a range of important factors such as past behaviour and habit (Gardner et al., 2012), emotion (Ferrer and Mendes, 2018) and culture/cultural context (Napier, 2017). They also tend to be quite simplistic whilst health behaviour is very complicated. Finally, as Cross et al. (2017: 6) point out, 'too often health communication efforts result in pointing the finger of blame at individuals or groups that "fail" to take up advice and change their behaviour without taking into consideration the complex contexts of everyday life'. Consequently some, like Short and Mollborn (2015: 78), would argue that a 'social determinants approach' to health behaviours needs to be taken which combines individually focused approaches to health behaviour with consideration of the context in which the behaviour takes place – this approach 'shifts the lens from individual attribution and responsibility to societal organization and the myriad institutions, structures, inequalities, and ideologies undergirding health behaviours'.

GO FURTHER 10.2

See if you can find any other models of behaviour change. Use the internet and the health promotion literature to help you identify one. Once you have found one try to critique it starting with the points outlined as general criticisms in this section. Is the model you have found subject to the same challenges? How could it be improved? What would you need to add or change?

SUMMARY

This chapter has considered the role of the individual in the promotion of health. It has explored the extent to which individuals are able to take control over their health and influence personal health outcomes, acknowledging some of the challenges and limitations involved. Health education has a part to play in the promotion of health; however, this approach also has limitations, as debated here. This chapter has also discussed the problem of victim-blaming and the role that digital technology has to play in the promotion of individual health. The positioning of the individual as responsible for health fits within a neoliberal public health agenda which has been critically deliberated in this chapter. In the next chapter we turn from the micro to the macro and explore the role of the state in the promotion of health.

SUGGESTED READING

Connor, M. and Norman, P. (2015) *Predicting and changing health behaviour: research and practice with social cognition models*. 3rd edn. Maidenhead, Open University Press.

Green, J., Cross, R., Woodall, J. and Tones, K. (2019) Education for health. In *Health promotion: planning and strategies*. 4th edn. London, Sage.

Naidoo, J. and Wills, J. (2016) Models and approaches to health promotion. In *Foundations for Health Promotion*. 4th edn. London, Elsevier. pp. 75–91.

THE ROLE OF
THE STATE

11

INTRODUCTION

The idea about who is responsible for the health of individuals and the community is contested, debated and not always straightforward. Are individuals wholly responsible for themselves, or should governments and other agencies also act to support the health and well-being of their citizens? The argument for state involvement is that many of the things that impact on individual and community health are outside of people's control with collective effort – driven by policy changes – often required to create conditions which support, rather than hinder, health. Yet, health promotion programmes and interventions tend to exclude such factors and instead focus on individual behaviour change. The role of the state and the value of tackling broader societal structures, as opposed to personal behaviours, will be outlined with reference to their contribution to the social determinants of health. The ideology of this position will be outlined and critiqued with successes shared in relation to several effective legislative changes. However, counterarguments that such approaches are paternalistic and a form of 'nanny state' will also be discussed.

SOCIAL STRUCTURE

In countries such as the United States, the UK and Australia, there has been a dominant view held that health promotion is about modifying and addressing individual behaviour – with modifying individuals' decision-making as a key component to improve outcomes. This is best summed up by the following quotation: 'most illnesses and premature death are caused by human habits of living that people choose for themselves' (Iglehart, 1990: 4). Despite this dominant and persuasive view, there are wider influences on individuals which can contribute to decision-making. Indeed, the notion of social structure is one of the most important terms in the social sciences. Some emphasise structure over people's ability to make their own choices (agency) and suggest that it is the social world that constructs people and their actions are predetermined by structural forces, such as the environment, culture (see Box 11.1) and political structures (Sibeon, 1999). At its extreme, those who emphasise structural forces would suggest that social structures and processes are so powerful that individual actions are relatively ineffectual (Donnelly, 2003).

BOX 11.1 CULTURE AND HEALTH (HUBLEY ET AL., 2021)

The concept of culture combines all or some of the following elements:

- norms: shared characteristics of a group;
- traditions: ideas, values and practices that have been held for a long time and passed on to the next generation;
- systems of thought and ideas: reinforced by language, religion and systems of medicine.

With this definition in mind, some of the ways in which culture can shape behaviours and choices may be as follows:

- *Life course*: family structure, patterns of influence among family members, the role of women, children, rituals and roles surrounding birth, growing up, relations with other people, sex and marriage, family formation, work, growing old, death.
- *Masculinity and femininity*: the roles of men and women in society, views of what makes a 'man' and 'woman', body image, gender stereotypes, divisions of roles and responsibilities between genders.
- *Patterns of living and consumption*: clothing, housing, child-rearing, food production, storage and consumption, hygiene practices, sanitation.
- *Health and illness behaviours*: concepts of health and illness, ideas about mental illness, care of sick people, traditional medicine systems, patterns of help seeking when ill, use of doctors and traditional healers, responses to pain, concepts about the biological workings of the body, growth, conception, pregnancy, birth, etc.
- *Patterns of communication*: language, verbal and non-verbal communication, taboos on public discussion of sensitive items, vocabulary of the language, oral traditions.
- *Religion and 'world view'*: ideas about the meaning of life and death, rituals surrounding important life events, ideals about the possibility and desirability of change.
- *Patterns of social influence, social networks and political organization*: influences in family and community, community leadership and authority, political structures, divisions and social inequalities.
- *Economic patterns*: types of employment, home based or workplace, casual or permanent, self-employed, family concern or employee, financial interdependency within the extended family, access to capital funds to initiate new ventures.

Dahlgren and Whitehead's (1991) model, shown in Figure 11.1, encapsulates some of the structural issues impacting on people. The model highlights the structural influences that constrain and enable health and also the individual lifestyle factors (choices) that people have some degree of control over. At the broadest level, Dahlgren and Whitehead (1991: 11) suggest that socio-economic, cultural and environmental conditions impact on health status. Indeed as seen in Chapter 5, it is demonstrated clearly how inequalities in these areas impact adversely on health outcomes including life expectancy.

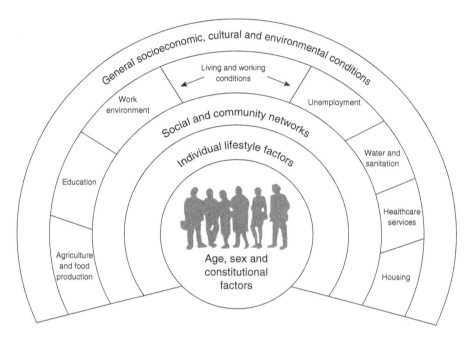

Figure 11.1 The main determinants of health

Source: Dahlgren and Whitehead (1991: 11) Reproduced by kind permission of Stockholm Institute of Future Studies

REFLECTIVE EXERCISE 11.1

'Are the decisions people make with respect to food, exercise, smoking, and the like largely a matter of individual choice or are they principally moulded by structural variables such as social class position and gender?' (Cockerham, 2007: 55) Consider the quotation and take some time to consider to what extent you agree with the ideas within it. How do structures influence what seem like people's individual choices? What implications does this quotation have for health promotion and how health inequalities are tackled?

HEALTH PROMOTION AND SOCIAL STRUCTURE

According to Green et al. (2019), one of the definitive features of health promotion has been an emphasis on the environmental determinants of health (structures), but, as mentioned, this is often reduced to focus on individual choices and behaviour. This is often referred to as 'lifestyle drift' (see Box 11.2). The recognition, however, that the major influences on individuals' health are outside of their immediate control and choice has resulted in a drive to create supportive environments where the 'healthy choice' is the 'easy choice' (Kickbusch, 1986; Milio, 1986). Several international declarations on health promotion have emphasised the structural factors influencing people's health – the Shanghai declaration on health promotion (WHO, 2016) strongly emphasises the role of structural forces on health over and above the role of individual decision-making and choice. However, in practice, there is a lot of emphasis on attempts to modify individual choices without a full recognition of the social context that individuals and community are living within.

BOX 11.2 LIFESTYLE DRIFT

Lifestyle drift is the inclination for policy that recognises the need to act on upstream social determinants only to drift downstream to focus on individual lifestyle factors (Popay et al., 2010). For an example of this in practice, see Case Study 11.1.

Psychological models of behaviour change are commonly used in health promotion, but these can be relatively futile as they fail to take into full account the broader social influences which can shape choices. For some time, health promotion has been criticised by some writers for being overly preoccupied by the ways in which individuals behave (Kelly and Charlton, 1995; Nettleton and Bunton, 1995). This criticism has been particularly directed at those interventions addressing lifestyle choices and on individual-level strategies to promote healthy living. These often include efforts to change individuals' diet, exercise routine, smoking behaviours, and so on.

Those challenging this individualistic view on health choices and decision-making suggest that this perspective oversimplifies disease causation and fails to address the social determinants of health, such as poverty, unemployment and poor housing (Davison and Davey Smith, 1995; Naidoo, 1986). Traditional health education (i.e. health education associated with authoritarian values integral to a preventive medical model (Green, 2008)), for instance, was condemned as being the embodiment of victim-blaming. Indeed, Crawford (1980) suggested that the ideology of blaming the victim underplayed, what he termed, the 'assault' on health caused by structural and environmental forces. Holding people responsible for their own health is particularly problematic in the case of those living in poverty as it is known that this is a significant risk factor for illness and early death. In addition, such a victim-blaming approach underplays just how difficult it can be to change and modify behaviours and also underplays how enjoyable some perceived 'unhealthy' behaviours can be: smoking, drinking alcohol and not exercising have their pleasurable qualities.

Instead of focusing on the structural and social determinants of health, the prescribed lifestyle approach – which advocates particular ways of behaving – puts particular health values on a pedestal to be attained (Nettleton, 1995), where lower socio-economic groups, for instance, are 'typically portrayed as those who fail to take up the exhortations of health promoters, who deliberately expose themselves to health risks rather than "rationally" avoiding them, and who, therefore, require greater surveillance and regulation' (Smith, 2000: 344).

This raises important questions in relation to values and perspectives (see Box 11.3). Such an outlook clearly has the potential to reinforce stigma and contribute towards 'deviance amplification', labelling or moral condemnation (Lowenberg, 1995; Nettleton and Bunton, 1995; Smith, 2000). Critiques from socialist perspectives assert that individualising health fails to take into consideration the complex social factors and pressures that accompany behavioural choice and ignores the broader context in which personal behaviours are embedded (Green and Raeburn, 1988; Laverack, 2004; Staten et al., 2005).

BOX 11.3 THE SMOKER AND THE SKIER

Why do we make a distinction between socially unacceptable and socially acceptable lifestyles, even though both may lead to disease and dysfunction? We excoriate the smoker but congratulate the skier. Yet both skiing and smoking may lead to injury, may be costly, and are clearly risky.

(Fitzgerald, 1994)

Reflect on this quotation and consider which lifestyles in society are considered acceptable and which are not? Think why this may be? Both the skier and the smoker have the *potential* to impact on healthcare usage but why do we stigmatise the smoker with lung cancer and not the skier with broken bones?

Schwartz (2004) asserts that choice undoubtedly improves our quality of life; however, the concept of 'free choice' can be somewhat of an illusion as the environment plays a major role in whether people are in a position to choose a healthy way of life. Structural conditions, for example, perform an important role in an individual's ability to exercise free choice. Material, environmental, social, political and cultural determinants can all influence people's capacity to take action (McKee and Raine, 2005). Indeed, a definition of health lifestyles, proposed by Cockerham (1993: 419), takes into consideration agency and structural conditions: 'health lifestyles refers to patterns of voluntary health behaviour based on choices from options that are available to people according to their life situations'.

REFLECTIVE EXERCISE 11.2

Imagine you are debating whether the state should intervene further in the health choices of its citizens. Review the arguments presented in parts of the chapter and decide which you feel would be the most convincing. Also, imagine a group arguing against your position – what counter-arguments would you consider to strengthen your position?

Restrictions on health choices by structural factors can be seen at more localised levels in settings (see Chapter 13). For example, enabling prisoners to make healthy choices can be a complex process. Squires and Measor (2001: 149), for example, note: 'Behavioural change is not facilitated by an institutional environment that has only limited access to exercise, relatively few dietary options, where smoking is endemic and an atmosphere of lethargy and intimidation, punctuated by outbreaks of violence and bullying, is all pervasive.' Prisons may also inhibit individuals from making healthy choices. Condon et al. (2008: 164), for instance, suggests that 'prison continues to restrict the ability of prisoners to make healthy choices and in some cases actively obstructs prisoners from making the healthy choices they wish to make'.

As an illustration, prisoners in previous research have demonstrated an understanding and awareness of what is meant by a healthy diet; however, prisoners have a limited choice over the foods provided to them (Gately et al., 2006; Ramaswamy and Freudenberg, 2007). In an extreme example, prison staff have expressed concerns about the provision and sale of fruit due to the possibility of prisoners using this to manufacture alcoholic drinks (Godderis, 2006; Hayton et al., 2000). Smoking provides a further example, as studies show that many prisoners are motivated to stop smoking, but often increase the number of cigarettes they smoke to cope with the 'suffocating boredom' of prison life (Belcher et al., 2006; Lester et al., 2003; Sim, 2002; Squires and Measor, 2001). A young prisoner, interviewed as part of a study exploring the resettlement needs of ex-offenders, summarised the issue:

> When you're inside, you're just bored or just stressed out, and you know you smoke and smoke and smoke. And when you're out here it's just I have the urge to smoke even though I don't even want one. I mean before when I got locked up yeah I didn't even buy cigs.
>
> (Burgess-Allen et al., 2006: 296)

Similar findings have been reported in regards to substance misuse, with male prisoners in an American study turning to drugs to relieve the stress, boredom and reality associated with prison life (Seal et al., 2004).

CASE STUDY 11.1: LIFESTYLE DRIFT IN ACTION IN PRISON SETTINGS

Some have suggested that health promotion practice in prisons is typified by lifestyle drift (Woodall, 2016). Several health promotion strategies and policies to address the health of the prison population have asserted the requirement to act on the social determinants of health. Such rhetoric is laudable and, given the inequalities faced by prison populations, such a strategy seems appropriate and potentially effective.

Nonetheless, in practice a downstream focus is clear with interventions often concerning smoking, physical activity and fitness, healthy eating, and so on (HM Prison Service, 2003). The reasons underpinning why lifestyle drift has occurred in this setting are not fully understood, although practical factors may be an issue. For example, lifestyle interventions are easier to devise than 'upstream' interventions (Carey et al., 2016) and the Scottish Prison Service themselves suggested that 'pragmatism' was a key factor in developing their approach to health promoting prisons. Moreover, in a culture where monitoring prison performance against benchmarks is common, lifestyle interventions are significantly easier to evaluate (Baum and Fisher, 2014). As an illustration, indicators developed to monitor the delivery of health promotion in prisons in England and Wales operated on a 'traffic light' indicator system which measures success against targets such as the completion of smoking cessation programmes and the number of referrals to prison exercise programmes (NOMS et al., 2007).

INTERVENTIONS TO ADDRESS SOCIAL STRUCTURES IN HEALTH PROMOTION

Encouraging individual change to modify health behaviours or to adopt alternative choices is unlikely to have a mass effect in shifting health inequalities and more effective change may come from legislative action. In tackling broader social forces that influence, there is an inherent ideological position being played out – that being, that it is social factors, not individuals, that create health outcomes for individuals. Some time ago, Tones (1986) attempted to demonstrate the factors influencing health choices. He argued that choices are based on individual decision-making processes and wider social and environmental forces. This is highlighted diagrammatically in Figure 11.2, where socio-political action and individually directed interventions are advocated to facilitate health choices. However, these are two distinct ideological approaches which imply different political orientations.

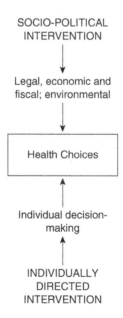

Figure 11.2 Factors influencing health choices

Source: Tones (1986: 6). Reproduced by kind permission of the Oxford University Press

A socialist, or left-wing position, in considering health promotion would see disadvantaged groups having limited power and choice in affecting the determinants that influence their health. Therefore advocates would call for collective solutions and interventions aimed at social justice to reduce inequalities in health (Davison and Davey Smith, 1995).

Left-wing views of health promotion support a systems or structural approach to health promotion, grounded predominantly in macro-level or environmental interventions which draws its focus towards the social, economic, political, institutional, cultural, legislative, industrial and physical environments of societies in order to modify behaviour change (Green and Raeburn, 1988). Nettleton and Bunton (1995: 44) summarise: 'Essentially the structural critique argues that attempts to prevent illness and to promote health have failed to take into account the material disadvantages of people's lives. This works at three levels: the political environment, the social environment and the physical environment.'

The structural approach avoids focusing on the individual and instead intervenes at a political or systems level (Stokols et al., 2003). Governments, therefore, act as stewards to create policy frameworks which encourage individuals to make healthier choices. This approach essentially evades blaming the victim (Jochelson, 2006; Lowenberg, 1995). Structural approaches, through legislation for example, can change behaviour on a great magnitude. McKinlay (1979: 23) has noted that this can be equal to several forms of individually targeted health intervention:

> It is probably true that one stroke of effective health legislation is equal to many separate health intervention endeavours and the cumulative efforts of innumerable health workers over long periods of time ... greater changes will result from the continued politicization of illness, than from the modification of specific individual behaviours.

THE ROLE OF THE STATE

The state is often considered as the overarching political body, such as a government, which has responsibility for its citizens. Policy is often utilised as a way of protecting citizens and efforts to improve their health. Most recently, the power of the state has been seen in relation to managing and controlling Covid-19 in almost every global nation. History has shown how effective state intervention has saved lives and improved the health of communities, but this has always come with a backdrop of heavy debate and disagreement as not everyone believes that state intervention is proportionate or even justifiable. By way of illustration, the first Public Health Act in Britain in 1848 gave the state control over the water and sewerage systems, but at that time it was seen as deeply controversial. Moreover, alcohol licensing legislation in 1872 which banned children from drinking spirits in pubs and limited opening hours for drinking was highly debated and seen as a challenge to liberty (Jochelson, 2006). Even more recently decisions by states to enforce seatbelt usage (see Case Study 11.2), restricting smoking in public places, encouraging healthy diets (see Box 11.4) and limits to advertising of tobacco products have created challenges and caused deep divisions of opinion (Green et al., 2019).

BOX 11.4 EXAMPLES OF STATE INTERVENTION TO ENCOURAGE HEALTHY DIETS (WHITSEL, 2017)

- Reduce sodium, trans fat and added sugar in the food supply.
- Improve food labelling.
- Nutrition standards for school meals.
- Nutrition standards in early care and education and out-of-school time programs.
- Eliminate unhealthy food marketing and advertising to children.
- Improve access to healthy affordable foods in the community (healthy food financing, school/community gardens).
- Continue to improve nutrition standards and nutrition education in government feeding programmes.
- Sugar-sweetened beverage taxes.
- Placement and maintenance of water fountains or dispensers in public places.

Interestingly many state or government decisions that impact on health are not from health departments necessarily – the broader policy environment can have huge impacts on the health of individuals.

REFLECTIVE EXERCISE 11.3

Make a list of governmental departments in your country and consider the policies that they implement and how they can impact on health. If you are unaware what the departments are, then you can search for them or use the examples below from the UK government:

- Department for Education
- Ministry of Defence
- Department for Communities and Local Government
- Department for Work and Pensions
- Department for Transport
- Department for International Development

CASE STUDY 11.2: THE IMPACT OF SEAT-BELT LAWS

Insisting that drivers and passengers in vehicles wear seat belts has been a very powerful approach that many countries have adopted. This has without doubt saved thousands of lives. Seat-belt legislation became common in many developed countries in the 1980s, but some countries have only recently passed the same laws. There is variability in the actual legislation in many countries. In some developing countries, there is no mandate for rear passengers to wear seat belts. Research shows that, despite being mandatory, seat belts are not always used or enforced by parents when they have children in the car. Reasons include: seat belts being uncomfortable, not working or absent; overcrowded cars; cars having airbags making seat belts unnecessary; short or bumpy journeys; and areas unlikely to have a police presence were also given as reasons (Green et al., 2007). This suggests that while legislation can be a useful tool that the state can use in protecting health and preventing injury, it requires enforcement and monitoring to ensure compliance.

One tool open to the state to modify health behaviours is the use of taxation as a way in which to place barriers on the purchasing of certain 'unhealthy' products (see Case Study 11.3). The basic notion being that if the cost is prohibitive, it will restrict people's ability to buy certain products. The best examples here are seen in relation to tobacco products, alcohol and some junk food. Evidence shows that price rises in unhealthy products leads to restrictions in people's purchasing and consumption (Hawkins and McCambridge, 2020).

CASE STUDY 11.3: SODA TAXES

The soda tax, a piece of public policy originating in the USA, was an illustration of state intervention in modifying people's consumption of sugar. Despite soda companies opposing the policy to raise taxes on sugary drinks to reduce consumption, many jurisdictions across the USA implemented this tax increase to prevent the consumption of sugary drinks and, indeed, saw reductions in consumption (Gostin, 2017).

Another state intervention tool comprises advertising bans to restrict exposure to certain unhealthy products and thereby reducing awareness or the influence advertising can have on decision-making. A historic example from the 1990s demonstrated the power of advertising and the impact of global corporations and why curbing their influence could offer positive outcomes. At the time, the average school child was watching 10,000 TV commercials per year – during one year Kellogg spent $32 million advertising a single high-sugar cereal product, but during the same period the US government spent only $50,000 per state on nutrition education (Callaghan, 2000).

REFLECTIVE EXERCISE 11.4

While watching TV, listening to the radio, or searching online, consider how many advertisements you are faced with. Which of these would you consider are the most persuasive and why? Consider which advertisements are promoting unhealthy products and which are promoting healthy products. Consider how this changes during different times of the day and reflect why this may be the case.

We have seen in recent times some radical action by some governments to support health and, more particularly, decelerate the spread of disease. During the 2013–2016 Ebola outbreak in western Africa, a series of government actions were undertaken to detect and lessen the transmission of Ebola. Countries with Ebola transmission were advised by WHO to begin exit screening at all international airports, land crossings and seaports. The advice included travel restrictions for all confirmed, probable, suspected or contact cases of Ebola. General bans on international travel, however, were not advised. Research showed that countries had variable levels of adoption of the WHO international travel recommendations made in response to the 2013–2016 Ebola outbreak based on, perhaps, political factors and risk perceptions (Rhymer and Speare, 2017). More recently, the Covid-19 outbreak in 2020 saw the Italian government place up to 16 million people under quarantine and announced the closure of schools, gyms, museums, nightclubs and other venues across the whole country to control the spread of the disease. Restaurants and cafes in the quarantined zones could open between 06:00 and 18:00 but customers had to sit at least 1 metre apart. The Italian government told its citizens to stay at home as much as possible, with those who break the quarantine facing three months in jail. Italy was the first European nation to enact such restrictions and, soon after, almost all other nations followed with some approach to protecting its citizens through restricting their autonomy and liberty.

CRITICAL PERSPECTIVES ON STRUCTURAL APPROACHES TO HEALTH PROMOTION

So far, this chapter has provided a strong argument for the role of state intervention in tackling health challenges. As noted, this view is an ideological one and does not come uncontested. The broader debate is where the line is drawn – to what extent should government and authorities intervene to protect or improve people's health through policy measures and to what extent should people have the right to make their own free choices? The debate is complex, although politicians and those in positions of authority are known to be hesitant to use the state to intervene in such health matters as it can jeopardise their own popularity (Zalmanovitch and Cohen, 2013). Banning, restricting and broadly legislating against behaviours is not always popular.

GO FURTHER 11.1

Think about the following and reflect as to whether you feel governments are right to intervene to protect and promote the health of their citizens in these ways:

- Banning smoking in cars when children are passengers.
- Banning junk-food advertisements on children's TV channels.
- Banning supermarkets from selling sugary drinks near the door, or sweets at the tills.
- Laws setting limits on working hours.
- Lower speed limits (20 mph) in high pedestrian areas.
- Betting companies to be restricted from advertising at sports clubs.
- Airports to restrict the amount of alcohol passengers can drink.

Some consider macro-health promotion activities (policy intervention, like taxation on unhealthy products) as an apparatus of an overly authoritarian and preaching 'nanny state' (see Box 11.5). They argue that the state should let its citizens choose how they wish to lead their own life (Lupton, 1995). In this individualist perspective, the enterprise of health promotion is challenged, with the only acceptable policy being based on free availability of epidemiological information and total liberty of choice (Davison and Davey Smith, 1995). The strength of the right-wing, or conservative, critique of health promotion lies in its libertarian antipathy to state intrusion into people's personal life (Fitzpatrick, 2001; Kelly and Charlton, 1995). Libertarian critics argue that lifestyle choices are decisions which individuals make, not governments, and that individuals have the autonomy and fundamental human rights to choose their own health-related behaviours (Jochelson, 2006; Minkler, 1999).

BOX 11.5 THE NANNY STATE

The nanny state is a term which is used to portray the state or governments overreaching into the lives of citizens. It is a term used to denote the influence on the state in, what some see, as private or personal decisions concerning health choices. Wiley et al. (2013) suggest that the term 'nanny state' itself is a loaded and evocative word that conjures negative images and is, therefore, frequently used by proponents of free choice in health matters.

The use of legal sanctions or fines or imprisonment or the manipulation of prices on alcohol or sugar is controversial as it involves forcing individuals to act against their will. However, most people would support this in some cases – for example, actions such as legislation on the wearing of seat belts, against selling cigarettes to persons under the age of 16 or regulations on safety of electrical and gas appliances. Others raise concern about the intrusive nature of this, which they see as paternalistic and interfering with rights and freedoms of individuals and where the government tells people what to do (Hubley et al., 2021).

CITIZEN VIEWS ON STATE INTERVENTION FOR HEALTH

Research outcomes on whether citizens support or reject state intervention in health promotion varies across demographic variables and between countries. Recent research in Australia (Grunseit et al., 2019) utilised a mixed-methods approach to data collection based on focus groups (n = 49) and a national survey (n = 2052). Just under half of the respondents felt that government has a large or very large role in maintaining people's health with 91 per cent suggesting that 'people themselves' have a large or very large role. The qualitative data mirrored the survey data showing support for government regulation despite the strong belief that people themselves are responsible for and in control of their own health. Two-thirds of the survey sample supported taxes on products which negatively affected health.

GO FURTHER 11.2

The research shows that certain demographics are more or less likely to support government intervention in health promotion matters. For example, those older than 55 years are more likely to oppose government intervention generally (Grunseit et al., 2019). In addition, reduced availability and advertising of unhealthy products to children enjoys broad acceptance across the community, while restricting access to alcohol to adults appeals less to women than men, but does not vary by income (Diepeveen et al., 2013).

What issues do you feel at play here? Why do these issues vary across demographic variables?

SUMMARY

This chapter has outlined the role of the state in promoting health, contrasting with Chapter 10 which examined the role of the individual. Given that health is determined by social and environmental factors that are outside of individual control, it stands to reason that intervention from the state, or governments, can be useful. Indeed, the chapter has shown how effective the state can be in improving people's health through using tools such as policy, taxation and regulation. Moreover, the chapter has demonstrated where state control may be critical, particularly in regard to disease management and surveillance. There are clear downsides, though, with people concerned about the intrusion of the state in individuals' affairs and choices. The notion of the 'nanny state', for example, was introduced – with critics arguing that the 'nanny state' can go too far.

SUGGESTED READING

Diepeveen, S., Ling, T., Suhrcke, M., et al. (2013) Public acceptability of government intervention to change health-related behaviours: a systematic review and narrative synthesis. *BMC Public Health*, 13: 756, 1–11.

Green, J., Cross, R., Woodall, J. and Tones, K. (2019) *Health promotion: planning and Strategies*. 4th edn. London, Sage.

Warwick-Booth, L., Cross, R. and Lowcock, D. (2021) *Contemporary health studies: an introduction*. 2nd edn. Cambridge, Polity Press.

PARTNERSHIP WORKING

12

INTRODUCTION

In all areas of life, relationships really do matter, whether that be on an interpersonal level or in addressing work problems or dealing with and managing global challenges. Partnership working is a key component of effective health promotion, featuring as a key principle throughout many declarations and appearing strongly in the sustainable development goals. This chapter outlines the reasons why partnerships are important – but challenging – in health promotion and describes how partnerships can be developed and sustained.

WHY PARTNERSHIP WORKING IS IMPORTANT IN HEALTH PROMOTION

As demonstrated earlier in this book, health issues are caused and influenced by a wide range of factors – including, housing, education, poverty, work and environmental conditions and individuals' social connectedness. The continuing appeal of partnerships lies in the fact that few challenges facing government, nationally and locally, fall exclusively within the confines of a single organisation, department or sector. Most health issues are cross-sectoral in nature and embrace multiple policy arenas, organisations and professional groups (Perkins et al., 2020). In recognising that health issues are caused by multiple factors, the potential solution to addressing these issues lies in working across boundaries and with others to create supportive conditions. This has been seen in relation to tackling complex, wicked health issues by using 'whole system' approaches. These approaches draw heavily on the notion of intersectoral collaboration, defined as:

> a recognised relationship between part or parts of different sectors of society which has been formed to take actions on an issue to achieve health outcomes or intermediate health outcomes in a way which is more effective, efficient or sustainable than might be achieved by the health sector acting alone.
>
> (WHO, 1997b: 3)

Partnership working offers multiple benefits. Arguably the most prominent benefit is the potential for improved health outcomes because of working together. In theory, partnerships are premised on the assumption that individuals or sectors working alone will achieve inferior outcomes to those working together (Jones and Barry, 2011). Moreover, partnership working is consistent with health promotion values given the inclusion of all members of society. Indeed, some argue that partnerships 'need to involve minority, grassroots and end-user groups' (Winer and Ray, 1994: 49) which resonates strongly with health promotion's philosophical position and mantra that health promotion is *everyone's* business:

> Partnership working and inter-sectoral collaboration are very much at the core of modern health promotion practice in which citizens, community groups, health professionals, governmental and non-governmental agencies work together to achieve agreed goals and objectives in promoting health and wellbeing.
>
> (Jané-Llopis and Barry, 2005: 48)

Notwithstanding these key points, there are several other benefits of partnerships described in Box 12.1.

BOX 12.1 BENEFITS OF WORKING IN PARTNERSHIP FOR HEALTH

- bringing together diverse ideas and views;
- drawing on a wide range of expertise and experiences to deliver effectively;
- avoiding duplication of work;
- sharing tasks and costs;
- increasing networks and capacity building;
- creating opportunities for shared learning to enhance professional development;
- increasing the likelihood of sustainability by building relationships for the future.

TYPES OF PARTNERSHIPS

Partnerships can vary considerably. For example, partnerships can work on different scales (i.e. national/local/global) and have varying levels of formality. Partnerships may also work across sectors, including public, private and voluntary organisations. Some have suggested a typology of partnerships which show varying levels of engagement and interaction between organisations, including: networking, co-operation, co-ordination, coalition and collaboration (Boydell, 2001). There are many variations of the types of partnerships in existence; Box 12.2 shows one such model.

BOX 12.2 DIVERSITY OF PARTNERSHIP MODELS

The networking model is the simplest model of partnership where organisations meet up regularly to share their practice and discuss areas of commonality. The purpose is for organisations to be able to take up opportunities that may arise, such as funding or delivering specific interventions.

The referral systems model is a partnership that is set up for the specific purpose of enabling inter-organisational referrals. One organisation refers onto another organisation that has specific expertise or skills to support individuals, for example.

The consortium model is a partnership set up for a mutually beneficial purpose, such as jointly bidding for resources or joining forces to act as a pressure group. The purpose is to act together, believing that the whole is greater than the sum of its parts and will garner more success.

The multi-agency working model is one where two or more organisations share resources to deliver work jointly. Partnerships based on this model need to be clearly planned, and relationships have to be carefully managed to ensure success.

(www.bridgesupport.org/blog/partnership-working-health-social-care/)

REFLECTIVE EXERCISE 12.1

Looking at Box 12.1, what are the advantages and disadvantages of each of these partnership models? Which model do you feel is likely to provide long-term, sustainable partnership working and why?

THE COMMUNITY AS A PARTNER

It would be short-sighted of anyone working in health promotion not to understand the value of the community as a key partner. Clearly the notion of 'community' means many things – based on geography, culture, circumstance, and so on. Many of the values highlighted in Chapter 6 resonate with the idea of working with the community in making decisions. This includes participation, empowerment and social justice. It is apparent that when communities feel involved in decision-making processes, they are far more likely to take greater ownership and accept the decisions made. Where people do not feel that they have been heard, it can cause frustration, disillusionment and reinforce feelings of marginalisation and disempowerment – clearly things to avoid as health promoters. There are, of course, varying ways in which communities can act as partners – ranging from being consulted on matters, to full-scale ownership on all decisions and how budgets are spent.

Perhaps one of the issues that have been seen in some health promotion initiatives wishing to engage communities as partners is the process of 'tokenism'; that is, giving the illusion of participation and partnership but without actually seeing it through fully.

IMPACT OF PARTNERSHIPS

Coalitions, community partnerships and collaboratives are increasingly being seen as a viable vehicle to create population-wide, macro-level changes. Indeed, 'the more people you have on your side the greater your influence' (Hubley et al., 2013: 181). This cannot be any clearer when tackling something that impacts on the global community, such as climate change (see Case Study 12.1).

CASE STUDY 12.1: UN CLIMATE CHANGE PARTNERSHIPS

The UN Climate Change partnership works collaboratively with governments, the private sector, foundations, international organizations, academia, NGOs, UN agencies and others. The collaboration draws upon partners' knowledge and expertise to promote positive, solutions-driven approaches to combat climate change, to highlight transformational climate action and to improve public understanding of the issue. The collaboration seeks meaningful relationships with partners that combine technical assistance and knowledge transfer with financial contributions to secure the implementation of the Paris Agreement for a clean, green climate-resilient future.

(https://unfccc.int/about-us/un-climate-change-partnerships)

Partnership working in health promotion occurs at an institution level or setting too – these initiatives are likely to be much more successful should they contain partners with diverse skills and ways of working.

REFLECTIVE EXERCISE 12.2

Take a health issue that you feel could be addressed in a school setting (e.g. mental health, obesity) and consider which partners need to work together, and why, to create effective change. Make a list of the key agencies, people or groups if you can.

International partnerships can be highly effective in creating change and improving health and well-being for populations. The WHO, through the Ottawa Charter, Sundsvall statement and Jakarta declaration, has been largely responsible for the development and leadership of a settings approach within health promotion. In relation to the health promoting prison movement, the WHO has also been pivotal in influencing policy and practice through bringing partners together. Prison health, as an example, is now firmly on the public health agenda of Europe and this has been mainly due to the work of the WHO in bringing together a range of diverse partners (Gatherer et al., 2005).

In comparison to other WHO regions, the work developed in Europe has been particularly prominent (Møller et al., 2007; Møller et al., 2009) and is seen as a model with which to expand globally. The American Public Health Association's (APHA) human rights committee, for example, is working to bring the lessons learned from successful European prison health initiatives to the Americas. Towards the end of 1995, an international meeting organised by the WHO and the UK government with senior prison health representatives from eight selected European countries agreed that the public health importance of prisoner health was neglected throughout Europe (Gatherer et al., 2005). The meeting convened to ascertain the validity and feasibility of health promotion in penal settings. Acknowledgement was given to several issues, including variations between countries in the provision of health promotion and the need to address the needs of prisoners' families and prison staff. The meeting endorsed prisons as settings for health promotion and recognised the potential for meeting target 14 of the WHO's European health for all strategy (WHO, 1995). Six conclusions emerged from the meeting:

1. The prison is a valid and feasible setting for health promotion.
2. Key elements of health promotion in prison include:

    - prevention of deterioration in health;
    - enablement and empowerment;
    - physical and mental components;
    - duty of care to the whole community;
    - a multidisciplinary and holistic approach.

3. All participants recognised health in prison as a priority area for action despite limited resources.
4. Prison services have a duty of care for prisoners and prison staff and to take account of the public health of the wider community.
5. It is important to listen to the views of prisoners and prison staff in order to meet their needs through a range of effective health promotion strategies.
6. A coordinating centre should be established.

The consensus for change generated from the meeting acted as a platform to launch the Health in Prisons Project (HiPP), the aim of which was to improve all aspects of health in prison through partnerships and changes in prison health policies (Gatherer et al., 2005). Prior to the establishment of the HiPP, prison health services throughout Europe were of limited interest to prison management and national health services (Gatherer and Møller, 2009). It is arguable that without the international collaboration and co-operation, prison health would not be as prominent as it is now.

CREATING EFFECTIVE PARTNERSHIPS

While there is no prescribed formula for partnership creations, there is some guidance on key processes necessary in order to make success more likely. For example, Hardy et al. (2000) suggest the following principles:

- Principle 1 – Recognise and accept the need for partnership.
- Principle 2 – Develop clarity and realism of purpose.
- Principle 3 – Ensure commitment and ownership.
- Principle 4 – Develop and maintain trust.
- Principle 5 – Create robust and clear partnership working arrangements.
- Principle 6 – Monitor, measure and learn.

In contrast, Hubley et al. (2021), describing how to form partnerships and alliances, suggest the following stages and approaches:

- *Prepare a list of possible partners* – What are their interests? What is their mission statement/vision statement?
- *Prioritise your possible partners* – Who could help you the most? Who is most likely to support your cause given their previous involvement in other issues? What positive features would they see in collaborating with you? With whom do you have contacts? How well are they regarded by other agencies? Do they have a track record of successfully implementing programmes?
- *Have an initial meeting* – At this early stage the first priority is to get to know one another, explore mutual interests, and learn about how activities are planned (e.g. the time of year they develop their annual work plans and how far ahead they plan their activities).
- *Agree on possible partnership* – Prepare a written agreement. Consider adopting a new name for the partnership that is relevant to its aims.
- *Establish a mechanism for partnership* – Set up collaborative structures and communication channels (e.g. regular meetings, planning group, working group, action group, mailing lists).
- *Plan and implement joint activities* – Design activities that use the strengths of each participating agency.
- *Review impact* and plan further activities.

There are other views on the factors for creating effective partnerships. One idea has been depicted diagrammatically in Figure 12.1, taken from Hermens et al. (2019) who was exploring the relationships between sport and health organisations, but the model has wider resonance for other areas. The model suggests the following three elements are required:

1. Personal elements – Personal commitment to the partnership and relationships, including trustful and engaged relationships facilitate successful partnership processes.
2. Institutional elements – The societal and political context in which partnerships operate are important. Partnership could only be maintained when local and national

policies were in favour of the partnership's work and goals, and when external funding was available. Organisational commitment from all constituents of the partnership is, of course, a necessary ingredient.

3. Organisational elements – Boundary-spanning leadership is required (see more details later in the chapter); task management – which includes creating a shared mission and role clarity; communication structure, especially opportunities for open communication; building on capacities, which is premised on the exchange of expertise between partners in order to achieve more than the organisations could on their own; visibility of the activities is the final domain with positive outcomes reinforcing motivation and consolidating vision and purpose.

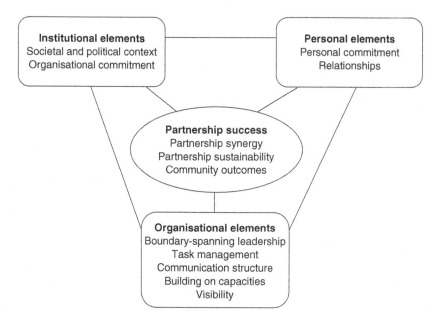

Figure 12.1 Elements of effective partnership working

Source: Hermens et al. (2019) reproduced by kind permission of the Sport Management Association of Australia and New Zealand

As already seen, there are several key ingredients that make partnerships more likely to occur and be sustained. Wildridge et al. (2004) suggest that a common vision or shared goal is a key element. This could be, for example, a partnership working towards the shared vision of addressing the aspects of the sustainable development goals or working towards a common goal of poverty reduction or reduction in health inequalities (Estacio et al., 2017). Stakeholder analysis is a key feature in this regard in identifying potential partners to work alongside. While some partners may be well known and recognised, other smaller agencies may not be, and analysing and understanding the motives and intentions of partners to be involved is essential in ensuring the correct blend of organisations and individuals working towards common goals.

As in any relationship, trust is paramount and is a cornerstone for building effective collaboration. Trust is one of the most important ingredients in partnership working and 'no amount of energy from the partners will compensate for its absence' (Child and Faulkner, 1998: 6). The longer partners work together, the greater the likelihood of increased levels of trust. Communication is also a critical element for successful partnership working – this can entail clear role definitions for the partners and regular communication on how the partnership is developing and the direction it is taking. In one highly effective health promoting partnership (Health Literacy Partnership in Stoke-on-Trent, UK), communication via email, regular meetings and an annual event to bring together the various partners was held to good effect (Estacio et al., 2017).

BOX 12.3 THE VALUE OF PRODUCTIVE MEETINGS BETWEEN PARTNERS (HUBLEY ET AL., 2013)

- Able to bring together a wide pool of skills and experience to consider the problem and ensure that as many different aspects as possible are considered when reaching decisions.
- Provides a participatory framework for planning and decision-making that involves all stakeholders.
- Decisions that are reached as a result of real group discussion are more likely to have the commitment of the whole group than those imposed from higher authority.
- Enables partners to obtain instant feedback about how the rest of a group feels about a particular issue or proposal.

Linked to effective communication is good management of partnerships – being able to have oversight of budgets and timelines and to ensure that the partnership has high levels of administration. Moreover, ensuring the joint ownership of decisions and having collective responsibility for the activities and outputs of a partnership is identified as a critical success factor (Wildridge et al., 2004).

Respecting partners' perspectives – which may be very different to your own organisations – is critical in making partnerships work. Understanding each partner's motives and incentives for the partnership is important and this can be done very openly through discussion alongside a recognition that language, working styles and approaches can be different. This can bring significant richness to the partnership, but can also cause difficulties if there is not clarity and understanding at the outset.

A willingness to learn from partners is a key factor in successful coalitions (Estacio et al., 2017). Indeed, the concept of learning organisations is a useful theoretical framework to inform successful partnership working. Learning organisations are defined as those which facilitate the learning of all their members and continually transform themselves (Pedlar et al., 1991). In short, a learning organisation is one where 'people continually expand to create the results they truly desire, where new and expansive patterns of thinking are nurtured, where collective aspiration is set free, and where people are continuously learning how to learn together' (Senge, 1994: 3).

Boundary spanners often can facilitate partnerships – these are people in organisations who manage the interface between the organisation and the outside environment and who span the boundaries between organisations, thus managing threats, handling information flows and monitoring communication. Effective boundary spanners in leadership roles create the frameworks within which shared meaning can be developed and trust can develop. They also tend to be good at assessing problems, and orchestrating people, resources and know-how to address those problems. As persuasive and likeable communicators, they can connect diverse people and cultures, because they understand both, or all, the agencies and sectors they work across. As such they not only work to 'span boundaries', they also understand the cultures and attributes of the separate components. As such, boundary spanners tend to be 'big picture' people, can think intellectually, strategically and long term, are enthusiastic and energetic, tend to be modest and to operate more 'in the background'. Moreover, they can identify internal senior 'champions' (Ansett, 2010) who help to support their cause.

In summary, there is a whole host of factors which ensure that partnerships work effectively. These have been summarised into 20 individual items covering six broad categories as shown in Box 12.4.

BOX 12.4 CRITICAL SUCCESS FACTORS IN PARTNERSHIP WORKING (WILDRIDGE ET AL., 2004)

ENVIRONMENT

- history of collaboration or co-operation;
- collaborative group seen as a legitimate leader;
- favourable political and social climate.

MEMBERSHIP

- mutual respect, understanding and trust;
- appropriate cross-section of members;
- members see collaboration as in their self-interest;
- ability to compromise.

(Continued)

PROCESS AND STRUCTURE

- members share a stake;
- multiple layers of participation;
- flexibility;
- clear roles and policy guidelines;
- adaptability;
- appropriate pace of development.

COMMUNICATION

- open and frequent;
- informal relationships and communication links.

PURPOSE

- concrete, attainable goals and objectives;
- shared vision;
- unique purpose.

RESOURCES

- sufficient funds, staff, materials and time;
- skilled leadership.

GO FURTHER 12.1

How can partnerships be constantly monitored to ensure they are working effectively and achieving their stated aims and visions? How should partnerships be evaluated? Should they be purely assessed on the extent to which they achieve their outcomes?

LEADERSHIP

A theme which has been mentioned in several places in this chapter is the importance of leadership when developing or maintaining partnerships. Leadership enables partnerships to 'work' successfully and has been suggested to have a positive effect on levels of partner participation (Jones and Barry, 2011). Robbins and Judge (2014: 204) define leadership as 'the ability to influence a group toward the achievement of a vision or set of goals'. Leaders therefore need vision, energy, authority and a strategic ability. They need to be able to influence, motivate and enable others to contribute towards the partnership's success.

While leadership is an important domain in all aspects of health promotion practice, it is perhaps none more so than in partnerships working. Leadership approaches should remain true to health promotion principles and maintain non-hierarchical and collaborative strategies (see Box 12.5).

BOX 12.5 DEMOCRATIC LEADERSHIP

This places collective ownership of decision-making within an organisation at a premium. It is a leadership style which seeks to foster democratic principles, including equal participation of partners. Those people adopting a democratic leadership style tend to have 'fairness' as a core personality trait. This style of leadership is often appreciated by people as it seeks to empower individuals and provide a sense that their views and perspectives are listened to and valued.

While some partnerships can be relatively straightforward to oversee, there are examples in health promotion of extremely complex partnership working requiring sophisticated leadership skills. The Healthy City initiative, as an example, had considerable complexity, multiple stakeholders and a very long-term vision. Leaders in health promotion were tasked to maintain the vision and manage networks, or even networks of networks (Dixey, Cross, Foster and Woodall, 2013). However, there have been increasing concerns about leadership within health promotion and the ability of an organisation or individual to bring people together under a common goal or focus (see Case Study 12.2).

CASE STUDY 12.2: WHERE ARE THE CHAMPIONS OF GLOBAL HEALTH PROMOTION?

ABSTRACT

For many years the World Health Organization (WHO) has provided the global direction and leadership that has helped to shape the way we view health promotion today. The future role of the WHO is now uncertain and the lack of global leadership for health promotion and identification of who will provide the future direction are issues that need to be addressed. The crucial question posed in this commentary is: Where are the individuals and organisations that will provide the global leadership and vision for health promotion in the future? We need named champions for the future leadership of health promotion practice – people and organisations who offer a leadership style that will maintain its global profile, be representative across

(Continued)

sectors and have the ability to maintain its political efficacy. The two key health promotion approaches, top-down and bottom-up, do not always share the same goals, and they demand different styles of leadership. This is an important consideration in our goal to find champions who can work with both approaches and understand how to accommodate them as a part of the future direction of health promotion. This commentary raises key questions to stimulate discussion and action towards addressing the lack of global leadership in health promotion. It discusses some of the key players, leadership characteristics and the contradictions in style that are inherent in achieving a goal of charismatic global champions.

Source: Laverack (2012)

REFLECTIVE EXERCISE 12.3

Take a look at Case Study 12.2 and consider how leadership in health promotion should be encouraged and galvanised. What should be the process for identifying key organisations or individuals to take forward the health promotion agenda? What organisations or types of individuals would be suitable for the role?

PARTNERSHIP CHALLENGES

In reality, partnerships are hard work to establish and maintain (Wildridge et al., 2004). They usually have a very high failure rate and are very difficult to measure and evaluate (Jones and Barry, 2011), so understanding why partnerships fail can be difficult to fully understand. Hubley et al. (2013) suggests that partnerships in health promotion face challenges because of differing concepts of health promotion, values, visions and aims, and issues whereby smaller organisations get swamped by larger ones.

Trust is a critical success factor for partnerships (Wildridge et al., 2004) and so it is obvious that mistrust is a key factor in partnership failure, with health promotion partnerships being particularly susceptible (Jones and Barry, 2018). As health promoters work across sectors there is the potential for partnership breakdown. This can be observed across statutory and voluntary partnerships, and/or the private and public sectors (Heenan, 2004). Indeed, cultural differences in ways of working can severely hinder partnership development and formation (Wildridge et al., 2004).

Power imbalances can derail a partnership, especially if some partners feel that distribution of resources or allocation of work and tasks are unevenly spread. Research demonstrates, for instance, that shared power ensures a partnership can work more effectively but misuse of power and power abuses prevent a partnership from functioning at all (Jones and Barry, 2018). Indeed, research shows that the process of building a partnership can be time-consuming, demanding and requires commitment, therefore it is crucial that those involved feel that their input is acknowledged and valued no matter how big or small the partner's share is (Heenan, 2004).

SUMMARY

Partnerships are the backbone of effective health promotion practice. Health promotion is interdisciplinary in its approach and therefore needs to draw on various sectors and expertise to reach its intended goals. Partnerships can create sustainable and effective interventions and can be instrumental and essential in tackling health challenges and in addressing health inequalities. That said, many partnerships do have challenges and limitations as demonstrated in this chapter.

SUGGESTED READING

Hubley, J., Copeman, J. and Woodall, J. (2021) *Practical health promotion*. Cambridge, Polity Press.

Jones, J. and Barry, M.M. (2011) Exploring the relationship between synergy and partnership functioning factors in health promotion partnerships. *Health Promotion International*, 26: 408–420.

Jones, J. and Barry, M.M. (2018) Factors influencing trust and mistrust in health promotion partnerships. *Global Health Promotion*, 25: 16–24.

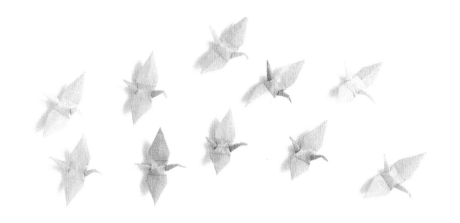

SECTION 5

WHERE IS HEALTH PROMOTION DELIVERED?

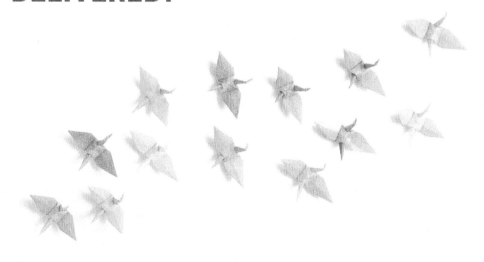

SETTINGS APPROACH

13

OVERARCHING THEORY

INTRODUCTION

We all interact in a range of settings and environments and, because of this, settings are often regarded as one of the key ways in which health promotion can take place. People connect with a range of settings either concurrently or consecutively throughout their lives. Children, for example, may spend their time in the school, family and community settings (concurrently), whereas people sentenced for criminal activities may spend time within a prison setting and then resettle back into the community (consecutively) (Dooris, 2006; Dooris and Hunter, 2007; Dooris et al., 2007). Either way, the time we spend in settings is significant.

The key idea of the settings approach, or healthy settings approach (see Box 13.1), is that investments in health are made in social systems where health is not their primary remit (Dooris, 2007). So, schools prioritise education and learning; workplaces focus on delivering services or maximising profits; and prisons are fundamentally concerned with rehabilitation and punishment. Despite this, there is clearly the opportunity to focus too on health and creating optimal conditions for health promotion.

Throughout recent times, settings have been mentioned as an important vehicle for health promoters. Some have suggested that the settings approach is one of the most successful and 'top rated' strategies to emerge from the Ottawa Charter (Torp et al., 2014). This is arguably because the settings approach offers a very practical and tangible way to 'do' health promotion (Dixey, Cross, Foster and Woodall, 2013).

It was the Ottawa Charter which highlighted the benefits of settings, stating that 'health is created and lived by people within the settings of their everyday life; where they learn, work, play and love' (WHO, 1986). This quotation has been long-standing, but recently redefined as 'created in the settings of everyday life – in the neighbourhoods and communities where people live, love, work, shop and play' (WHO, 2016). This chapter will look specifically at the theory and concepts underpinning a settings approach and will show both the benefits and challenges of using 'settings' for health promotion.

WHAT'S IN A NAME?

A range of terms have been used to identify settings-based health promotion (see Box 13.1). Much of the semantic differences are unintentional with terms often used interchangeably. The terms used for health promotion in higher education has differed internationally. Europe and Latin America use the phrase 'health-promoting universities', while in the UK 'healthy universities' and in the USA a mixture of 'healthy campus' or 'healthy campus community' is used (Sarmiento, 2017). That said, others have been clearer on terminology and vocabulary (see Kokko et al., 2014).

BOX 13.1 KEY TERMINOLOGY

A range of terminology has been used to denote settings-based approaches to health promotion. 'Health setting', 'health-promoting settings', 'settings for health', 'settings for health promotion', 'the settings approach' and 'the settings-based approach' are all terms which are commonly in use.

Barić (1998) differentiates between a 'health promoting setting' and a 'healthy setting'. In the case of a healthy setting, campaigns and interventions are considered on a higher organisational level with the aim to reach all of its citizens. In contrast, within a 'health promoting setting' planning will be more explicit and formal and characterised through distinct organisations like schools, workplaces and hospitals to reach the population (Barić, 2000). Kokko et al. (2014: 499) also note the differences between a 'healthy setting' and 'health-promoting setting'. The former term, they suggest, gives the indication of a static or ideal setting. In contrast, the term 'health-promoting setting' invokes 'the dynamic and conditional nature of health promotion activities and conditions and the process of making them healthful' – it does not assume a permanent healthy state but, rather, considers the actions that are necessary to continuously adapt the setting to changing circumstance.

TYPES OF SETTINGS

Settings have traditionally been seen as physical organisations where people come together to interact, but this notion has shifted as virtual settings, discussed in Chapter 15, are becoming more common in supporting health and well-being. Originally, the WHO (1998: 19) adopted a definition of a setting for health as follows:

> The place or social context in which people engage in daily activities in which environmental, organisational and personal factors interact to affect health and well-being … where people actively use and shape the environment and thus create or solve problems relating to health. Settings can normally be identified as having physical boundaries, a range of people with defined roles, and an organisational structure.

A critical point made in the definition is the importance of environmental and organisational factors that impact on health as well as the individual and personal factors.

Figure 13.1 shows some of the common health-promoting settings. It is worth considering who is encompassed within each of the settings – when people think of health-promoting schools, for instance, they often think primarily of work with children; however, teachers, caretakers and parents also are integral to that setting as well.

Figure 13.1 provides a timeline of when settings were first recognised and conceived and shows how some settings have a longer history and pedigree than others. The WHO's first healthy settings initiative was the 'Healthy Cities' project, set up in 1987 and involving some 11 European cities (Green et al., 2019). The 'Healthy Cities' project has been attributed for the subsequent development of other settings-based initiatives and inspiring the diversity of settings-related work now seen globally (Dooris, 2013). There are Healthy Cities Networks in all six WHO regions – in the European region, for example, there are now over 1400 healthy cities and towns as members and in Asia, the Alliance for Healthy Cities (AFHC) coordinates information exchange and good practice in this region (Hu and Kuo, 2016).

It is interesting to consider why certain settings have emerged more quickly than others – why schools and cities, for instance, have developed more rapidly than prisons and hospitals? Perhaps in settings where there exists a clear logic between settings-based health intervention and individual and societal gains – for example in schools – there is a stronger momentum and commitment. Conversely, these arguments may be more difficult to make in a setting where ideological views differ, for instance the role of prisons or workplaces.

Clearly all settings are different in the way that they operate and how they are structured. Hospitals, prisons, schools and workplaces, for instance, have clear systems and structures in place and these contrast from other settings that have informal, flexible and open structures, such as homes, communities, cities and islands (Dooris, 2004; Poland et al., 2000; Whitelaw et al., 2001). Some have described settings as being 'elemental' and 'contextual' to suggest differences in the structure and scale of settings – elemental settings are situated within contextual settings. So, for example, a healthy city may contain important elements, such as health-promoting schools, hospitals, workplaces, prisons and markets. This idea has been adapted by Scriven and Hodgins (2012) who has shown interconnections and linkages between settings.

Others have provided a more visual representation and suggested that settings operate like 'Russian dolls' (Dooris, 2006: 5) whereby settings situate within and alongside each other. This perspective is gaining increased traction, especially as the notion of 'planetary health' (Hancock et al., 2017) is emerging rapidly as a response to the contemporary challenges impacting on health, such as climate change (as discussed in Chapter 4). Figure 13.2 shows how conceptualising settings as 'Russian dolls' can be a helpful way to note the relationships, interconnections and nesting arrangements between settings.

It is also worth remembering that no two settings are alike and therefore it is important to be aware of the diversity that lies behind the apparent homogeneity (Poland et al., 2009). So, for example, when discussing 'health-promoting schools', practitioners

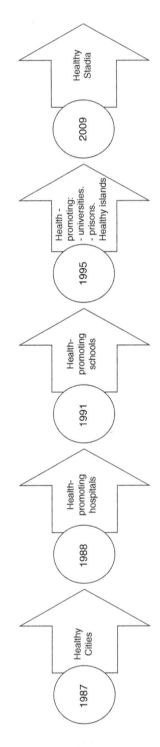

Figure 13.1 A selected history of settings

1987 — Healthy Cities

1988 — Health-promoting hospitals

1991 — Health-promoting schools

1995 — Health-promoting:
- universities.
- prisons.
Healthy islands

2009 — Healthy Stadia

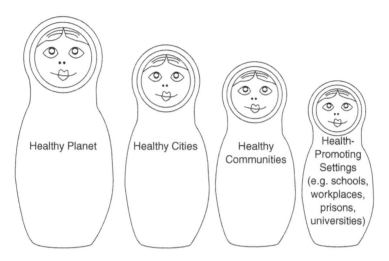

Figure 13.2 Settings as 'Russian dolls'

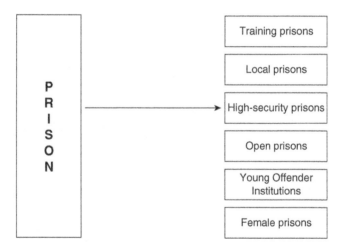

Figure 13.3 No two settings are alike: a prison example

and decision-makers working in health promotion need to recognise that schools themselves greatly differ. To advance both the concept and practice of the settings approach, a more detailed analysis of settings is needed. So, using the prison setting as an example, more sensitive policy and practice is encouraged which reflects the remit and function of the prison itself. In enabling this to take place, the overarching notion of 'the prison' should be disaggregated (see Figure 13.3). Whilst there are certain overlaps and commonalities between each prison, strategies and approaches would attempt to reflect the category and type of establishment and state realistic outcomes to be achieved.

GO FURTHER 13.1

Take a setting of your choice, say a school, and consider the different variations of that setting. How are these variations of settings under the same 'title' similar and different? What implications does this have for developing a settings approach and the way in which policy and practice is developed and undertaken? What is the danger of a 'one size fits all' approach?

WHAT THE SETTINGS APPROACH IS (AND WHAT IT ISN'T)?

There is a crucial difference between health-promoting settings and conducting health promotion in settings. This is an important point that is often confused and can lead to ineffective, unsustainable healthy settings practice. One-off, ad-hoc or opportunistic activities conducted in a location where a 'target audience' is not an attribute synonymous with a true settings approach. This, however, is common and often seen when national campaigns are conducted in settings almost on a monthly basis. So, for example, there may be a focus in January on 'Dry January' which challenges people to remain alcohol free for 31 days, aiming to raise awareness of the effects of alcohol. Or, in April, there is a 'stress awareness week' with workplace settings often raising the causes and consequences of stress. Or in November, there is a focus around diabetes prevention during 'World Diabetes Day'. This list goes on.

Conducted on their own and in isolation from broader activities, such as changes to policies or structures within the settings themselves, there is a danger of 'project-ism' (Dooris, 2001: 58). This is where organisations can find it difficult to translate isolated and discrete health promotion activities into more penetrative settings based work (Whitelaw et al., 2001). The major challenge is the transition from separate projects to mainstream activities involving whole organisational change and commitment (Dooris and Thompson, 2001).

In contrast, a 'health-promoting setting' adopts an ecological approach (see Box 13.2) in which the whole environment and culture is committed to promoting health in a way that is coherent and integrated (Tones, 2001). This could include the physical structure and composition of the setting; the policies and strategies; the culture and ethos; and the activities that happen within that environment. So, as an example, rather than delivering an annual 'stress awareness week' in a workplace, policies and practices are developed to ensure that stress is mitigated through flexible working; appropriate working conditions and annual leave entitlement, opportunities for staff to contribute to decision-making processes; and with mental well-being as a cornerstone of the workplaces ethos.

REFLECTIVE EXERCISE 13.1

Select a setting of your choice and consider how you, as a health promoter, would inform and advise the physical design and architecture of that building. What would the setting physically look like? How would it promote health, but retain the setting's purpose and function? Also, consider how the ethos and values of a settings approach could be instilled into the organisation – again, keeping in mind, that the setting must function to fulfil its primary remit.

There have been proposals to develop an agreed set of activities which, if implemented, would classify an organisation as a health-promoting setting. On an operational level, this would provide clarity and guidance to those organisations that wanted to develop a settings approach. However, Poland et al. (2000) suggest that implementing an identical set of rules in similar settings is often ineffective and inappropriate, as local autonomy is needed when understanding needs and circumstances. Shareck et al. (2013: 46), drawing on Poland and Dooris (2010), identify six guiding principles of the approach. They are:

- adopting an ecological and whole system perspective
- starting where people are and respecting people's lived experiences
- rooting practice in the social context of settings
- deepening the socio-political analysis in order to locate action in the broader context of power relations
- building on assets and successes already prevailing in settings
- building resilience and capabilities for sustained change.

Others have suggested that it may be more desirable to consider shared principles and values that health-promoting settings have. For instance, this could include:

- A holistic and socio-ecological understanding of health;
- Focus on populations, policy and environments;
- Equity and social justice;
- Sustainability;
- Community participation;
- Enablement and empowerment;
- Cooperation;
- Consensus and mediation;
- Advocacy;
- Settings as social systems;
- Sustainable integrative actions;
- Settings as part of an interdependent ecosystem.

(Dooris, 2001: 52)

BOX 13.2 SOCIO-ECOLOGICAL APPROACHES TO HEALTH PROMOTION

An ecological model for health promotion, discussed in more depth in Chapter 3, is where health behaviours are seen as being determined by a whole range of factors – personal, community, environmental, economic and political issues. In order to modify behaviours of people and communities, attention needs to be given to these multiple levels if change is to occur. Ecological approaches stand in contrast to focusing on the individual one on hand or social structures on the other – indeed, it combines both for effective health promotion.

Health promotion orientation	Determinants of health and illness	Health promotion focus	Examples of interventions
Individual approaches	Individual health behaviour	Modify individuals' health-related attitudes, beliefs and behaviour	Health education
System and environmental approaches	People's physical and social environments	Improve environmental safety and strengthen social supports for health	Passive interventions (taxation, legislation)
Ecological approach	*Degree of fit between people's biological, behavioural and sociocultural needs and the environmental resources available to them*	*Integrate behavioural and environmentally based health promotion strategies*	*Combination of active and passive interventions spanning individual, organisational and community levels*

Some authors have offered a spectrum of activities within a settings approach. Whitelaw et al.'s (2001: 346) typology of settings-based health promotion consists of five types of settings-based activities. This is an attempt to show the differing approaches and strategies that could be considered in the settings approach (see table in Box 13.2). The latter two approaches are clearly more consistent with the 'ideal' interpretation of the settings approach (Green et al., 2019) – perhaps considered as more of a 'gold standard'. The spectrum of activities resonates strongly with a broader structure *versus* agency debate and comes back to whether individuals or wider social structures and processes are responsible for promoting health. In practice, variability of activity exists. Johnson and Baum (2001:

286) demonstrated a variety of interpretations in the meaning of a health-promoting hospital. They suggest that: 'Some hospitals do little more than move beyond providing health information and education to patients, while other initiatives achieve a significant re-orientation of their activities and institute significant organizational reform supported by strong policy and leadership.' This issue is not limited to hospitals, as variation of practice seems to exist across settings.

Table 13.1 Overview of the 'types' of settings-based health promotion according to Whitelaw et al. (2001: 346)

Setting type	Description
'Passive' model	The problem and solution lie with the behaviour and actions of the individual. Setting plays a passive role only providing access to population group. Traditional health education activities are at the heart of the work.
'Active' model	The problem lies within the behaviour of the individual; however, the solution is broadened to encompass features of the system in which the individual exists.
'Vehicle' model	The problem lies within the setting, the solution in learning from individually based projects. This is still focused on topic-based activities but does so with an expectation of moving beyond individual behaviour change to impacting on broader settings features.
'Organic' model	The problem lies within the setting, the solution in the action of the individuals. This approach focuses on strengthening collective participation; the focus is not on tangible health gains but reflects a desire for improved ethos or culture within the setting.
'Comprehensive/ structural' model	Both the problem and the solution lie within the setting. This approach sees that individuals are powerless to make any changes therefore enduring change can only come from within the system. The emphasis therefore targets broad settings policies and bringing structural change.

Source: Whitelaw et al. (2001) reproduced by kind permission of Oxford University Press

GO FURTHER 13.2

Using Whitelaw's typology, select a setting of your choice and apply the five setting 'types' to a chosen health issue. This will enable you to identify a range of interventions working from a 'passive' to a more 'comprehensive' settings strategy. We have provided an example below using workplaces and the aim to improve mental health and well-being.

(Continued)

Improving mental health and well-being in a workplace using Whitelaw et al.'s typology of settings-based health promotion

Setting type	Description of activity to improve mental health and well-being
'Passive' model	The workplace engages in 'stress awareness week' and delivers education and awareness sessions during this time.
'Active' model	An email is regularly sent to all employees raising awareness of the causes of stress and advice on how stress can be managed. In addition, a working group of employee representatives is established to share their concerns regularly with senior managers on stressors within the organisation.
'Vehicle' model	Educational activities and information on stress are freely available to employees. To complement this, mental health champions are trained in the workforce so that employees can share their mental health concerns with peers confidentially.
'Organic' model	Open dialogue between employees and managers is actively encouraged with regular forums to engage in discussions on a range of workplace well-being issues. Staff concerns are listened to and acted upon.
'Comprehensive/ structural' model	Policies and procedures with the workplace are re-designed to ensure that stress is minimised (e.g. reviewing workload management) and activities to promote well-being (e.g. flexible working policies) are integral to the ethos of the organisation. Employee assistance interventions (counselling, legal and debt advice) is comprehensively provided and advertised to staff.

CONNECTING 'OUTWARDS', 'UPWARDS' AND 'BEYOND' HEALTH

Settings must connect 'outwards', 'upwards' and 'beyond' health if the approach is to be successful (Dooris, 2013). Connecting 'outwards' relates to settings working in joined-up ways in order to maximise health, recognising that health issues do not respect physical or virtual boundaries. There are some clear marriages between settings that could work more effectively – most notably, the linkages between the prison setting and community setting. This is a particularly critical period as research shows that male prisoners are 29 times more likely to die during the week following release compared to the general population (Farrell and Marsden, 2008).

Connecting 'upwards' would see settings staying with 'the big picture' (St Leger, 1997: 101), recognising the wider determinants impacting on the health of those within the setting. Dooris (2013) suggests that settings should also take on an advocacy role to achieve national and international-level leverage (see Case Study 13.1).

CASE STUDY 13.1: SETTINGS INFLUENCING AND ADVOCATING FOR POLICY CHANGE

The European Healthy Stadia Network lobbied UEFA (Union of European Football Associations) to ensure that the consumption of alcohol at stadia was 'responsible' by advocating a series of recommendations for change. These included:

- Stopping sale of alcohol at the end of half-time.
- Agreement on what maximum strength alcohol may be sold at UEFA matches (restricting this to drinks with alcohol content of no more than 3 per cent).
- Agreement on maximum number of alcoholic drinks to be purchased at UEFA matches per visit to drinks concession (two drinks per person, per visit).
- UEFA-led campaign promoting responsible consumption of alcohol at all food and beverage (F&B) concessions selling alcohol, with specific advice on rehydration through water.
- Availability of free, clean drinking water for rehydration upon request at all UEFA matches.
- Up-to-date training of all F&B serving staff (full-time and part-time) to recognise signs of overconsumption of alcohol and protocol on declining sale of alcohol to intoxicated fans.
- In-depth training of stewards and security staff on overconsumption of alcohol by fans within the stadium.

(Philpott, 2018)

Connecting 'beyond health' concerns settings making connections with other agendas, such as the broader sustainable development agenda. This is emphasised fully in the Shanghai declaration on promoting health in the 2030 Agenda for Sustainable Development where reference is made to several issues, such as globalisation and migration that are closely intertwined with the healthy cities approach:

> Together with city leaders we must address the toxic combination of rapid rural-to-urban migration, global population movements, economic stagnation, high unemployment and poverty as well as environmental deterioration and pollution. We will not accept that city residents in poor areas suffer ill-health disproportionately and have difficulty accessing health services.

(WHO, 2016)

BOX 13.3 'SUPERSETTINGS'

Some have sought to enhance the notion of settings in health promotion further and have proposed the idea of 'supersettings' (Bloch et al., 2014). While the extent to which this is different from a 'true' or ideal version of settings-based health promotion is debatable, it is premised on the synergistic effects of activities carried out in multiple settings. Supersettings are characterised by interventions that are co-ordinated, planned and integrated, and moreover involve the community in planning. As an example, childhood obesity is more effectively addressed when a range of settings work synergistically – so, the school setting, community setting, shops and sports clubs work together to tackle the issue. A supersetting initiative is 'owned' by a range of stakeholders who have equal say in the direction and content of the work – without such co-operation, the supersetting fails to maximise the potential to improve health of communities. The approach offers potential to address health issues that are too complex and challenging to be delivered in isolation.

WHAT INHIBITS THE SETTINGS APPROACH FROM TAKING PLACE?

Not all settings desire or even want to engage in the health-promoting settings philosophy. In fact, there are several examples of organisations and places that are the antithesis of 'healthy'. In most cases, there are reasonable barriers precluding health promotion from taking place. First, health promotion is often under-resourced, underfunded and an activity on the periphery of the organisation's priorities (Caraher et al., 2002; Johnson and Baum, 2001). There are always limitations in support structures (e.g. finance, time, training, expertise) within settings (Whitelaw et al., 2001). Second, organisations often view health promotion as constituting additional work that diverts attention from the 'core business' of that setting – this perception can be an inhibitor to action. Third, there can be challenges in translating the philosophy of the approach into tangible activities (Whitelaw et al., 2001). Fourth, there can be genuine forces acting against the health agenda in settings – prison, for instance, will always have elements that will compromise health. Fifth, there can be challenges associated with health promoters being perceived as credible agents of change (Whitelaw et al., 2001) or with possession of a credible evidence base to convince individuals of the benefits of a settings approach.

THE LIMITATIONS OF THE SETTINGS APPROACH

We see three drawbacks of the settings approach that limit its potential as a crucial strategy and approach to promoting health. First, consider those members of society who do not interact in settings. There are several sub-sections of communities that do not have sustained contact with settings – for example, the unemployed, illegal immigrants, children who truant from school and the homeless. Early settings-based approaches focused efforts on 'legitimate sites of practice' (Green et al., 2000: 25) and by only focusing on large-scale, identifiable and easily accessible organisations there was a drawback in making inequalities wider, not narrower.

As the settings approach has developed, it has stimulated practice in 'non-traditional' arenas (Poland et al., 2000; Tones and Tilford, 2001) – it may have been unthinkable, for instance, in the 1980s to consider the idea of a health-promoting prison, or nightclub or stadium, but these are now more commonplace. This continued shift towards focusing attention on 'non-traditional' settings will undoubtedly offer those once marginalised by a settings approach to have some contact with professionals to address key determinants of their health (Poland et al., 2000). The challenge ahead seems to be that those working within health promotion must continue to consider emerging settings to tackle health issues.

REFLECTIVE EXERCISE 13.2

Using the timeline in Figure 13.1, predict where future settings-based health promotion will take place. Undoubtedly there will be a rise in virtual environments (see Chapter 15), but what other physical spaces do you think will be utilised to promote health effectively?

CASE STUDY 13.2: BINGO!

The bingo hall has been utilised as a setting for health promotion after recognising that women from socio-economically disadvantaged backgrounds who face health and social inequalities are more likely to use a bingo hall as part of their social activity. Although regarded as a 'passive' settings intervention, the Well!Bingo physical activity intervention for older women comprised structured exercise sessions, intervention messages and a social component. The 12-week intervention consisted of three different instructor-led exercise sessions in the bingo club each week (chair-based exercise, dancercise and line dancing) held before bingo games started. The practical and social familiarity of the setting were seen as important constituents which facilitated engagement and attendance (Evans et al., 2018).

The second drawback with the settings approach is in the evaluation of its effectiveness. Some have noted that settings have 'an uneven and under-developed evidence base' (Dooris et al., 2007: 335). There are exceptions to this – for example, the establishment of an evidence base for health-promoting schools where clear benchmarks and standards have developed (South and Woodall, 2012). Settings approaches can be very difficult to evaluate and it can be difficult to compare between settings given the diversity and understanding of the approach. This creates particular issues in the transferability of research evidence (Dooris, 2005). Some of the challenges that have inhibited the generation of a convincing evidence base for settings-based health promotion include:

1. The funding structures for evaluative work are often focused on specific diseases and risk factor interventions. This would run counter to a comprehensive settings-based evaluation.
2. There are challenges with evaluating ecological and whole-system approaches. If the settings approach is about integration within organisations, it can be argued that the greater the success, the more difficult the evaluation becomes.

Finally, the settings approach has often lacked the commitment and full support of global organisations, like the WHO (Woodall, 2016). Some have suggested that the WHO has had a fading role in global health (Lidén, 2014) and in relation to settings-based health promotion, questions have been raised in relation to the WHO's role in facilitating co-ordination between settings and providing ongoing support (Dooris, 2013). It has been argued that global organisations, such as the WHO, could do more to promote and enhance a settings-based approach.

SUMMARY

This chapter has outlined the theory of settings-based health promotion. The settings approach is not about targeting individuals, but instead creating conditions for health within organisations and places that people come together. There are differing views on the activities that can be conducted within settings, but there are models and typologies that can be used to aid thinking and practice. One-off activities or interventions with a convenient location is not in itself characteristic of a settings approach. Health-promoting settings have health as an integral part of the organisation's culture and ethos. Effective activity is ensured when settings 'join up' and work mutually to ensure holistic and integrated activities. While there is a critique of the settings approach which suggests that it is limited in addressing the health of some groups, particularly those who find themselves 'outside' of traditional settings, it has been regarded as one of the most practical ways to 'do' health promotion.

SUGGESTED READING

Green, J., Cross, R., Woodall, J. et al. (2019) *Health promotion: planning and strategies*. 4th edn. London, Sage.

Poland, B.D., Green, L.W. and Rootman, I. (2000) *Settings for health promotion: linking theory and practice*. Thousand Oaks, CA, Sage.

Scriven, A. and Hodgins, M. (2012) *Health promotion settings: principles and practice*. London, Sage.

HEALTHY SETTINGS IN ACTION

14

INTRODUCTION

The previous chapter provided the background theory and concept of a settings approach. This chapter will demonstrate further 'where' health promotion can be conducted, using specific examples. To this extent, it provides an overview of 12 settings for health promotion – some well known and understood and others far less so. The chapter is unapologetic in its whirlwind overview of these settings; rather, the purpose is to broaden the horizons of where health promotion can be undertaken. For those wishing to understand more about these settings, the 'Suggested Reading' at the end of the chapter points in the direction of more in-depth reviews.

The chapter first discusses 'contextual settings' – cities, communities, families – which are seen as being difficult to define with fluid boundaries and undefined structures, and latterly 'elemental settings' – marketplaces, schools, workplaces, hospitals, prisons, universities, nightclubs, sports clubs, airports – which often have more easily defined physical boundaries, rules and structures. Of course, and to reiterate, this is only a relatively short overview of some examples of 'where' health promotion can be undertaken (the previous chapter, for instance, highlighted examples of healthy stadia and healthy bingo halls!).

HEALTHY CITIES

The healthy cities movement is perhaps the longest-standing and most researched of all the settings. The idea emerged almost simultaneously with the establishment of the Ottawa Charter in the mid-1980s, with cities regarded as one of the key ways in which the pillars of the Ottawa Charter could be operationalised. In short, the rationale for establishing healthy cities is that 'people's physical, mental and social wellbeing is the core business of cities' (International Institute for Global Health, 2018: 150). With the increasing complexity of health, especially in urban environments, and the wider recognition of the need to act using a multi-sectoral approach, the city is seen as a prime vehicle to potentially address the health of individuals on a relatively large scale.

Initially the healthy cities project was established as a pilot, but has since gone on to become a growing global movement. According to the WHO (2018b) a healthy city aims to:

- create a health-supportive environment;
- achieve a good quality of life;
- provide basic sanitation and hygiene needs;
- supply access to healthcare.

There has been a whole range of activities and initiatives delivered under the healthy cities banner – some targeted at specific groups in cities (children, older people, immigrants, travellers, etc.), other approaches focusing on lifestyle issues (for example, cycling and walking projects) and others targeted more broadly on the social determinants impacting on health. This includes efforts to address unemployment; ensuring good housing; and, more broadly, the regeneration of urban areas (Fawkes et al., 2012). The settings approach, as discussed in the previous chapter, has several limitations – including the size and variability of settings. The healthy cities approach is just the same – the smallest healthy city is l'Isle-aux-Grues in Québec, Canada, with a population of a few hundred, whereas the largest one, Shanghai, China, exceeds 16 million people (de Leeuw et al., 2018). This clearly provides challenges and means that a 'one size fits all' approach is relatively futile.

It is the shared principles and values of the approach that binds the healthy cities concept. The WHO (2009c) has for some time summarised these as: equity; participation and empowerment; partnership; solidarity; and sustainable development. These values have been discussed in-depth in Chapter 6. The principle of participation and ensuring the democratic engagement of citizens was recently reaffirmed as a core value (International Institute for Global Health, 2018), with the active participation of citizens in the process of decision-making being an essential prerequisite for a healthy city.

HEALTHY COMMUNITIES

The idea of a 'healthy community setting' is quite abstract and difficult to define. Communities are often defined by place or geography, but this is not always the case as is seen in Chapter 15 where virtual communities are discussed. Laverack (2014b) suggests that community settings generally have a spatial dimension (i.e. some form of geographical boundary, like a neighbourhood or village) and also a non-spatial element, referring to relationships and social connections.

Communities and neighbourhoods are often regarded as being at the core of health promotion practice, but relatively little has been written about their standing as a 'setting' (see Biddle and Seymour (2012) and Naidoo and Wills (2016) for exceptions to this). One of the primary focuses within communities and neighbourhoods is often the development of appropriate infrastructure to support health and well-being. This could include access to appropriate services; access to green space; safer road crossings; better street lighting, etc. Housing and accommodation issues are also issues that are frequently high on the agenda. Yet, there is increasing recognition of the value of individuals within communities feeling more connected and having a greater say in how their community is organised (Public Health England, 2015). Good social relationships within communities are good for health and therefore should be fostered within this setting (Naidoo and Wills, 2016). In addition, there has been a greater recognition that the answer to health inequalities in communities can be addressed from within, using community assets and skills. Morgan and Ziglio (2007: 18) define a health asset as:

> any factor (or resource), which enhances the ability of individuals, groups, communities, populations, social systems and/or institutions to maintain and sustain health and wellbeing and to help to reduce health inequities. These assets can operate at the level of the individual, group, community, and/or population as protective (or promoting) factors to buffer against life's stresses.

A useful menu of approaches that can enhance the health of community settings has been provided by South et al. (2019) who have produced a 'family' of interventions which would be characteristic of a community-centred approach to health promotion (see Figure 14.1). These include:

1. strengthening communities;
2. volunteer and peer roles;
3. collaborations and partnerships; and
4. access to community resources.

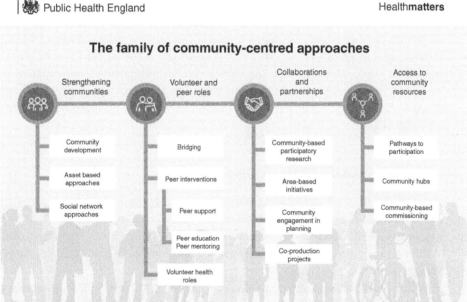

Figure 14.1 The 'family of community-centred approaches'

Source: www.gov.uk/government/publications/health-matters-health-and-wellbeing-community-centred-approaches/health-matters-community-centred-approaches-for-health-and-wellbeing

By encouraging the development of activities under these 'community-centred' domains, evidence shows that this increases the potential for health outcomes and health equity with the potential to reduce health inequalities.

HEALTHY FAMILIES

Research has shown how the focus of the family can be a practical and effective setting for health promotion (Robertson et al., 2018; Soubhi and Potvin, 2000). However, it is arguable if health promotion practice or policy has fully utilised or embraced families as a viable setting for health promotion interventions (Novilla et al., 2006). As a general theme, there are limitations in providing a 'one size fits all' approach to addressing health in settings and the same can be applied for family settings. Indeed, traditional family structures are now being accompanied by structures that are more diverse and heterogeneous. Children may be raised by married parents, cohabiting parents, single parents, step-parents or same-sex parents (Golombok, 2015), for example.

The family has a very powerful influence on a range of health-related factors, such as diet, physical activity, alcohol and smoking and social connections. Research has particularly shown how these influences can impact on the health of children within families (Christensen, 2004). Some have offered a conceptual model for the health-promoting family and this can be seen in Figure 14.2. Within the model, the family sits within a wider social and community context and the effects of these determinants on health cannot be understated. Nevertheless, the model also shows how family health practices (both present and historical) and the 'family ecocultural pathway' (comprising family values, goals and needs) interact together, alongside the genetic predispositions that the family may be exposed to and the existing health status of the child. In addition, the agency of the child is also presented in the model showing how their individual choice can influence the family unit in both positive and negative ways. As a tangible example, research has shown how children can act as 'change agents' in the promotion of positive oral health practices with their siblings and wider-family (Woodall et al., 2014).

HEALTHY MARKETPLACES

In some communities and regions, marketplaces are at the forefront of social life and are reflective of the local culture of the people – they can also be an attraction for tourists and visitors (WHO, 2003). Healthy food markets have been implemented in all WHO Regions, although they were launched and remain concentrated in the WHO Western Pacific Region (WHO, 2019f). People use markets with the expectation that the food they buy is safe and nutritious (Green et al., 2019) and it is obvious, therefore, that the focus on the activities within a healthy marketplace is on food safety and the prevention of food-borne illness and disease (see Case Study 14.1). In developed countries,

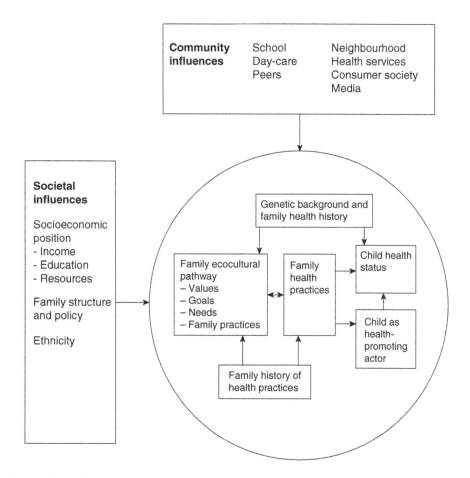

Figure 14.2 The health-promoting family

Source: Christensen (2004) reproduced by kind permission of Elsevier Science & Technology Journals

food regulation frameworks are clear and enforced whereas this may be less apparent in resource-poor countries.

The WHO (2019e) suggest that a healthy food market is one that seeks to protect health by eliminating disease and other hazards at all places along the farm-to-consumption continuum. However, the opportunity for marketplaces to also look beyond food safety is clear with the potential to address working conditions, encourage sustainable and environmentally friendly practices, and create opportunities for social well-being and intergenerational activities within communities. Markets can also act as a conduit for educational activities and for raising broader awareness of issues (Morales and Kettles, 2009). Some have therefore suggested that 'markets not only helped preserve the physical health of the people, but also the social and economic health of the community' (Morales and Kettles, 2009: 22).

CASE STUDY 14.1: BUGURUNI MARKET

One example of the development of a healthy food market is Buguruni Market in Dar es Salaam, Tanzania. Prior to work to develop the healthy market, Buguruni Market had a single pit latrine and one water standpipe. The market lacked central administration and maintenance, there was no pest control programme and, moreover, food inspections were infrequent. Vendors from the market, alongside governmental and non-governmental organisations, established the Buguruni Healthy Marketplaces Task Force. As a consequence of the task force there have been significant developments, including:

- improvement in road access;
- construction of a solid waste storage bay;
- construction of toilet and hand-washing facilities;
- development of a system for the collection and sorting of solid waste for subsequent disposal.

The success of the Buguruni Market has been seen in the development of the healthy market concept being introduced into several other markets in Dar es Salaam and other cities in Tanzania (Green et al., 2019).

In the past number of years, the healthy marketplace idea has expanded widely and now encompasses street-food vendors; taco trucks; sidewalk fruit vendors; and 'pop-up' kitchens at festivals and other events (Morales and Kettles, 2009). The rise in these 'new' marketplaces for health has increased awareness of sustainability and food provenance and has perhaps created the need to re-define the concept and practice of health promotion in these settings.

HEALTHY SCHOOLS

Schools, for some time now, have been considered as being one of the most important 'settings' in health promotion practice (Whitehead, 2011) and have been consistently present in conferences and charters on health promotion. This success has manifested in examples of health-promoting schools in all parts of the world. The health-promoting school recognises that a child's learning at school is the product not just of what is taught through the planned formal curriculum, but also the totality of their school experience and interaction. This would encompass the physical and social environment, relationships and practices in the school (the hidden curriculum), the activities organised by the school (the informal curriculum) and contact with the school health service (the parallel curriculum) (Green et al., 2019).

According to the WHO (2019f), a health-promoting school:

- Fosters health and learning with all the measures at its disposal.
- Engages health and education officials, teachers, teachers' unions, students, parents, health providers and community leaders in efforts to make the school a healthy place.

- Strives to provide a healthy environment, school health education, and school health services along with school/community projects and outreach, health promotion programmes for staff, nutrition and food safety programmes, opportunities for physical education and recreation, and programmes for counselling, social support and mental health promotion.
- Implements policies and practices that respect an individual's well-being and dignity, provide multiple opportunities for success, and acknowledge good efforts and intentions as well as personal achievements.
- Strives to improve the health of school personnel, families and community members as well as pupils; and works with community leaders to help them understand how the community contributes to, or undermines, health and education.

REFLECTIVE EXERCISE 14.1

To what extent should schools be responsible for the health of pupils? There have been several studies that have pointed to schools as the lynch-pin to tackle child health issues, such as obesity. In response to this, Ofsted (the Office for Standards in Education, Children's Services and Skills) in the UK suggested: 'Teachers simply cannot take on the job of health professionals, nutritionists, parents and other new roles that are demanded of them on an almost daily basis. The answer to the obesity crisis lies in homes, communities, health services and schools acting in concert' (Ofsted, 2018: 19). What are the arguments for and against this view? To what extent can a settings approach in health promotion aid organisations 'acting in concert'? How could this happen in reality?

HEALTH-PROMOTING WORKPLACES

People spend at least forty years of their lives, one third of the day, five days a week and over forty weeks of the year in a workplace setting (Hubley et al., 2013). They therefore offer a prime opportunity for health promotion and evidence shows a range of positive effects as a result of workplace health promotion, including improvements in the status of employees' health; increased health consciousness; changes in health behaviour; better working atmosphere; better communication and co-operation among employees; and reduction of risk factors that affect health (Brandenburg, 2012).

The European Network for Workplace Health Promotion has defined workplace health promotion as the combined efforts of employers, employees and society to improve the health and well-being of people at work. This vision of workplace health promotion places particular emphasis on improving the work organization and working environment, increasing workers' participation in shaping the working environment, and encouraging personal skills and professional development (WHO, 2019g).

However, many workplaces do not engage in health-promoting activity. The barriers to conducting health promotion in workplaces have been summarised by Rojatz et al. (2016). They suggest the following:

- external conditions (e.g. global economic downturns) hindering the likelihood of workplaces engaging in workplace health interventions;
- limited managerial support and an unfavourable health-promoting 'organizational culture/climate';
- lack of 'resources' to implement interventions (time, money, staff and infrastructure);
- the incompatibility of the intervention with staff working hours/processes;
- the workplaces' lack of 'experience with health promotion';
- poor staff participation rates, especially when interventions are scheduled during holiday periods.

Often, those working in health promotion within workplace settings will need to draw on their communication skills (see Chapter 20) in order to convince organisations about the benefits of a health-promoting workplace. This communication strategy often needs to be premised on economic gains for the organisation, including increases in productivity and enhancements to the corporate image. While it may be disappointing to frame health in this way, rather than for the intrinsic or moral benefits of the approach, it is characteristic of a settings approach where alternative demands within the organisation frequently place health promotion activity on the periphery.

HEALTH-PROMOTING HOSPITALS

It can be surprising to learn that the *modus operandi* of a hospital is not generally health or health promotion. Green et al. (2019) have argued that many hospitals must re-orientate if they are to be health-promoting organisations, making a transition from curing disease to promoting health; from patient compliance to empowerment; from a narrow concern with patients to including relatives, staff and the wider community; and from being inward-looking to being outward-looking.

There has been widespread commitment to the health-promoting hospital concept and networks established initially in Europe, but now globally. There are also several endorsed principles and recommendations for health-promoting hospitals (see Box 14.1). However, the concept has not had the same penetration as health-promoting schools or healthy cities.

BOX 14.1 THE VIENNA RECOMMENDATIONS ON HEALTH-PROMOTING HOSPITALS

1. promote human dignity, equity and solidarity, and professional ethics, acknowledging differences in the needs, values and cultures of different population groups;
2. be oriented towards quality improvement, the wellbeing of patients, relatives and staff, protection of the environment and realization of the potential to become learning organizations;

3. focus on health with a holistic approach and not only on curative services;
4. be centred on people providing health services in the best way possible to patients and their relatives, to facilitate the healing process and contribute to the empowerment of patients;
5. use resources efficiently and cost-effectively, and allocate resources on the basis of contribution to health improvement; and form as close links as possible with other levels of the health care system and the community.

Research has suggested four broad types of health-promoting hospitals (Johnson and Baum, 2001). Type 1 are hospitals that are 'doing' a health promotion activity or project on a one-off or ad hoc basis. Type 2 are hospitals that 'delegate' the health promotion activity to a specific department or member of staff. This often results in the activities being marginalised and not seen as the responsibility for the 'whole' organisation. Type 3 are hospitals that are organisationally committed to the settings approach and have this as an integral part of the organisation's activities, focusing on patients, staff and visitors. Finally, type 4 are hospitals that demonstrate all of the type 3 characteristics but extend this further to ensure a wider focus on the surrounding community.

REFLECTIVE EXERCISE 14.2

As a more advanced activity, look back at Chapter 13 and compare and contrast Whitelaw's (2001) theoretical view of settings-based health promotion and the explanation of the four 'types' of health-promoting hospitals identified by Johnson and Baum (2001). Where is there overlap and difference between these models? What would your critique be of these models and which do you think offers greater conceptual and practical clarity for health promoters?

HEALTH-PROMOTING PRISONS

Prisons have a concentration of people with very poor health, including poor mental and physical health. In October 1995, an international meeting with senior prison health representatives from eight selected European countries agreed that the public health importance of prisoner health had been neglected (Gatherer et al., 2005). The settings approach to health promotion was recognised as a way of addressing the health of the prison population after observing the effectiveness of the settings approach in schools, workplaces, hospitals and cities. However, despite the global endorsement for healthy cities and health-promoting schools, the health-promoting prison has to date failed to penetrate beyond a few countries (Woodall and Dixey, 2015).

There are clearly several issues that prevent a health-promoting agenda from being present within this setting. The notion of being excluded from society, having autonomy and choice removed, and having restrictions placed on movements are just a few examples.

REFLECTIVE EXERCISE 14.3

If prisons are to embrace the healthy settings philosophy, they must ensure that values such as control, choice and empowerment are embedded within the organisation (Woodall et al., 2013). To what extent is this a contradiction in terms? As an example, consider how a healthy diet could be maintained and compromised in the prison environment.

There have been many difficulties in moving from the strategy, or theory, of what a health-promoting prison should be and how to deliver this in practice. One response to this has been to apply the principles of the Ottawa Charter to action within the prison context (see Figure 14.3).

Those tasked with translating the strategy of the health-promoting prison into practice have needed to tread a delicate and difficult policy path in which wider public and political opinion is an ever-present force (Tabreham, 2014). Improving prison health does not generally gather political capital or public endorsement. This may be compounded by the fact that many of the health issues that manifest in the prison population often emanate in behaviours that may be associated with social stigma and criminality (Whitehead, 2006). Wider public perceptions about who is 'deserving' of support has created challenges in providing equivalent health services in prison (Baybutt et al., 2010), including health promotion where ideas such as the 'empowerment' of prisoners sit uneasy in parts of the public and political domain.

HEALTH-PROMOTING UNIVERSITIES

Health-promoting universities have been synonymous with the settings approach in health promotion, but the concept and practice has been relatively slow to adopt (Newton et al., 2016). These challenges are not necessarily distinct from other 'settings' and include competing organisational priorities and a lack of evidence of the success of the approach. The commitment of a health-promoting university is to promote the health and well-being of staff, students and the wider community through co-ordinated and integrated policies and practices that embrace health-promoting values (Dooris, 2001). Activities delivered under the health-promoting universities umbrella have been diverse and wide-ranging. In the UK, this practice is captured and shared via a website which offers 'real-life' examples of initiative and programmes. These include activities and policies to raise awareness of alcohol; encourage active commuting on university campuses and initiatives to encourage

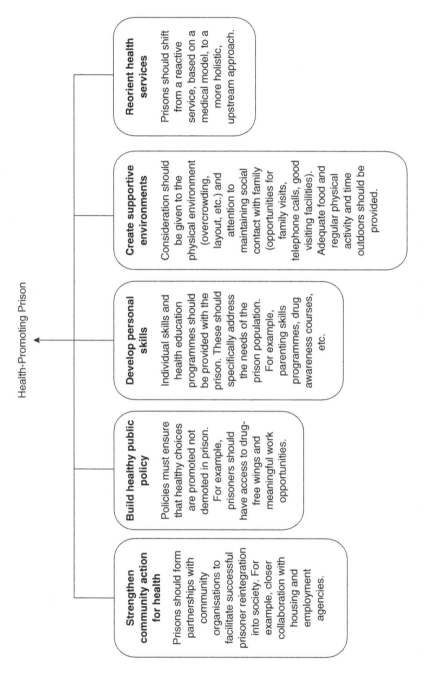

Health-Promoting Prison

Strengthen community action for health

Prisons should form partnerships with community organisations to facilitate successful prisoner reintegration into society. For example, closer collaboration with housing and employment agencies.

Build healthy public policy

Policies must ensure that healthy choices are promoted not demoted in prison. For example, prisoners should have access to drug-free wings and meaningful work opportunities.

Develop personal skills

Individual skills and health education programmes should be provided with the prison. These should specifically address the needs of the prison population. For example, parenting skills programmes, drug awareness courses, etc.

Create supportive environments

Consideration should be given to the physical environment (overcrowding, layout, etc.) and attention to maintaining social contact with family (opportunities for family visits, telephone calls, good visiting facilities). Adequate food and regular physical activity and time outdoors should be provided.

Reorient health services

Prisons should shift from a reactive service, based on a medical model, to a more holistic, upstream approach.

Figure 14.3 The Ottawa Charter as a framework for action within the health-promoting prison

Source: Woodall and South (2012: 173)

universities to consider ease of access to sustainable and healthy food choices (see https://healthyuniversities.ac.uk/toolkit-and-resources/case-studies/).

HEALTHY NIGHTCLUB

Going out with friends, dancing and engaging in nightlife activities can have significant health and social benefits. Nevertheless, there is also a potential for adverse health effects caused by alcohol, drugs, unsafe sex and exposure to loud noise (Bellis et al., 2002). In responding to this, the concept of a health-promoting nightclub has been growing for some time and is now well established, with international conferences on the topic having been regularly held for the past two decades. Arguably the focus on healthy nightclubs has been reduced in recent times, caused by reductions in people choosing to attend nightclubs. Nevertheless, there is still momentum for such an approach with recent successes in lobbying against cheap alcohol promotions and the consumption of highly caffeinated drinks.

The development of a safe nightlife is a growing priority for many towns and cities across the world. The Club Health project is a collaboration involving partners from 15 EU Member States and Norway to support local, national and European policy-makers and practitioners to develop healthier and safer nightlife environments. To date, the project has produced guidance to be used by governments, local authorities, health professionals, police, non-governmental organisations, the nightlife industry and other parties working to protect health and promote safety in nightlife environments. The vision of the project is to reduce diseases (especially addictions and sexually transmitted infections), accidents, injuries and violence within nightlife settings.

GO FURTHER 14.1

The previous chapter highlighted how effective activity is ensured when settings 'join up' and work mutually to ensure holistic and integrated activities. Using the example of a health-promoting university and healthy nightclub, describe how these two settings could work together to effectively tackle health issues and health inequalities. What would be the 'added value' in these two settings working synergistically to address, for instance, safe sex or substance and alcohol use?

HEALTH-PROMOTING SPORTS CLUBS

Health-promoting sports clubs are becoming more globally prominent with examples of good practice reported across many parts of the world (Kokko et al., 2016). Given the enthusiasm for sport and the centrality of sports clubs in many communities, they are regarded as a key site for tackling health inequalities and, in particular, addressing the issues facing young people as well as spectators, supporters and the wider community

(Dobbinson et al., 2006; Lane et al., 2017). There has been growing focus also on the importance of professional sports clubs in influencing the health promotion agenda. Some sports clubs have been effective in reaching sub-sections of the community where engagement with health promotion has traditionally failed (Pringle et al., 2013). Professional sports clubs represent a good illustration of a settings approach, whereby activities can be undertaken within the environment to influence individuals' behaviours and knowledge and where the structures and policies of the setting itself is geared towards creating healthy environments; for instance, the responsible serving of alcohol, sun-protection policies and healthy catering (Dobbinson et al., 2006).

HEALTHY AIRPORTS

Reflecting the impact of an ever-increasing globalised world, one of the more contemporary settings for health promotion has been airports. Airports can impact the social, physical and economic environment. Indeed in communities surrounding airports, noise and environmental pollution are acute issues impacting on individuals and families (de Leeuw et al., 2018). Airports as healthy settings have been conceptualised more broadly and, perhaps more usefully, as the notion of an 'aerotropolis' – which encompasses the wider environmental and geographical footprint of an airport.

REFLECTIVE EXERCISE 14.4

In what ways can airports and the wider 'aerotropolis' impact positively on individual and community health? Think about: the potential for employment; the effect of provision within the airport itself (for example, food and catering, hospitality, opportunities for rest, minimising stress and anxiety through built design); the positive impact of transport infrastructure and increased connectedness; the impact on the local economy and culture; the social benefits of travelling to holiday destinations or connecting with family and friends.

Table 14.1 The healthy airport

Dimension	Example
Environment	• Engages in planning processes that result in health promoting aesthetic built environments • Provides a clean, safe, high-quality physical environment for all people inside the airport boundaries and in surrounding communities • Ensures that systems that are in place to protect individual and collective safety and security are implemented in least obtrusive ways in accordance with their specific purpose

(Continued)

Table 14.1 (Continued)

Dimension	Example
Ecosystem	• Creates, maintains and aligns with governance, policies and practices for a sustainable ecosystem • Protects as much as possible the natural ecosystems within and beyond the airport boundaries • Addresses sustainability principles • Reduces its environmental footprint (particularly with regard to carbon emissions and waste generation) to the greatest extent possible, on a trajectory to carbon neutrality • Reflects local communities' sensitivity/connection to landscape and environment (e.g. local flora, fauna and open spaces)
Community	• Builds on consultative/participatory community engagement to ensure fairness and equity in risks and benefits • Ensures an inclusive, respectful and mutually supportive community through consultative processes • Actively pursues its ability to build positive social change outside the boundaries of its general business
Participation	• Implements governance structures that enable a high degree of public participation in and control over the decisions affecting one's life, health and well-being • Provides avenues for all airport users and members of communities affected by the airport's operations with effective means of providing feedback on the airport's operations and involvement in decisions that affect them
Basic services and facilities	• Ensures that hygienically prepared food and beverages are available that meet a wide range of preferences and prices • Ensures that potable plain water is available free of charge throughout the airport • Ensures that all activities at the airport are conducted with adherence to high standards of workplace health and safety • Ensures that conditions of employment for all persons working at the airport are meeting appropriate international/national standards • Offers healthy food choices, including meeting the needs of all diet requirements when travelling and in the airport • Ensures equitable affordable transport options for workers and visitors
Experiences and resources	• Provides a range of passive and active recreational spaces and activities for residents, workers and visitors • Provides a wide range of opportunities for relaxation and physical and mental activity for persons waiting at the airport • Provides free family-friendly activities for travellers and people waiting • Provides accessible and acceptable connectedness to internet and (social) media
Economy	• Creates and sustains a lively economy that supports a diversified skill set within local industry and provides opportunities for advancement • Makes a vital and innovative contribution to the economy of the region around the airport • Provides equitable employment
Heritage	• Maintains and promotes the historical, social, economic, geographic and cultural contexts of the region • Provides many tangible links with the historical, cultural and biological heritage of the region in which it is located
Form and design	• Has a physical form that is compatible with and enhances all the other elements of a healthy airport • Integrates coordinated high-level infrastructure planning with the local urban (political, social and environmental) context

Dimension	Example
Public health and sick care services	• Engages in activities that promote and maximise the health of individuals, peoples and communities • Provides appropriate public health and sick care services that are easily accessible by all who need them, particularly travellers and employees
Connectedness	• Is designed to make people feel welcomed • Is designed to blend into the region and culture • Recognises its glocal (the interface between global and local) footprint in all of the above qualities
Nuisance and impact	• Works proactively and in collaboration with potentially affected individuals to reduce health risks and build (health) resilience • Aims to meet and exceed the strictest standards in noise, air, water and soil pollution

Source: de Leeuw et al. (2018). Reproduced by kind permission of the Centre for Health Equity Training, Research & Evaluation (CHETRE)

There are 12 dimensions which together provide the underpinning foundations of a healthy airport. These are presented in Table 14.1

SUMMARY

The potential for 'where' health promotion can be conducted is limitless. This chapter has sought to provide a brief overview of 12 different settings ranging from the well established (such as cities and schools) to those in their relative infancy (such as airports). The examples provided here, albeit brief, show that the settings approach is a useful framework to fully consider 'where' practice should take place. The following chapter moves into the virtual world, showing the potential for health promotion in the increasingly digital world.

SUGGESTED READING

Naidoo, J. and Wills, J. (2016) *Foundations for health promotion.* 4th edn. London, Elsevier.

Poland, B.D., Green, L.W. and Rootman, I. (2000) *Settings for health promotion: linking theory and practice.* Thousand Oaks, CA, Sage.

Scriven, A. and Hodgins, M. (2012) *Health promotion settings: principles and practice.* London, Sage.

VIRTUAL SETTINGS FOR HEALTH

15

INTRODUCTION

As has been seen in the preceding two chapters, settings have been long defined and practised in physical environments and contexts often with clearly defined boundaries. However, the Ottawa Charter's suggestion that 'health is created and lived by people within the settings of their everyday life; where they learn, work, play and love' (WHO, 1986) could, quite easily, be applied to virtual environments where many of us now spend a high proportion of our time (O'Neil, 2019).

The exponential growth of the internet, and social media particularly, has created opportunities for health promotion to locate in 'virtual' settings (Cross et al., 2017). This chapter will show the importance of health promotion in virtual environments, including applications (apps) and social networking sites, such as Twitter and Facebook. The chapter focuses on these virtual settings for health promotion and many of the arguments in favour of adopting this approach overlap with related terms such as 'eHealth', 'mHealth', 'connected health' and 'Health 2.0' (Lupton, 2015). Specifically, the chapter shows the opportunities and value of Web 2.0 for health promotion and moreover demonstrate why it has such potential in health promotion. Nevertheless, and as with all settings, the drawbacks and challenges of the virtual world being conceptualised as a healthy 'setting' will be explored.

WEB 2.0

The focus in this chapter is on Web 2.0, a term used from 2004 to encapsulate interactive, user-generated and user-controlled web-based content and applications (apps). The predecessor of Web 2.0 was the original Web 1.0 which is often regarded as being more static and less interactive, with content largely in the form of written text (Korda and Itani, 2013) – it is characteristic of a 'one-way' information exchange with limited opportunity for collaboration or exchange of ideas between users and professional or between users themselves.

At its very best, Web 2.0 is exciting, innovative, participatory and collaborative. It encourages open dialogue and the exchange of ideas, as well as information and viewpoints from a range of professional and lay people (Chou et al., 2013). Web 2.0 was a term coined to encapsulate this dynamic, user-generated online experience and online social networking sites, such as Facebook, Twitter, Instagram and YouTube (see Box 15.1), are now characteristic of Web 2.0 (Loss et al., 2014). Social networking sites can be accessed 'on the move' and at any time using smartphones, tablets, laptops and computers.

The usage and popularity of online social networking is staggering. While the preference for sites changes, the growth in this area has been exponential as access to the internet has become far more readily available.

BOX 15.1 SOCIAL NETWORKING SITES AND THEIR DEFINING FEATURES

There are many popular social networking sites, such as Facebook, Twitter, Instagram and LinkedIn. According to Verduyn et al. (2017) these sites have three common characteristics:

1. Users have a personal profile which often includes photographs and information about people's current status or whereabouts.
2. The sites publicly show people's visible lists of connections - people the individual is 'following' or people that are following them in Twitter, for example, or the list of friends in Facebook.
3. Social networking sites have a constantly updated 'live' newsfeed, populated by posts and content from people's connections.

People may use multiple social networking sites to fulfil a range of different purposes - this could be for personal and professional reasons.

THE BENEFITS OF VIRTUAL SETTINGS FOR HEALTH PROMOTION

Technological enhancements and online communication have revolutionised the way many of us live our lives. Work, education, leisure and social interaction have increasingly moved away from geographically bounded locations to the virtual world. Indeed, research shows that people spend more time interacting each day virtually than in person (Verduyn et al., 2017). Many people now work from home, enrol on distance learning courses, or spend leisure time in online communities (Loss et al., 2014). The reality is that we now live in a fast-paced, 24-hour world, where people demand instantaneous information via their smartphones, tablets, laptops and computers. Given this context, it is clear that health promoters must embrace this and consider the virtual space as a legitimate setting for health.

REFLECTIVE EXERCISE 15.1

Which social networking sites do you use and not use? What are the reasons behind your decision-making? What are people's motives for engaging in social networking? Is it for connecting with others? Making new friends? Following trends and celebrities? To feel socially included or to avoid FOMO (the fear of missing out)?

The extent to which health promotion has kept pace with the digital age is debatable, many practitioners still often relying on other ways to communicate health information. Several commentators have argued that the cornerstone of health promotion practice, the Ottawa Charter (WHO, 1986), should be redefined and re-conceptualised since the expansion and popularity of the virtual world. Debates within health promotion have suggested that the original values and principles espoused in the Ottawa Charter in the mid-1980s need to be updated given the changing technological world and both the opportunities and challenges this provides (Nutbeam, 2008; Tilford, 2016). While such debates may seem relatively trivial, we would argue that a clear framework for practice within virtual environments would encourage consistency of practice and provide guidance on the ethics and evaluation of working in this setting.

Notwithstanding a clear framework for practice, there are promising signs that virtual contexts can impact positively on health. A systematic review found several benefits of social media – including Facebook, Twitter, Wikipedia, YouTube, blogs, etc. – for health purposes (Moorhead et al., 2013). These can be summarised as follows:

1. Social media provides access to a vast array of health issues.
2. Social media can widen access to those who may not easily access health information.
3. Social media can deliver information in a range of innovative and interesting ways.
4. Dialogue and collaboration.
5. Access to peer, social, and emotional support.
6. Providing anonymity (or not).

Elaboration on each of these benefits will now follow.

Social media provides access to a vast array of health issues

Use any search engine, or log on to any social networking site, and the array of health information at the fingertips of the user is immense. Where seeking out information on particular issues is difficult and time-intensive, this material can be obtained in less than a second. Not only does social media offer access to myriad health issues, but the vast quantity of information means that content can be found that is customised to the specific recipient. The pre-contemplating dieter, the new mother struggling to breastfeed or the relapsed smoker, for instance, can all find specific information relating to their circumstance and situation. The added benefit of potentially being able to interact with others searching for similar content or able to share lay experiences is a further advantage to virtual environments. Moreover, where information may not be readily available a social media post requesting further insight will often yield useful material or contacts.

Social media can widen access to those who may not easily access health information

Providing health information or raising awareness or consciousness of issues via social media is low cost and has the potential to reach a mass audience. Few, if any, social networking sites charge the user for posting or subscribing which means that start-up costs for health campaigning is very cost-effective. This means that the potential 'returns' can be great.

The notion of something 'going viral' online means the exponential growth in audience views when users share content. Being able to do this would hold benefits for health promotion if a health education message becomes shared via Facebook or re-tweeted in Twitter. This kind of phenomena can be regularly observed when celebrities champion a particular cause, but also when lay people capture the essence of an issue in a very provocative or engaging way.

Social media may also have the advantage of reaching those who may not easily access 'traditional' health information in crisis situations. Research is showing, for example, the advantage of social media for disease surveillance and control – particular examples include the use of social media to communicate information regarding Ebola, natural disasters, avian bird flu and influenza. This approach provides real-time information and support that can easily be followed using the news feed on social media sites.

The notion that young people are a group that may benefit particularly from social media content is true given that lots of data suggest that this demographic use social media more than others. However, patterns of usage are constantly changing with 'silver surfers' – those aged over 50 who use the internet – growing in their social networking uptake.

Social media can deliver information in a range of innovative and interesting ways

Photographs, videos, wikis, quizzes, vlogs, blogs and the provision of live update information is a huge benefit of social media for health promotion which when used appropriately can create an engaging backdrop to raise awareness or promote activities. People's preferences for how content is displayed is, of course, variable, but there is likely to be a virtual post or website that engages people. Some will prefer video content whereas others may prefer blogs or quizzes to hold their attention.

The historical reliance in health promotion to use written-based communication via leaflets has been a cornerstone of practice – but consistently these have proved limited in engaging particular audiences (Murphy and Smith, 1993). Social media allows for creative ways to engage people outside of these usual modes of delivery. In some instances, words can be replaced completely through visual imagery or videos. A YouTube video by Sussex Safer Roads Partnership reached a mass audience to encourage seat-belt use – the 1.30 minute video uses no words or written text, but powerfully communicates the message using visual imagery and emotive sound (see www.youtube.com/watch?v=h-8PBx7isoM).

Mobile-phone apps have also supported the growing use of social networking for health promotion. There are tens of thousands of health-related apps for mobile digital devices (Lupton, 2015) – designed by private providers, charities and the public sector. These can cover all sorts of content from physical activity, to monitoring alcohol intake, to breast-feeding. Evidence has shown the value of apps in achieving a range of health outcomes (Lee et al., 2018). The ability for apps to track and monitor information and to provide real-time information and data is considerable. Interactive quizzes and games built into the app technology also broadens appeal and potentially the uptake and usage.

Dialogue and collaboration

Social media holds many characteristics of mass-media communication, but also features of personalised one-to-one messaging. The link between social networking and social capital is perhaps one of the biggest strengths of virtual settings. The ability to stay in touch with others is comparatively easy within social networking sites than in physical environments – a brief message or a tagged photograph, or even a quick 'happy birth-day' posted to somebody, for example, keeps connections between people and prevents friendship or connection from dissolving. This allows people to comfortably maintain and expand social networks and thereby increase social capital (Verduyn et al., 2017). Message boards and discussion forums, easily facilitated by social networking sites, can bring peo-ple together. People congregate online with various social backgrounds and experiences to discuss shared issues of importance.

Looking broadly at what encompasses 'health' (see Chapter 1) we know that relation-ships, and indeed intimate relationships, are supported by social networking. There is little doubt that social networking in contemporary society is a prominent part of people's life which facilitates friendships, flirting, sexual encounters and also break-ups (Loss et al., 2014). Clearly the 'strength' of these bonds can be called into question and whether they are as effective as face-to-face interaction is for further discussion and research.

Access to peer, social and emotional support

Social networking means that there is *always* someone available to respond to people's concerns. Given the global accessibility of the internet, people living in different time zones can connect very easily. People can very readily share information and lend support via social networking – this could be with existing friends, or with strangers who people have never met before.

The potential for social media to address social isolation is one clear area that can be facilitated and research is beginning to explore this relationship. Social contact at par-ticular times of the year is sometimes sought by people – perhaps around anniversaries of deaths of significant others or other significant events (see Box 15.2).

BOX 15.2 HOW THE HASHTAG COMBATS LONELINESS: #JOININ

There is growing interest in the way in which social media can combat loneliness and increase social connectivity. Research has shown, for instance, that image-based social media in particular (e.g. Instagram) can reduce people's feelings of loneliness and boost happiness (Pittman and Reich, 2016).

People can feel more isolated and lonelier at particular times of the year, none more so than at Christmas. The British comedian Sarah Millican has for a number of years hosted the hashtag on twitter #joinin - the purpose is to create a supportive virtual community of people who are feeling alone. Within this space, people lend support to each other and start online conversations which alleviates feelings of isolation.

Providing anonymity (or not)

One of the attractions of virtual settings is that they are non-judgemental so people can provide personal information without feeling threatened (Hubley et al., 2013). Social media can, if desired by people, offer the opportunity to be anonymous and not to disclose particular information. This can be very desirable to people who may want to go into personal details about their circumstances, with a safety net that they cannot be identified. This, of course, stands in contrast to face-to-face help-seeking whereby the person's anonymity can be compromised by disclosing such information. Finding ways to manage workplace stress using social networking, for instance, may be desired by some in contrast to using services and support in the workplace or community. It may also facilitate a greater openness and honesty with the guarantee that the post could not be traced by their employees.

CASE STUDY 15.1: SOCIAL MEDIA HEALTH PROMOTION IN SOUTH AFRICA: OPPORTUNITIES AND CHALLENGES

BACKGROUND

Health promotion is an effective tool for public health. It goes beyond preventing the spread of diseases and reducing the disease burden. It includes interventions encompassing the creation of supportive environments, building public health policy, developing personal skills, reorienting health services and strengthening multi-sectoral community actions.

AIM

The aim of the review was to conduct an analysis on the opportunities and challenges of the use of social media for health promotion in South Africa.

METHODS

A search of review articles on health promotion using social media conducted using Medline and Google Scholar. Secondary searches were conducted using references and citations from selected articles.

RESULTS

Social media has the potential of being an effective health promotion tool in South Africa. It presents an opportunity for scaling health promotion programmes because of its low cost, its ability to have virtual communities and the ease of access eliminating geographical barriers. It also allows real-time communication between various stake-holders. It allows information to spread far and fast and leaving irrespective of the credibility of the source of information. There is a need to take into account country-specific socio-economic issues, which may perpetuate unintended consequences related to the digital divide, data costs and the varying levels of health literacy.

CONCLUSION

Considering the opportunities presented by social media, the National Department of Health needs to review its health promotion strategy and include the use of social media as an enabler. They also need to explore intersectoral measures to address issues which threatening equitable access to credible health promotion information.

Source: Kubheka et al. (2020)

CAN VIRTUAL SETTINGS *REALLY* BE CONSIDERED AS SETTINGS FOR HEALTH PROMOTION?

The attraction of virtual settings and social networking sites is very clear, given their potential to reach a vast global audience. Virtual environments can, as shown, enable people to change their behaviour and have an immense capacity to raise awareness of particular issues and topics. The benefits of this are not to be underplayed; however, we outline a series of arguments why virtual settings offer challenges for health promotion.

First, it is very clear that virtual settings for health currently reinforces an individualistic view of health promotion and seems to dilute a focus on the social determinants influencing health behaviours (Lupton, 2015). The notion that health is something that is controlled by the individual, that self-responsibility is key to a 'healthy life' and that individuals have free agency in their health actions is reinforced. The theory (see Chapter 13) illustrates that 'true' health-promoting setting considers and addresses the political and environmental context alongside individual behaviour change. Without this component, the setting simply is a convenient vehicle for a particular target audience – what Whitelaw et al. (2001) refer to as a 'passive model'. Lupton (2015: 179) notes: 'Digitized health promotion that seeks to move away from changing individual behaviour to broader initiatives such as community development and challenging the political status quo remains in the minority.' Others have also argued that virtual settings have been extremely limited in their ability to influence the political and environmental structures and only a few tangible examples of how the virtual environment itself has been made 'healthier' (Loss et al., 2014). As an example, the environment online is often the antithesis of 'healthy'. In extreme cases, social networking sites glorifies self-harm or suicide and causes mental and emotional distress.

Second, the internet is largely a business with online content often funded through sponsorships and endorsements. The use of subtle and sophisticated online advertisements has reached such sophistication that even the most savvy internet user can be misled. This can often impact on more vulnerable groups – children, for example, may not be able to distinguish an advertisement from entertainment content and can be unconsciously influenced by companies selling fast food, slimming and tobacco companies (Freeman and Chapman, 2007). However, children may, in fact, be more conscious of these implicit effects within virtual settings than adults, given that many children are now more digitally literate and sophisticated than their parents and grandparents (ASA, 2013).

Third, there is huge potential for virtual settings to 'join up' effectively with physical environments and settings, but so far this potential has not been fully realised (Loss et al., 2014). The theory of settings-based health promotion suggests that the approach will be best realised when there are synergistic effects across settings, but there are few examples where this has happened. Taking school settings and virtual settings as an illustration, pupils often use social media to learn and explore the world without adult constraint and yet social media and mobile phones are often banned in schools (Ahn et al., 2011). There is a clear contradiction here. Where the virtual world and school setting has come together, it has commonly created adverse effects – at worst that can include cyber-bullying, but more implicit is the impact on self-esteem of individuals based on the number of 'likes' or the comments made by others on their social media posts.

Fourth, the argument that a settings approach can exacerbate, rather than address, health inequalities is perhaps starkly shown when virtual settings are considered: 'The well-educated and well-off have access to and use the Internet to a much greater extent than those who are less well educated and who are less well off' (Korp, 2006: 82). People from disadvantaged groups are often doubly disadvantaged in that they often lack both health literacy (see Box 15.3) and digital literacy, resulting in less knowledge and fewer skills in using digital technologies for health-promoting purposes (Lupton, 2015).

BOX 15.3 HEALTH LITERACY

1. Functional health literacy – concerned with improved knowledge of health risks and health services and compliance with prescribed actions.
2. Interactive health literacy – developing personal and social skills to act independently on knowledge and to improve motivation and self-confidence to act on advice received.
3. Critical health literacy – high-level cognitive skills supporting effective social and political action based on information provided.

Source: Hubley et al. (2021)

Digital access and inequality is also a geo-political issue, with some countries still without the appropriate infrastructure to support fast broadband. In addition, there are linguistic and cultural barriers to access (Warwick-Booth et al., 2019). All of these issues raise questions as to who is excluded from this valuable setting for health. Indeed, one study noted that health promotion material within virtual environments were predominantly designed and maintained by organisations or individuals from high income countries (Gold et al., 2011). Also, research showed that during the Ebola crisis in 2014 there were more tweets about Ebola in the USA than in Guinea, Liberia, and Sierra Leone where the epidemic was taking place. The major challenge facing health promotion is the issue of equity and addressing inequalities in health. While virtual settings have an important place, it needs to be supplemented by other methods if we are to reach the communities who have the most need.

Fifth, the extent to which critical health literacy is required in this setting over any other is clear. The debate about the quality and credibility of information available online has been a long-standing concern (Korp, 2006). This field is constantly changing, but evidence has shown that breast cancer information online (one of the most searched health issue) was frequently inaccurate (Hubley et al., 2013). It is not easy to determine good-quality information from pseudo-science or, as noted earlier, sophisticated attempts to mask the advertisement of products as entertainment. Health promotion activity is often more closely 'regulated' and scrutinised in physical settings – in schools, for instance, teachers and parents would be aware of what was being delivered and would raise concerns if the credibility of the information was dubious. Prisons are routinely inspected and assessed in the health information it provides to prisoners. In virtual environments, the oversight and regulation of information is far less apparent and arguably far more complicated and time-consuming (ASA, 2013).

REFLECTIVE EXERCISE 15.2

What advice would you provide to enable people to distinguish credible, high-quality online health information from material that may be from less trustworthy sources? Think about the ways in which you identify and use health information online and how you determine the legitimacy of web content. How would you advise a young person *versus* an older person, as an example?

Sixth, there have been several concerns of the impact of spending time on social media and the physical inactivity that this can promote (Loss et al., 2014). The evidence is currently mixed and inconclusive in relation to whether social media promotes sedentary behaviour or promotes isolation from the 'real' world. Perhaps linked to this is emerging evidence and research that envy of others can be a consequence of social networking sites (Verduyn et al., 2017). How many of us have seen the pictures and posts on social networking sites of holidays, fantastic relationships or amazing moments and not been envious? How this impacts on individuals is yet unknown, but there may be clear psychological influences.

Finally, the internet and virtual environments have become highly adept at influencing our choices based on our search and internet history. The use of algorithms to create digital spaces where people are directed as to what to watch and buy is potentially problematic. The broader ethical concerns that this creates requires health promoters to consider carefully how best to use or avoid such functionality.

SUMMARY

The potential of virtual settings for health promotion is abundantly clear, but the extent to which this is simply versions of old-style health communication using new media is highly debatable (Lupton, 2015). The principles of health education and peer support are clearly seen in social networking for health purposes. The theory surrounding this is long-standing and so it could be that the internet offers health promoters nothing 'new'. We wouldn't necessarily subscribe to this position and would see mass potential of virtual environments for health promotion.

Arguments put forward in this chapter suggest that there is still some distance for health promoters to travel if virtual spaces are to be considered as a health-promoting setting. In short, social networking in particular fosters an individualistic notion of health and, as yet, has not managed to gain traction on tackling wider determinants of health. Moreover, there is still some way to see virtual settings 'joining up' with physical settings too. Overall though, the concept of a virtual setting for health promotion offers great excitement and, indeed, the pace of change suggests that there will be constant changes in this environment. There is already talk of Web 3.0 – a paradigm shift in online interaction where artificial intelligence will become more central to developments (O'Neil, 2019). This will inevitably bring new opportunities and challenges for health promotion.

SUGGESTED READING

Cross, R., Davis, S. and O'Neil, I. (2017) *Health communication: theoretical and critical perspectives*. Cambridge, Polity.

Hubley, J., Copeman, J. and Woodall, J. (2021) *Practical health promotion*. 3rd edn. Cambridge, Polity.

O'Neil, I. (2019) *Digital health promotion*. Cambridge, Polity.

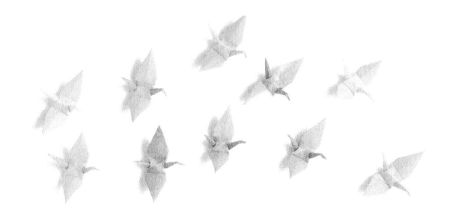

SECTION 6

HOW IS HEALTH PROMOTION PRACTISED?

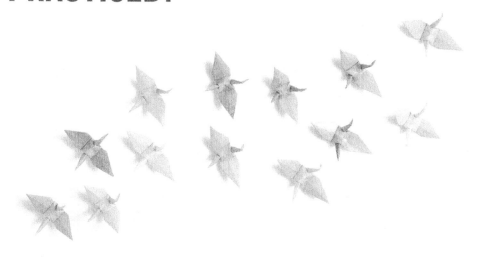

PROFESSIONAL COMPETENCIES AND CORE SKILLS

16

INTRODUCTION

The previous section of this book has explored the concept of settings as an approach to promoting health and in terms of where health promotion might/can take place. In this chapter we move on to consider what skills and competencies are required of the health promotion practitioner in order to be effective. This chapter will do two things. Firstly, it will outline, describe and discuss the attributes and skills required for professional practice in health promotion. In doing so we will refer to recognised national and international standards, and frameworks in health promotion practice. Secondly, the chapter discusses some of the challenges of working in health promotion. We conclude by considering the health promoter as an agent of change.

SKILLS AND ATTRIBUTES

At the outset it is important to define what we mean by 'skills' and 'attributes' and what the differences are. Skills and attributes differ. *Skills* can be learned and typically develop during training, education, work or through life experience. Skills can be developed and improved upon. Dreyfus's (2004) model outlines five different stages of skills development illustrating how we move from being a novice to being an expert which is relevant here (see Box 16.1). *Attributes*, on the other hand, are more inherent or natural, perhaps an intrinsic part of our personalities; for example, being empathetic or outgoing. It is important to note that there is some overlap between skills and attributes at times; however, for simplicity, we will consider these as separate entities and note where there are intersections.

BOX 16.1 THE FIVE-STAGE MODEL OF ADULT SKILL ACQUISITION

Stage 1: Novice - at this stage the person is a complete beginner and will likely be unskilled needing a significant level of education, guidance and instruction.

Stage 2: Advanced Beginner - at this stage the person will be developing skills and experience and learning new things but is still likely to need instruction and guidance.

Stage 3: Competence - at this stage the person will have had more experience and have developed more confidence in their own ability to perform the skill.

Stage 4: Proficiency - at this stage the learner has advanced further in the skill and is able to grapple with increased complexity.

Stage 5: Expert - at this stage the person will have achieved expertise and the skill will have become intuitive (or natural) to them.

Source: Dreyfus (2004)

Before you go any further take some time to do Reflective Exercise 16.1.

REFLECTIVE EXERCISE 16.1

Take some time to consider what *skills* and *attributes* you think an effective health promoter needs to have in order to achieve success. What do you think a health promoter should be able to *do* (skills)? What *attributes* do you think would be beneficial for a health promoter? Make a list for each. If you can, try to identify the top three skills and three top attributes - those that you think are most important. As you read the next section of this chapter compare the discussion with your list and the skills and attributes that you prioritised in your top three. How does your list compare?

THE HEALTH PROMOTION SKILL SET

Here we outline what we see as the key skills for health promotion. We will discuss six key areas: communication, tackling health inequalities, working ethically, using the evidence-base, working in partnership and management.

Communication

Without doubt the health promoter needs to be an effective communicator. Briefly this means having good interpersonal communication skills such as being able to listen to people as well as being able to communicate well with different groups of people using a variety of different means and methods. Communication is discussed in more detail in Chapter 20, 'Communicating Effectively', so refer to that chapter as well. As Gottwald (2012: 136) argues, 'establishing a rapport and being empathetic, communicating clearly, and negotiation are basic skills required for health promotion practitioners'. Linsley and Roll (2020: 26) identify three broad areas of skills needed for health promotion which relate to communication skills more generally. These are:

1. the ability to engage and communicate with people;
2. the ability to show empathy and encourage others; and
3. skills in listening and questioning.

They go on to argue that these skills need to be supported by the ability to think creatively, to problem-solve and to be flexible. Of course, some people are more naturally proficient at communication than others so this set of skills is linked to personal attributes; however, we can also learn to be better communicators. For example, Scriven (2017) outlines a number of specific skills for personal effectiveness in health promotion including writing skills (i.e. report-writing).

Tackling health inequalities

Tackling health inequalities is a key theme of this book. An appreciation of the fundamental role that inequality and inequity have to play in the development (or not) of health is vital for the health promotion practitioner. This requires focusing on the social, behavioural, economic, environmental and political determinants of health (Wills and Jackson, 2014) and on the up-stream causes of ill health (see also Chapter 1, 'What Is "health"?' and Chapter 5, 'Inequalities in Health' (Hubley et al., 2021)). Being able to understand the complexity of health is a necessary requirement for tackling health inequalities (Gottwald and Goodman-Brown, 2012). The skills required to tackle health inequalities include, for example, leadership, partnership working, being able to understand and appraise evidence, and being able to prioritise.

Working ethically

Developing knowledge and skills in ethical reflection on practice is a necessary and important skill for health promoters (Masse and William-Jones, 2012). All of the competency frameworks that have been developed for health promotion, and are presented later in this chapter, have ethics at the core of them (a competency framework is a structure that sets out the individual competencies that are required from someone working in a specific profession, institution or organisation). Health promotion often brings forth ethical dilemmas that need to be considered and dealt with so practitioners have to possess and develop skills in identifying and addressing these in practice. This also requires reflective skills, which include the ability to consider the impact of our actions on other people and how we might do things differently or better. Carter et al. (2012: 1) discuss four main issues of ethical consideration. Firstly, 'the potential for health promotion to limit or increase the freedom of individuals'; secondly, 'health promotion as a source of collective benefit'; thirdly, 'the possibility that health promotion strategies might "blame the victim" or stigmatise those who are disabled, sick or at higher risk of disease'; and fourthly, 'the importance of distributing the benefits of health promotion fairly' (see Carter et al., 2012 for a more detailed discussion).

Using the evidence base

Chapter 17, 'Searching and Appraising the Evidence', discussed this skill set in more detail; however, it is important to highlight here how necessary this is for successful health promotion. Making judgements about what it is most effective in promoting health is key to improving it. This requires a range of skills including epidemiological and analytical skills. Being able to understand information and the limitations of it is vital. So, appreciating and understanding demographic and epidemiological data and information, and how to make use of it in order to improve health, is a key skill for health promotion (Hesman, 2014). It is essential that the value of evidence is appreciated by the health promoter, and that they 'are able to understand and appraise research, apply relevant theory and research findings to their work, and identify areas for further investigation' (Evans et al., 2017: 5).

Working in partnership

Working in partnership with people is an essential skill in health promotion as well as being an underpinning principle of practice (Wild and McGrath, 2019). The emphasis in health promotion is on *working with* rather than *doing to* (Laverack, 2007). The resulting focus on participation and empowerment requires the ability to develop and create meaningful relationships with other people and being able to work effectively with a range of key stakeholders. Collaborative and co-ordination skills are therefore also necessary. As Scriven (2017) points out, health promotion frequently involves multi-agency and multi-disciplinary working so being able to work in a team is an important skill. 'Collaboration and working together is more likely to increase motivation and avoid conflict' (Gottwald, 2012: 112). These are also essential ingredients for working in empowering ways. Promoting shared decision-making, which is a two-way process where the health promoter might present the risks and benefits of changing behaviour and the person concerned would share their own perspective (lived experience, beliefs and values, challenges and opportunities, etc.), is also vital (Piper, 2009). A consensus is then reached about a way forward rather than using persuasive or coercive means. Working in this way promotes collaboration and reduces the unequal power distribution within relationships. It also values people's contribution putting their views and experience at the centre of the process.

Management

Scriven (2017: 115) conceptualises management as being 'about adopting practices which ensure effectiveness and efficiency in your work' – being *effective* means producing effects and accomplishing goals whilst being *efficient* means producing results with little wasted effort or resources. Management includes planning and priority-setting, problem-solving and identifying solutions, organisation and evaluation. The effective health promoter therefore needs to be able to manage well – to manage information, project work, time, people, processes and change (Scriven, 2017).

Desirable attributes for promoting health

Attributes are inherently linked to values. As Hubley et al. (2013: 23) state, 'values are attributes that are held in high regard by individuals, communities, societies and social movements'. Values can be a very individual phenomena; however, there are a particular set of core values that sit well with people who want to promote health. Tilford et al. (2003) identified these as:

- A holistic view of health
- Equity
- Equality
- Empowerment
- Autonomy
- Justice/fairness
- Partnership working
- Participation
- Choice
- Respect
- Sustainability
- Inclusiveness

Some of these clearly link to personal attributes and to the skill set for health promotion that we discussed earlier in this chapter. Treating people with respect and dignity is central as it enables trust to be established which is very important for building relationships (Mabuza, 2018). This includes respect for autonomy and for differences of opinion and also having empathy with other people's perspectives and situations. Other attributes include being non-judgemental, accepting, encouraging, motivating, supporting and guiding. Being reflective is also necessary and can likewise be regarded as a skill, as discussed earlier. Being creative and innovative is an asset in health promotion as well in order to identify new ways of working with individuals and communities to support their health and well-being. A personal interest in, and emphasis on, health rather than illness is, of course, essential (Wild and McGrath, 2019). Now take some time to carry out Reflective Exercise 16.2.

REFLECTIVE EXERCISE 16.2

Return to the lists of skills and attributes that you wrote for Reflective Exercise 16.1 and reflect on it in the light of this chapter. Would you add anything to your lists? Would you remove anything? Would you change or re-order your top three skills and attributes? If so, why? What made you change your mind about what skills and attributes were important for promoting health?

COMPETENCY FRAMEWORKS

Cross et al. (2017: 189) criticise the broad approach that competency frameworks take arguing that they tend to 'promote an expert-led *doing unto* rather than true engagement with communities or facilitating action'. Nevertheless, there have been a number of competency frameworks established that outline the skills, attributes and knowledge deemed necessary to practise health promotion to good effect. Knowledge is not easily defined as a skill or an attribute but it is essential for the health promotion practitioner and a solid knowledge base is a fundamental requirement for people who are promoting health. Of course, knowledge can be developed and built upon and would not necessarily be described as a skill, but the importance of having a sound knowledge base cannot be contested (Hanson, 2007). Those working in health promotion will need generalist as well as specialist knowledge. Specialist knowledge will relate to the specific area that the person is working in so they may, for example, need to be more knowledgeable about certain issues such as tackling obesity or reducing road traffic accidents, or particular ways of working such as community development or social marketing. Theoretical knowledge is also necessary for effective practice (Green et al., 2019). Given that health promoters can work in very different settings and roles, and have various education and employment backgrounds, developing competency frameworks enables the values, principles, skills and knowledge required for health promotion practice to be outlined and/or defined (Health Promotion Forum of New Zealand, 2012).

The notion of competence is important in any profession and therefore also for those working to promote health. 'Competencies are the combinations of knowledge, attitudes and skills needed to plan, implement and evaluate health promotion [...] practice activities in a range of settings' (Scriven, 2017: 141). Competence is achieved in a number of ways such as through 'interest, personal aptitude, education, and professional experience' (Hanson, 2007: 144). Laverack (2007) identifies six core competencies for health promotion practitioners (see Table 16.1).

As argued by the Health Promotion Forum of New Zealand (2012: 4), 'our understanding of health and wellbeing, and the determinants of health is growing and changing. Competencies are important for provider organisations and health promoters to help us look forward and strengthen our ability to meet future challenges'. Some countries, typically where the health promotion profession is more well-defined and structured, have produced specific health promotion competency frameworks to support the

Table 16.1 Core competencies for health promotion practitioners

1. Programme design, management, implementation and evaluation	The ability to plan effective health promotion programmes including the management of resources and personnel. This involves an understanding of programme cycles, budgeting, and the planning and evaluation of bottom-up approaches in top-down programming.
2. The planning and delivery of effective communication strategies	Communication strategies are an integral part of many health promotion programmes to increase knowledge levels and to raise awareness. A high level of competence is needed for the development of programmes that target individuals, groups and communities, including one-to-one communication, the design of print materials and the use of the mass media.
3. Facilitating skills	Training (e.g. for skills development, usually within a workshop setting) is a key part of many health promotion programmes. Good facilitation skills are essential for health promoters and are an important part of programme design.
4. Research skills	Health promotion programme design and evaluation is based on sound research including the use of participator techniques, qualitative and quantitative methods and systematic reviews.
5. Community capacity-building skills	Community empowerment is central to health promotion. This is a process of capacity-building and health promoters must be competent in a range of strategies that they can use to help individuals, groups and communities to gain more power.
6. Ability to influence policy and practice	Health promoters have the opportunity to influence policy and practice in their everyday work, for example, through technical advisory groups and through helping communities to mobilise and organise themselves towards gaining power. Health promoters must develop competence in the use of strategies to influence policy, developing partnerships and sound working relationships.

Source: Laverack (2007: 5) reproduced by kind permission of Open University Press.

development of the health promotion workforce. Health Promotion Canada (2015) has published a competency framework specific to health promotion that outlines the knowledge, abilities, skills and values that are deemed necessary for health promotion practice as listed here:

1. Health promotion knowledge and skills
2. Situational assessments
3. Plan and evaluate health promotion action
4. Policy development and advocacy
5. Community mobilization and building community capacity
6. Partnership and collaboration
7. Communication
8. Diversity and inclusiveness
9. Leadership and building organizational capacity

See www.healthpromotioncanada.ca for more detailed information.

In another example, *Ngā Kaiakatanga Hauora mō Aotearoa*: Health Promotion Competencies for Aotearoa New Zealand (Health Promotion Forum of New Zealand, 2012) presents a set of competencies specific to the Māori context which includes nine competency clusters:

1. Enable
2. Advocate
3. Mediate
4. Communicate
5. Lead
6. Assess
7. Plan
8. Implement
9. Evaluate and Research

See www.hauora.co.nz for more information on this competency framework.

The similarities between the two sets of competencies (from Canada and New Zealand) are clear – they are broadly more or less the same. The Australian Health Promotion Association also produced a competency framework in 2009 – the Core Competencies for Health Promotion Practitioners. 'Core' competencies were defined as 'the minimum set of competencies that constitute a common baseline for all health promotion roles' (Australian Health Promotion Association, 2009: 2). The major competencies required for entry-level health promotion roles in Australia are outlined as follows:

1. Programme planning, implementation and evaluation competencies including

    a. Needs assessment competencies
    b. Programme planning competencies
    c. Competencies for planning evidence-based strategies
    d. Evaluation and research competencies

2. Partnership building competencies
3. Communication and report writing competencies
4. Technology competencies, and
5. Knowledge competencies.

For more detailed information see www.healthpromotion.org.au.

In an effort to produce a more global (or international) set of health promotion competencies (rather than country by country) there has been a large body of work carried out over several years led by Professor Margaret Barry and colleagues on behalf of the International Union of Health Promotion and Education which latterly resulted in the IUHPE Core Competencies and Professional Standards for Health Promotion (IUHPE, 2016). This set of competencies resulted from consultation with many different stakeholders including practitioners, policy-makers, employers and health promotion education providers in Europe as well as from the global health promotion community. The resulting competencies comprise nine domains:

1. Enable change
2. Advocate for health
3. Mediate through partnership

4. Communication
5. Leadership
6. Assessment
7. Planning
8. Implementation, and
9. Evaluation and research

These are underpinned by two further domains – knowledge and ethical values so there are 11 domains of competency in total within this framework. These competencies define what is required at graduate entry level to the health promotion profession. The competencies are outlined in detail in the full version of the framework which is available at www.ukphr.org – visit this for further detail. You will note that there are 68 competency statements in total which highlights the complexity of health promotion practice (Van Den Broucke, 2018).

As Mereu et al. (2015: 33) argue, defining competencies in health promotion 'makes it possible to inform students, professionals, employers, and political decision-makers about what is expected from [the] profession and its values'. However, a lack of awareness of health promotion competencies is a challenge in practice and Battel-Kirk and Barry (2019) have identified this as a 'major limiting factor in the implementation' of the competencies in, for example, Italy and Northern Ireland.

GO FURTHER 16.1

You are tasked with writing a job description for a health promoter and need to find the best person for the job. Given the discussion that has taken place so far in this chapter, consider what you will be looking for in that person. Use the following headings to structure the job description:

- A *general description* of the type of person you are looking for
- *Essential* skills and attributes (those that are vital to the role)
- *Desirable* skills and attributes (those that are not essential but would be an asset for anyone in post)

Now use the internet to find a job description for a health promotion, health improvement or public health role. How does your job description compare with the 'real world' one?

For successful health promotion to occur Hanson (2007) argues the health promoter must be an expert, an advocate, a deliverer, a participant, a change facilitator and a decision-maker, factors that link to different types of competence as discussed. All of these roles have been discussed within this chapter to varying degrees so far. Next we will consider some of the challenges of health promotion working in practice.

THE CHALLENGES OF WORKING IN HEALTH PROMOTION

There are many different challenges that might arise when working in health promotion and you will already be aware of some of these having read other chapters in this book. For example, there might be unintended consequences that result from health promotion intervention which might be positive or negative. Health promotion messages can be undermined by conflicting information, confusing use of data, or the over-enthusiasm of the (potential) impact of a vaccine (as we have witnessed during the global coronavirus pandemic of 2020). Hann and Peckham (2010) illustrated this in respect to the 2008 HPV vaccination campaign in the UK and Pap smear testing. They highlighted several difficulties around how women were recruited into the cervical cancer screening programme, how the Pap smear results and information about risk and the efficacy of the HPV vaccination were communicated to women. Most importantly Hann and Peckham (2010) pointed out how women who are most at risk of developing cervical cancer are the least likely to take up screening opportunities. More recently (as of August 2020) we have witnessed some of the confusion that has arisen from the seemingly contradictory advice and guidance given about Covid-19. There are also potential challenges with accessing, evaluating and using evidence (Woodall and Rowlands, 2021). These are discussed in more detail in Chapter 17, 'Searching and Appraising the Evidence'. Knowing when, and at what level, to intervene is tricky. Case Study 16.1 outlines some possible levels of intervention to tackle obesity.

CASE STUDY 16.1: TACKLING OBESITY AND THE INTERVENTION LADDER

Do nothing - do not intervene at all or just monitor the situation

Provide information - make information about healthy eating and physical activity available

Enable choice - enable people to lose weight by providing healthy cooking lessons or exercise on prescription

Guide choices through changing the default policy - provide healthier options as standard in workplace and school canteens

Guide choices through incentives - guide choices through fiscal measures such as making healthier food cheaper or providing free exercise equipment

Guide choices through disincentives - put disincentives in place so that people do not do certain things, i.e. raising the price of less healthy food ('fat tax')

Restrict choice - removing unhealthy food choices from restaurant menus

Source: Adapted from Nuffield Council on Bioethics (2007)

There are also challenges concerned with manipulation, coercion and persuasion. As Woodall and Rowlands (2021) argue, health promoters sometimes 'tread a fine line between educating, persuading and manipulating behaviour'. In addition, the use of fear and shock tactics to change behaviour has been debated at length in the health promotion literature and the ethics of such approaches have been called into question (Cross et al., 2017; O'Neil, 2019). Telford (1998) outlined 13 different ethical dilemmas in health promotion practice – see Box 16.2 for details.

BOX 16.2 ETHICAL DILEMMAS IN HEALTH PROMOTION PRACTICE (TELFORD, 1998)

STRATEGY DILEMMAS

1. Persuasion – persuasion can sometimes be viewed as empowerment and yet it is not
2. Coercion – can coercive intervention be justified in order to benefit some people (i.e. by using legal measures to shape behaviour)?
3. Targeting – focusing on certain groups of people can cause or increase stigma
4. Harm reduction – are there situations where this is justified (i.e. the use of drunk 'tanks' in city centres where people can dry out)?

INADVERTENT HARM DILEMMAS

5. Labelling – may also stigmatise people
6. Depriving – depriving people of pleasurable activities such as eating unhealthy food
7. Culpability – who is responsible/to 'blame'; should some behaviour/s be permitted even if other people do not approve?

POWER AND CONTROL DILEMMAS

8. Privileging – does the intervention privilege certain groups above others?
9. Exploitation – does the intervention exploit any groups or persons?
10. Control – could the intervention be used to control people?

SOCIAL VALUES DILEMMAS

11. Distraction – does the focus on certain groups of people distract from the bigger issues (social and environmental)?
12. Promises – does the intervention promise change that will not benefit everyone?
13. The health as a value dilemma – is this compatible with other values?

GO FURTHER 16.2

We have highlighted the importance of skills in evidence-based practice in this chapter (see also Chapter 17, 'Searching and Appraising the Evidence'). Working in an evidence-based way presents a number of challenges. Take some time to consider what these might be and then compare your ideas with those presented by Hesman (2014) – see Box 16.3. How might each of these be addressed?

In addition to the many challenges in health promotion practice that we have already discussed there are also possible difficulties with using evidence-based approaches. See Box 16.3 for further information.

BOX 16.3 POTENTIAL LIMITATIONS OF EVIDENCE-INFORMED APPROACHES (HESMAN, 2014: 45)

- Innovative approaches may not get adopted as there is no evidence to support them
- Problems for which no clear solutions have been shown to be effective may get sidelined
- Evidence is not always taken up and is sometimes used inappropriately or out of context
- Evidence that is perceived as more subjective, for example how well people feel themselves to be, may be undermined
- Decisions about funding research may be politically driven
- Evidence cannot compensate for a lack of political will to deal with a problem.

As will be common in many types of profession, constraints in health promotion practice will include limited time (Gottwald, 2012), differing stakeholder agendas (Scriven, 2017), finite resources (Hubley et al., 2021) and potential lack of political will (Cross et al., 2017). No doubt you will be able to think of other potential constraints as well. All of these need to be taken into consideration. Earlier we highlighted the importance of having skills in building and maintaining successful partnerships; however, this can also bring challenges. See Box 16.4 for some examples.

> # BOX 16.4 POTENTIAL DIFFICULTIES WITH PUBLIC HEALTH PARTNERSHIP WORKING
>
> - Organisational or institutional change can damage long-term commitment and planning
> - Competition for funding (seeking it from the same source)
> - Lack of resources, such as money and person-power
> - Lack of commitment from top levels of the partnership
> - Domination by one or two people
> - Differences in input/contribution from different agencies
> - Professional jealousy and lack of sharing of information and expertise
> - Different goals, values and ways of working or different levels of experience and expertise.
>
> Source: Adapted from Scriven (2017: 139)

BEING AN AGENT OF CHANGE

Promoting health requires change at many different levels and in many different ways. A key feature of the health promoter is the ability to effect change, or to be an agent of change (Hanson, 2007; Piper, 2009). Whether that is working with someone to facilitate behaviour change at an individual level or working with policy-makers or legislators, change is a necessary part of the health promotion process. Managing change is therefore an integral part of what it means to promote health. Being a change agent means 'initiating and implementing changes in health promotion or public health policy or practice' (Scriven, 2017: 122) which, as stated, can occur at any level. Scriven (2017: 123) goes further and argues that 'understanding how to implement and manage change successfully is a fundamental part of a health promoter's role'. However, change is not always embraced by people or within organisations and there may be many reasons why this is the case. Effecting change can therefore be a major challenge for health promoters. Scriven (2017) suggests five ways of overcoming resistance to change: 1) education and communication; 2) participation and involvement; 3) facilitation and support; 4) negotiation and agreement; and 5) political influencing. See Table 16.2 for further information and application.

SUMMARY

This chapter has explored the skills and attributes that are required for effective health promotion. Clearly the health promoter needs to be interested in, and value, health for its own sake but there are a wealth of other factors that will increase the likelihood of effectiveness. Some of these can be developed and finely honed (broadly defined as 'skills') and some of these are considered to be more inherent in individuals (broadly defined as 'attributes'). The skills and attributes discussed are more or less represented in the competency frameworks that are presented in this chapter. The commonalities between these frameworks showcase the fundamental aspects of what is required for successful health promotion practice. The next chapter, Chapter 17, 'Searching and Appraising the Evidence', picks up on the research skills that have been cited as vital to the health promotion role in this chapter.

Table 16.2 Methods for overcoming resistance to change

1.	Education and communication	Resistance to change may occur due to lack of information or understanding, or even misinformation. Communicating with people and educating them about a change before it takes place is important to avoid these. This can happen in a variety of ways such as group discussion and written forms of communication or by using social media. A downside to this is that it can be time-consuming and sometimes change needs to happen quickly (for example, as it did during 2020 and the global coronavirus pandemic).
2.	Participation and involvement	If people are actively involved in the process of designing and implementing any change they are less likely to resist it. This makes sense as many of us do not like being told what to do! Working in this way means that the facilitator of change must be prepared to listen and learn, and must avoid tokenism. People's contributions have to be taken seriously.
3.	Facilitation and support	Resistance can be reduced or avoided by working in ways that involves helping people to identify what change/s are needed and then providing the necessary support to plan and manage the change themselves. Support can take various forms - practical or emotional, for example.
4.	Negotiation and agreement	Resistance can be dealt with by offering incentives to change. This is more appropriate when people stand to lose something from as a consequence of changes taking place.
5.	Political influencing	If one or two powerful people are resisting change then this approach can be appropriate - targeting persuasive efforts at the people who are in control of things.

Source: Adapted from Scriven (2017: 125)

SUGGESTED READING

Laverack, G. (2007) *Health promotion practice: building empowered communities.* Maidenhead, Open University Press.

Linsley, P. and Roll, C. (2020) Core skills for health promotion. In *Health promotion for nursing students.* London, Sage. pp. 23–34

Scriven, A. (2017) Skills of personal effectiveness. In *Promoting health: a practical guide.* 7th edn. London, Elsevier. pp. 115–129.

SEARCHING AND APPRAISING THE EVIDENCE

17

INTRODUCTION

The skills necessary to search for evidence and then appraise this for its quality and appropriateness are vital for making evidence-based decisions. Such skills are not usually regarded as a core feature of a health promoters' repertoire, but we argue here that such attributes are increasingly necessary in the information age in which we now live. This chapter will describe the evidence challenges that face health promotion and rehearse some of the key debates. It also provides guidance on how health promoters can search for and appraise research evidence to aid decision-making.

EVIDENCE-BASED HEALTH PROMOTION

Evidence-based health promotion is 'the systematic integration of research evidence into the planning and implementation of health promotion activities' (Wiggers and Sanson-Fisher, 1998: 141). In effect, it is about making sensible decisions based on the information available. Health promotion has tried to establish more credibility through gathering evidence of what works in programmes, projects and interventions (Green et al., 2019); doing so is critical in order to make the best decisions and to learn from experience.

Using 'evidence' is mentioned in several WHO declarations on health promotion – the notable exception being the Ottawa Charter – with this idea becoming more apparent in later conferences (Groot, 2011). The Nairobi Call to Action, for example, urges the use of 'the existing evidence to prove to policy-makers that health promotion is fundamental to managing national and global challenges such as population ageing, climate change, global pandemic threats, maternal mortality, migration, conflict, and economic crises' (WHO, 2009b). For some time, however, health promotion has struggled to establish a firm and credible evidence base. Some have even suggested 'hostility' towards health promotion interventions by medical professions as health promotion has struggled to accumulate a robust evidence-base of what works and why (South and Tilford, 2000). Despite this, there is growing momentum for the importance of evidence-based practice within the wider public health arena and considerable current interest in evidence-based health promotion (Green et al., 2019).

The increasing emphasis on evidence-based practice has come from a wider commitment to justify expenditure, accountability and ensuring that resources are deployed to maximum effect. Governments in high-income countries and low- and middle-income countries as well as donor agencies have had less resource in recent times and, therefore, budgetary allocations for public health and health promotion interventions need to be based on solid evidence (Owusu-Addo et al., 2017). There are broader questions, though, like what evidence is, how to effectively gather evidence and how to understand and interpret it.

WHAT IS EVIDENCE?

In our everyday lives we use evidence all of the time. Think, for example, about the last time you bought a new domestic product – the chances are you used evidence in the form of written reviews, recommendations from friends or expert advice.

REFLECTIVE EXERCISE 17.1

Think about the last time you made a significant purchase on a product or an item (like a TV, car, mobile phone, etc.). How did you arrive at the choice that you did? What evidence informed your decision-making process? What evidence did you class (subconsciously maybe) as being more relevant or important than others?

In health disciplines and in medical sciences, there are some very well-established views on what constitutes evidence. These views often describe different types of evidence and categorise them as higher- and lower-quality. This is often seen as a hierarchy with 'gold standard' research designs producing more reliable or effective evidence than others (see Figure 17.1). It was initially created by the Canadian Task Force on the Periodic Health Examination to help decide on priorities when searching for studies to answer clinical questions (Petticrew and Roberts, 2003) and was only later considered for its implications for public health and health promotion evidence.

Quantitative design such as experiments, cohort studies and case-control studies are used to answer questions about cause and effect. As an example, we may need to know if a health promotion intervention (cause) is effective in producing positive health outcomes (effects). The randomised control trial (RCT), has been regarded as the 'gold standard' and sits very firmly towards the top of the hierarchy (Woodall and Rowlands, 2021). Chapter 19 describes this design in much more detail. The evidence hierarchy has been debated and argued for some time across a range of disciplines (Petticrew and Roberts, 2003). It is an extremely helpful idea for assessing clinical studies, but is less helpful for complex interventions that occur in natural, or real world, settings and contexts. Health promoters often need to rely on qualitative information to help them make decisions. This could come from published qualitative studies, or through discussing, first-hand, issues of importance to individuals and communities. There has also been a trend to draw on 'expert' evidence to help answer questions of interest to health promoters (see Case Study 17.1).

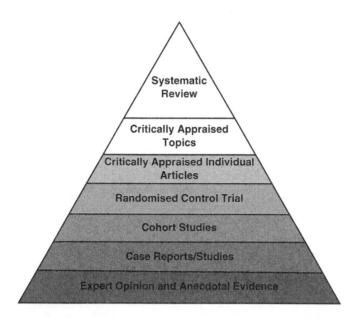

Figure 17.1 Evidence hierarchy

CASE STUDY 17.1: EXPERT EVIDENCE

Evidence hierarchies recognise the value of professional and expert knowledge to generate information for decision-making purposes (Green et al., 2015). Expert information is utilised in a diverse range of disciplines where accessing more 'traditional' types of empirical data may be insufficient or too challenging (Caley et al., 2014). Expert knowledge is defined as 'substantive information on a particular topic that is not widely known by others' (Martin et al., 2012: 30). Petticrew and Roberts (2003) suggest that expert knowledge can be particularly useful in understanding the process and mechanisms of implementing an intervention. While experts are regarded as proving credible sources of information, the use of experts to inform decision-making processes is contentious and has been challenged. One prevailing argument is that expert judgement may be veiled with bias or expert opinion may be self-serving (Martin et al., 2012).

Expert knowledge can be ascertained in several ways and common group approaches include expert panels and Delphi methods (Martin et al., 2012). Expert hearings or symposia are approaches designed to facilitate the process of deliberation on an issue or series of issues (South et al., 2010) and were used in a study by Woodall et al. (2015) to stimulate dialogue and to gather expert evidence on peer-based approaches in prison settings. Rather than a traditional focus group discussion, the process of deliberation provided a mutual dialogue between researchers and delegates that involves considering different points of view and coming to a reasoned decision (Abelson et al., 2003).

Using a range of evidence within health promotion in order to inform policy and practice decisions is now understood and this has meant abandoning hierarchies of evidence towards typologies of evidence (Woodall and Rowlands, 2021) or evidence that is fit for purpose. Wharf-Higgins et al. (2011: 291) notes that:

> Evidence comes in many types of formats, including academic research, informal or formal evaluations of community-based programs and policies, stories and experiences of public health staff and community leaders. Diverse types of evidence are used by staff to shape programs and make policy decisions, and all should be considered valid.

Some have suggested that health promotion should adopt a "horses for courses" approach to making decisions – in other words using the best research design or a multiple of designs for the question posed. Indeed, many sources of evidence are often required to address and understand complex interventions (Woodall and Rowlands, 2021).

REFLECTIVE EXERCISE 17.2

Consider these questions below and consider what types of research design would be best placed to answer these:

- Does a dementia awareness programme increase knowledge of dementia?
- Are peer education approaches to improve emotional well-being acceptable to school children?
- What process and challenges are faced when implementing smoke-free environments in prisons?

EVIDENCE CHALLENGES IN HEALTH PROMOTION

Despite the position that health promotion needs to adopt and embrace different research designs to address evidence-based questions, there remain several challenges (see Box 17.1). These dilemmas directly influence how practitioners access, use and implement evidence.

BOX 17.1 THE EVIDENCE CHALLENGE

In some areas of life the question of whether what is being done works is relatively simple to answer. When I do my weekly food shopping at the supermarket, or travel to work on the train, or go out to see a film at the cinema, I know

> whether the service I am using is 'working'. My judgements might be imperfect, and sometimes they will be qualitative and complex, but I will be able to make them relatively simply. There is much more difficulty in making claims about whether health promotion 'works' or not.
>
> (Cribb and Duncan, 2002: 82)

An initial challenge may be that there is insufficient high-quality evidence to make a useful decision on the delivery of an intervention. This poses a challenge in how best to proceed as the evidence does not conclude whether the intervention is likely to succeed or not. At this point the practitioner may consider two options. First, it could be that the best way to proceed is to commission research or seek funding to understand the effectiveness of the intervention before it can be rolled out and implemented. Second, the practitioner may consider implementing the intervention but on a small scale, usually termed a 'pilot', to prevent too much resource being used on a potentially ineffective intervention. This can raise a range of ethical issues, certainly if it is unknown whether the intervention will be beneficial.

A further issue for the practitioner assessing evidence is how much evidence is sufficient to make a decision. Would one, well-designed and robust study be enough to base a decision? Or would further research be needed to verify these results? In addition, how should evidence-based decisions be made when the evidence is very mixed? Several studies, for instance, may show positive effects but other studies could demonstrate opposing conclusions. Such decision-making needs to be transparent and based on an assessment of the overall weight of evidence available. Linked to this, it may be that practitioners do not have sufficient knowledge, skills and experiences to be able to fully understand how research is conducted and how conclusions are made. Without such skills, there is the potential to misinterpret the evidence. There is, fortunately, some good guidance on appraisal of evidence which can support practitioners (discussed later in this chapter).

A final dilemma may be the stifling of innovative practice at the expense of adopting an evidence-based approach. If decisions can only be made on a firm evidence base, then how can creative and innovative ways to promote health, which may have an absence of evidence and research, be encouraged? It may be that a wedded fixation with evidence-based decision-making has its limitations and that it may be prudent to allow some innovative practice to be conducted *alongside* careful evaluation of the delivery. A useful quotation summarising the dilemma is given by Perkins et al. (1999: 13):

> It is important not to get so bogged down in evidence that we can neither think nor act creatively; but it is also important that we do not inflict our inspirations on the world of practice (and next year's budget!) without some reality checking against the evidence.

REFLECTIVE EXERCISE 17.3

Imagine you are a health promotion practitioner working on behalf of a large multinational company. You are asked to make an evidence-based decision as to whether or not classes or seminars on health topics such as fitness, nutrition, tobacco cessation or stress management would be beneficial for employee health and well-being. Consider how you would address or manage the following:

- A lack of robust evidence on the topic, with few well-designed studies to base your decision.
- Identifying mixed or variable evidence – for instance, some studies showing highly beneficial outcomes; some studies showing no differences and some showing negative outcomes for employees.
- The evidence shows the effectiveness of delivering the intervention, but the details of the programme and how it was delivered is lacking and therefore replication is difficult.
- The evidence and the views of experts in the field of workplace health promotion differ considerably.

THE EVIDENCE-BASED HEALTH PROMOTER

There is significant rhetoric about evidence-based practice and making evidence-based decisions, but fewer discussions about the practicalities of this and how to engage and collect evidence to inform practice. In some countries national agencies support health promoters and produce evidence 'briefings' aiming to update practitioners in easy to digest bite-sized chunks (Woodall and Rowlands, 2021). In addition, many research funding agencies insist on producing accessible briefing materials for practitioners to distil key findings. Nonetheless, we would see the development of searching and appraisal of evidence as being fundamental to good health promotion practice. There are several steps and processes in evidence-based decision-making, highlighted in Box 17.2. The remainder of this chapter will begin to highlight some of these processes.

BOX 17.2 THE STEPS AND SKILLS IN THE PROCESS OF EVIDENCE-BASED DECISION-MAKING

1. Identifying evidence-based questions
2. Finding evidence that addresses the stated questions
3. Understanding the quality of the evidence

4. Determining if the evidence can be transferred to the practitioners' local context and client group.
5. Ability to communicate and disseminating evidence to other practitioners.

Source: Woodall and Rowlands (2021)

IDENTIFYING A QUESTION

Generally, practitioners start out with a broad area which they wish to explore or investigate in order to inform the decision they need to make. In order to develop a more focused question(s) the process of refinement is essential. According to Aveyard and Sharp (2009), questions can be refined using some of the following techniques:

- Talking to experts
- Sharing and discussing ideas with colleagues
- Using tools like spider diagrams or mind maps
- Running quick searches on the internet

SEARCHING FOR EVIDENCE

Once a question has been identified, an effective approach to search for the literature is required. The retrieval of literature can be undertaken in a range of ways from rapid evidence assessments to literature reviews and, perhaps at the pinnacle, systematic reviews (see Box 17.3).

BOX 17.3 SYSTEMATIC REVIEWS

Systematic reviews bring together all the published and unpublished material on a particular issue. Good reviews can be one of the most efficient ways to become familiar with research and practice (Brownson et al., 2009). Both the selection of studies and extraction of data should conform to explicit criteria so that the process is rigorous, transparent and essentially replicable. The development of the methodology for conducting systematic reviews has been focused particularly on healthcare interventions, pioneered by the Cochrane Collaboration (Green et al., 2019). Ensuring that the selection of articles is free from bias and replicable is fundamental to the systematic reviewing process. Guidance on undertaking systematic reviews developed by the Centre for Reviews and Dissemination (2009) suggests that criteria for inclusion

(Continued)

should be developed from consideration of the following key elements (referred to by the acronym PICOS):

- Population
- Interventions
- Comparators
- Outcomes
- Study design

Whichever approach is used, a search strategy will enable the identification of relevant material (Aveyard and Sharp, 2009). Haphazard approaches to searching for evidence rarely provide successful outcomes and this approach, according to Aveyard and Sharp, can create lots of potential problems:

- The literature could be out of date.
- The literature may not be from trusted sources.
- Key literature could be missed.
- You may not find the harder-to-access literature which may be crucial in helping you answer the question.

Evidence that underpins decision-making is likely, although not exclusively, to be obtained via academic sources like journal articles and research literature. This is because these sources are often regarded as being more robust, credible and reviewed by experts in the field (known as peer review). Access to journal articles has been traditionally done in three ways:

1. access via the journal website;
2. accessing a paper copy via a library;
3. accessing the journal via an academic database.

Access to these sources is not always easy, although information availability is becoming easier given recent developments in publishing practices (see Box 17.4)

BOX 17.4 OPEN ACCESS (OA) PUBLICATIONS

OA publications are free, unrestricted online access to research evidence. They ensure that research is easily accessible to practitioners, policy-makers and researchers without a cost. Traditional publishing models mean that journals usually have a subscription cost which means that research can be inaccessible to many. Some excellent examples of OA journals which frequently feature health promotion studies include *BMJ Open*, *BMC Public Health* and *Global Health (PLOS ONE)*.

The starting point for finding evidence is a search strategy – this enables a focused approach to the literature search and provides clear boundaries. Doing this is critical to avoid the results of the search being too overwhelming. Search strategies include key terms which are used to search the literature. These key terms can include free text words and their synonyms and also specific subject headings used by specific academic databases (e.g. Medical Subject Headings (MeSH)). It is important to consider the search terms within the strategy as this avoids missing key literature and research. It is important to be creative and think about the words that researchers may use to describe something – using a thesaurus is a great way to start this process. It is also worth considering variation on spellings (e.g. 'World Health Organization' and 'World Health Organisation') to ensure all possibilities are covered.

REFLECTIVE EXERCISE 17.4

You have been asked to review the evidence in relation to how burnout can be reduced in workplaces. What search terms and words would you use to ensure that you fully covered all aspects of the literature? When you have identified your list of terms, you can compare and review your list with a government review which is in the public domain (Bagnall et al., 2016).

Limits and filters can be applied to the search strategy – so, for example, the search is focused on the past ten years of *published* literature (see Box 17.5); only concerned with studies in English; or the search strategy could be limited to particular study designs (so only including systematic reviews or only RCTs). This latter filter would be unusual to see in health promotion practice, given the debates outlined earlier.

BOX 17.5 UNPUBLISHED, OR GREY, LITERATURE

The search process may also include exploring grey literature – this is regarded as evidence which is unpublished, so could include research reports, working papers, conference proceedings and theses. There are several ways to do this – internet searches can effectively yield grey literature, as can requests via professional networks and affiliations or using social media, such as Twitter, to request information not readily in the public domain. There may be some important research that, for whatever reason, has not yet been published and therefore you may wish to consider this when undertaking a comprehensive search. There are, of course, reasons why people may not include grey literature as without going through a peer-review process it is questionable if the research is of a high standard.

Once a search strategy has been developed, there are many academic databases to search which host a range of research (see Box 17.6). Different methods exist for accessing each database and every system has its own nuances or particulars (McKibbon and Marks, 1998). Most use Boolean operators which is the use of AND, OR and NOT, which helps with refining the search and making it as specific as possible.

BOX 17.6 EXAMPLES OF ACADEMIC DATABASES

- Cochrane Central Register of Controlled Trials (CENTRAL)
- Cochrane Database of Systematic Reviews (CDSR)
- Embase
- MEDLINE
- PsycINFO (psychology and psychiatry)
- ASSIA (Applied Social Sciences Index and Abstracts)
- Social Policy and Practice, Social Care Online
- Sociological Abstracts

Of course, depending on the time available and other resource issues, it may be difficult to access literature via academic databases. While these databases do offer the best possibility of accessing the available evidence, there are other arguably more expedient approaches. Google Scholar, for example, has a very familiar and simple interface that makes searching very easy; it also retrieves more than journal articles and includes pre-print archives, conference proceedings and institutional repositories (Shultz, 2007). The problem with Google is that it can lack the specificity of search that a subject-specific database can provide (Aveyard and Sharp, 2009).

Academic databases are the most effective way of accessing evidence and research literature; however, there are other strategies that should be considered alongside this:

- Hand searching – this means going through the contents of individual journal publications.
- Searching reference lists of relevant articles.
- Making contact with authors directly.

In some situations, literature searching can be never-ending and knowing when to stop is important. In most cases, it will not be possible to find every possible piece of research on a given topic and therefore judging when is enough is critical. That said, in some situations, albeit relatively rare, there may be no evidence at all on a particular topic or area of interest. You may wish to reflect on how specific the search strategy is and whether broadening this out may be helpful to identify *relevant* material (see Box 17.7).

BOX 17.7 WHAT TO DO WHEN THERE IS NO EVIDENCE ON A TOPIC?

Let's say you are interested in understanding what works to improve mental well-being for people who are homeless in Kuala Lumpur. Your search has yielded no useful literature or research. You may wish to ask yourself instead:

- What is it that is specific to Kuala Lumpur? Would evidence from a different geographical location still be useful and, if so, which places?
- Is there literature on other aspects of health in this population, not just mental well-being?
- Could there be research on other populations that shows what works to improve mental well-being? Would this be at all helpful?

APPRAISING EVIDENCE

Literature searching can yield thousands of studies. This means that there needs to be a process of screening the literature for relevance and a process of assessing the quality of the literature retrieved. This can be done using established checklists for different study designs, including quantitative and qualitative research (see NICE, 2019) and also using your own skills in determining the research quality as not everyone has time to follow lengthy checklists and appraisal tools. This process is important as practitioners should be able to go beyond what the descriptive findings of the research state to a more critical understanding of how the research was designed and conducted (Woodall and Rowlands, 2021). Research may provide conclusions, but the studies could be poorly designed which may raise significant questions about their trustworthiness.

GO FURTHER 17.1

Imagine that you were asked by a friend about the safety of electronic cigarettes. They have come to you because you have an interest in health promotion. First, where would you search for this information? Second, if the studies you found were supported by manufacturers of electronic cigarettes or studies were conducted on animal populations (not humans), how strongly would you recommend this evidence?

In terms of assessing research quality, there may be some initial clues and signs that should provide an initial insight into the work. This is regardless of study design or methodology. Such questions may include:

1. Where is the research published? Is it in a recognised peer-review journal that is well regarded in the field?
2. Who is/are the author(s)? What affiliation(s) do they have?
3. Do the author(s) disclose any conflicts of interest?
4. Who is funding the research?
5. Are the aims of the research clear and sensible?
6. Does the study have ethical approval from a recognised organisation?
7. Is the approach to conducting the research appropriate? Are the methods for gathering information in line with the study aims and objectives?
8. How were participants included and excluded in the research? Do these decisions seem reasonable?
9. Is the process of analysing the data transparent and clear?
10. Do the conclusions from the study match the data collected?

There are, of course, some very specific questions you may need to ask based on the actual study designs. A qualitative study, for example, may encourage additional questions such as those suggested by Greenhalgh and Taylor (1997):

1. What was the researcher's perspective and has this been taken into account?
2. What methods did the researcher use for collecting data – and are these described in enough detail?
3. What methods did the researcher use to analyse the data – and what quality control measures were implemented?
4. Are the findings of the study transferable to other contexts and settings?

However, appraising a randomised control trial may encourage different questions, including:

1. Is the control and intervention described clearly and adequately?
2. What is the method of randomisation of participants to the intervention and control groups?
3. Are both groups treated *exactly* the same apart from the intervention itself?
4. Is the blinding of the intervention done appropriately (should it be feasible)?

GO FURTHER 17.2

Identify a research paper that covers a topic or issue that concerns you or that you have interest in. It could be a qualitative or quantitative study or a systematic review. Using a recognised checklist from NICE (2019) critically appraise the study. At the end of the activity, ask yourself if the evidence presented in the paper is something you could base a policy or practice decision upon.

TRANSFERABILITY OF EVIDENCE

An intervention may be very effective according to the research literature. However, it is important to know if the intervention will transfer into a specific context. Rarely do we find research conducted in settings identical to where decisions need to be made. So, as an example, even research conducted in school settings may not be applied to *all* schools as schools can be diverse and heterogeneous. Practitioners must assess whether the research is, or is not, transferable to their specific circumstance. Several factors may come into play in this decision-making process, including the geographical location of the research and cultural factors. When research papers provide detailed descriptions of the design, development, delivery and context of an intervention this can aid the decision-making process, but often these details are omitted.

SUMMARY

Making evidence-based decisions is an important aspect of health promotion practice, although in reality this can be highly challenging. The challenges posed by traditional evidence hierarchies has been unhelpful in health promotion – designs which are often regarded as 'gold standard' cannot be easily applied to health promotion where interventions are normally complex and multifaceted.

SUGGESTED READING

Aveyard, H. and Sharp, P. (2009) A beginner's guide to evidence-based practice in health and social care. London, McGraw-Hill Education (UK).

Cribb, A. and Duncan, P. (2002) *Health promotion and professional ethics*. London, Blackwell.

Green, J., Cross, R., Woodall, J. et al. (2019) *Health promotion: planning and strategies*. 4th edn. London, Sage.

PLANNING AND DESIGNING HEALTH PROMOTION PROGRAMMES

18

INTRODUCTION

The previous chapter argued the importance of evidence-based health promotion, particularly for underpinning effective health promotion programmes. In this chapter we move on to consider how we design and deliver health promotion programmes and interventions (we use these two terms interchangeably here). We will outline the various key stages and processes when delivering health promotion 'on the ground'. A range of theoretical frameworks for planning health promotion are presented and described including a simple approach to planning, Hubley et al.'s Health Promotion Planning Cycle, Dignan and Carr's Planning Model, and Ewles and Simnett's Framework for Planning. Useful aids for effective planning, monitoring and tracking are also presented, such as problem trees, logical frameworks and Gantt charts. The chapter ends with a case study illustrating some of the challenges for health promotion programme planning.

WHY PLAN?

Planning is an important part of everyday life. Planning helps us to achieve what we set out to and enables us to establish whether or not we have been successful. Before we go any further, take some time to do Reflective Exercise 18.1.

REFLECTIVE EXERCISE 18.1

Think about a time when you have had to plan something, perhaps a holiday or a family event. Why was planning important? What did you need to include in the plan? What might have happened if you hadn't made a plan?

Planning is a central part of success and there are many reasons why we need to plan in health promotion. Some of these are practical, such as delivering more successful interventions, whilst others might be more esoteric such as making the world a better place. Other reasons include developing evidence-based practice, demonstrating cost-effectiveness, meeting targets and being economically accountable which is especially important in an economic climate of austerity (Evans et al., 2017).

In health promotion 'the purpose of planning is to identify goals and the most effective means of achieving them. Programmes are more likely to be successful if planning is approached in an inclusive way, involving all the major stakeholders' (Green et al., 2019: 181). Baldwin (2020: 223) concurs with this and states that planning for health promotion is an essential process that can 'be guided by planning frameworks, theories and tools, and adapted to suit local needs' as will be discussed further in this chapter. However, health promotion interventions are sometimes 'criticised for being unstructured, opportunistic, *ad hoc*, and failing to comply with established systematic processes' (Whitehead, 2010: 61). The importance of being systematic when planning health promotion interventions has been emphasised by many, for example Green et al. (2019). Systematic planning is about knowing what your intervention is about and why it is being done, knowing why it is important and who it's intended for; knowing who is going to carry it out (do it) and where it will be delivered; and, finally, knowing how you will know it has been successful.

There are many different health promotion planning models presented in the wider health promotion literature and it is not feasible to outline each in turn in this chapter. Instead we will focus on a select few by turn. Each follows a logical sequence and you will see that there are some common elements to them, namely needs assessment, implementation and evaluation (Nutbeam et al., 2010).

PROBLEM TREES

Let's start with needs assessment, a very important part of the health promotion planning process whichever health promotion planning model you happen to be using. Chapter 7, 'Assessing Health Needs: Principles and Practice', outlines many of the facets of needs assessment and presents different ways of assessing health needs. As you will have appreciated from reading Chapter 7, identifying needs is often multidimensional and multifaceted (Baldwin, 2020). Another useful way of assessing need is to develop a 'problem tree'. A problem tree can help you to identify the range of factors that need to be considered and is a useful tool for helping analyse a specific public health issue. The roots of a problem tree represent the causes of the health issue; the branches of the tree represent the effects of the health issue and the trunk of the tree is the issue itself. The root causes of a public health issue can run very deep and examining these will often lead to the identification of the causes of the causes (Marmot et al., 2020). Likewise, the effects can be far-reaching from the proximal, more immediate effects to the distal, more long-term effects. Problem trees are not just used in health promotion but for a range of issues where causes and effects need to be established. See Figure 18.1 for an example of a simple problem tree.

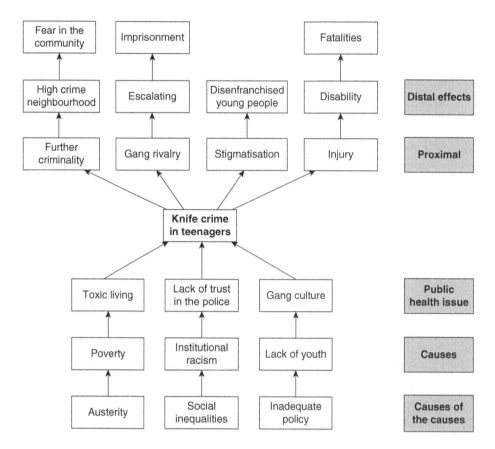

Figure 18.1 A problem tree about knife crime in teenagers

A problem tree can be a useful way to represent an issue and the roots can be used to determine what causal aspects to focus an intervention on. A problem tree can also be used to develop a solution tree by changing negative statements into positive ones (Naidoo and Wills, 2016).

WHAT NEEDS TO BE CONSIDERED WHEN PLANNING A HEALTH PROMOTION INTERVENTION?

The following questions provide a useful guide as to what needs to be considered in the planning and design of a health promotion intervention:

* *Who are the relevant partners (key stakeholders)?* Anybody who has a vested interest in the health issue or health promotion programme would be involved here, including the intended beneficiaries themselves (Evans et al., 2017). This is central to the partnership working that is key in health promotion. A stakeholder is anyone

who might be involved in, or affected by, the intervention (Linsley and Roll, 2020). This should, ideally, include the community itself (Baldwin, 2020). Working with relevant stakeholders can occur in many different ways but is essential for success (Baldwin, 2020).

- *Has the activity worked elsewhere (what is the evidence-base)?* Health promotion research and literature is a very valuable source of information about what works (and what does not work), as is the experience of other people working in health promotion and public health. Finding out what has worked in tackling the public health issue you are concerned with before starting to plan will help you to save time and to avoid 'reinventing the wheel'! Whilst the context and target community might be different there are often valuable lessons that can be learned from programmes that have been implemented elsewhere.

- *What resources will you need in order to do the activity?* This will include physical resources as well as personnel. Physical resources such as infrastructure, technology and health education materials will likely be needed. People will often be the most valuable resource, and this will include the intended recipients of the intervention as well as other 'experts'. It is also useful to think about time as a resource. Many changes in health outcomes only become manifest in the longer term.

- *How acceptable is the intervention to the intended recipients?* It is important to consider the target group and, as Evans et al., (2017: 137) argues, to pay attention to their 'values, beliefs, behaviour patterns, customs and culture, aspirations and attitudes'. This is why community participation is so important (Baldwin, 2020) – you need to know and understand your intended recipients in order to attain the best possible buy-in from them and, subsequently, the best possible results.

- *Are there any legal or ethical considerations or implications?* Consider whether the means you are using contain any elements of persuasion, coercion or manipulation; and if the methods are appropriate to the situation at hand (Green et al., 2019). Ethical practice is fundamental in health promotion and there are likely to be ethical dilemmas at many of the decision-making stages during the planning process. For example, at the outset how will you justify the prioritisation of one public health issue at the expense of another?

- *How are you going to establish whether or not the intervention has worked/been effective?* Finding out if you have been successful is a key part of planning health promotion programmes. You'll need to know if you have achieved what you set out to and whether or not the desired outcomes have come into effect. This is all about evaluation, evaluation, evaluation! (See Chapter 19, 'Health Promotion Research and Evaluation' for more on evaluation, and the later discussion in this chapter.)

Baldwin (2020) suggests that there are four core principles for planning health promotion interventions. These are evidence-based practice, strong evaluation and ownership, and relevance to the community or population of focus. Each of these mirror the underpinning principles of health promotion that we have discussed elsewhere in this book and are reflected in the previous set of questions.

WHAT IS A PLANNING MODEL?

Planning programmes or interventions is central to health promotion and having a clear strategy or process is really important in order to guide things. It is vital to consider all the stages of planning a health promotion programme, so as not to miss out anything of importance (Linsley and Roll, 2020). A number of health promotion planning models exist that will be described and discussed in this chapter which are useful for keeping track of the key stages of the planning process. Using a planning model helps with setting a clear plan of action about what needs to be achieved, how it will be done and what resources are needed (Naidoo and Wills, 2016). Planning and evaluation are often cyclical in nature even though models are sometimes presented in a linear way (Issel, 2014).

Hubley (2004) suggested four questions to help guide the planning process as follows:

- Where are we now?
- Where do we want to go?
- How will we get there?
- How will we know when we get there?

A SIMPLE APPROACH TO PLANNING

Hubley's (2004) four questions as set out earlier are manifest in the simple approach to planning. See Figure 18.2 for illustration.

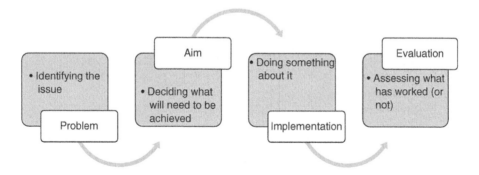

Figure 18.2 A simple approach to planning

The simple approach to planning sets out four key stages of the process starting with the identification of the problem or issue, followed by deciding what the aim is (or what will need to be achieved), then how this will be done (choosing methods) and doing it (implementation), and finally, evaluating what has been done and finding out whether it has worked or not.

Hubley et al.'s Health promotion planning cycle

Hubley et al. (2021) provide another relatively simple planning model called the health promotion planning cycle. As you can see from Figure 18.3 this model begins with a health promotion needs assessment or situational analysis followed by identifying the health promotion strategies that will be used, then implementation, and, finally, evaluation, reflection and learning. The cycle then starts again. Figure 18.3 provides further detail at each stage.

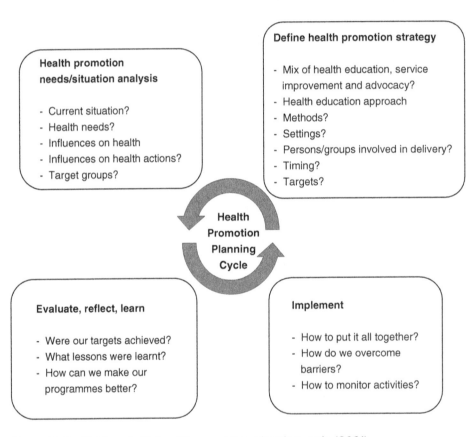

Figure 18.3   Hubley et al.'s health promotion planning cycle (2021)

Source: Hubley et al. (2013) reproduced by kind permission of Polity Press

Dignan and Carr's planning model

Dignan and Carr (1992, cited in Green et al., 2019) provide a health promotion planning model which has similarities with the simple planning cycle and Hubley et al.'s (2021) health promotion planning cycle – see Figure 18.3. Dignan and Carr's model begins with a needs assessment (or community analysis) at which point a specific issue

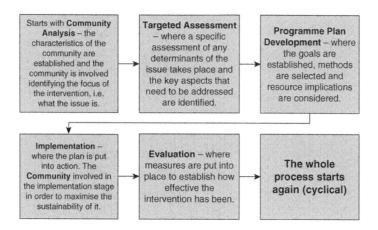

Figure 18.4   Stages of Dignan and Carr's planning model

Source: adapted from Dignan and Carr (1992)

is identified that will be addressed. Questions at this stage will include 'What is the current situation?', 'What health needs are there?', 'Who are the intended beneficiaries?' and 'What is influencing health behaviour?' There are many ways of assessing need and determining what issue to focus on (see Chapter 7, 'Assessing Health Needs: Principles and Practice', for further information). After the community analysis has taken place the programme plan is developed and implemented. At the development stage aspects like the setting, the method/s, involvement of stakeholders, timing, outcomes and targets, and approaches will have to be considered. At the implementation stage the following questions would be asked – 'How do we put it all together?', 'How will we overcome any potential barriers to implementation?' and 'How will the activities be monitored?' Finally, evaluation takes place and the cycle then starts over again. At the evaluation stage useful questions include 'Were our targets achieved?', 'What lessons did we learn?' and 'How can we improve for next time?'

Ewles and Simnett's framework for planning and evaluating health promotion interventions

This model is a flowchart for planning and implementing health promotion interventions and is one of the more popular planning models in use (Whitehead, 2010). The model provides a linear planning process broken down into seven key stages. Figure 18.5 details the seven steps in this health promotion planning model. The arrows on the model indicate the flexibility of the model and how, in practice, we might need to retrace our steps and go back to make sure that the plan is going to work. For example, you might need to go back to step 4 and revisit the resources available if you realise at step 5 that you do not have the appropriate resources to make a plan. Once again you will see that needs assessment is an integral part of the process and that, at the end of the planning cycle, evaluation is also absolutely key.

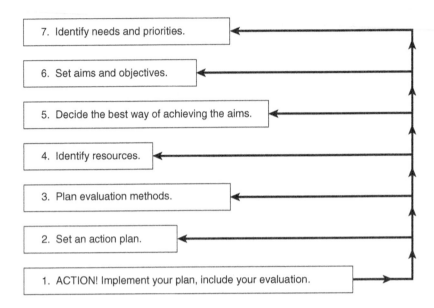

Figure 18.5 Ewles and Simnett's framework for planning and evaluating health promotion and public health practice interventions and projects

Source: Scriven (2017)

SETTING AIMS AND OBJECTIVES

In each of the four planning models we have looked at it is important to identify the overall aim of the intervention alongside the objectives of it. Aims are 'general statements of intent that indicate overall priorities and purposes without going into specific detail' (Hubley et al., 2013: 283). For example, an aim might be to reduce road traffic accidents or to promote vaccination uptake. Objectives, on the other hand, are more detailed and play an important role in shaping the intervention from the outset. These are statements of 'proposed change over a fixed

BOX 18.1 SMART OBJECTIVES

- Specific – having clear, defined outputs
- Measurable – knowing when these outputs have been achieved
- Achievable – knowing that these outputs can be reached
- Realistic – being realistic about what can be achieved
- Time-bound – having a clear time-frame

Source: Adapted from Cragg (2006: 195)

time period' (Hubley et al., 2013: 284). Objectives should be SMART – 'Specific, Measurable, Achievable, Realistic and Timely' (McKenzie et al., 2016, cited in Baldwin, 2020: 217) – also see Box 18.1. Aims and objectives are vital to the planning process and necessary for evaluation; if they are poorly stated or too vague then it will cause difficulties (Bowden, 2017).

Objectives should be precise and measurable and should reflect what would be achieved by an intervention if it is successful (effective). Using the SMART acronym will help to develop strong objectives. In the Australian context Baldwin (2020: 217) offers some examples of SMART objectives as follows:

- To increase consumption of fruit and vegetable intake by adolescents in our community by 40 per cent by 2021
- To increase the number of transport options to health services for all older persons in our community by 50 per cent by 2022
- To decrease reported sunburn rates in school children in our community by 30 per cent by 2021.

Now take some time to do Reflective Exercise 18.2.

REFLECTIVE EXERCISE 18.2

Consider the following aims, or you can think of a broad aim of your own:

- To reduce childhood obesity
- To promote cervical screening
- To reduce gender-based violence
- To promote safer road use by pedestrians and drivers

Now try to develop three or four objectives for your aim using the SMART acronym detailed above.

GO FURTHER 18.1

Using the internet try to find an example of a health promotion programme plan that has been used to address a specific public health issue. See if you can identify the different stages of the planning process using one of the frameworks that have been presented in this chapter. Use the SMART acronym to assess the objectives of the programme. Are they 'Specific, Measurable, Achievable, Realistic and Timely'?

METHODS AND RESOURCES

The aims of your intervention will determine what type of methods will be used. For example, if your aim is about raising awareness about a public health issue then there are several different methods that can be used to achieve this aim including interpersonal communication and mass media (Scriven, 2017). As Linsley and Roll (2020: 156) state, 'the planning and implementation stages of any health promotion intervention are vital for ensuring successful outcomes'. Evans et al. (2017: 138) provide a useful set of questions that can guide the choice of methods and resources:

- Do they use clear language that is suitable for my target group?
- Are they non-racist, non-sexist (inclusive)?
- Are there any legal issues concerning consent?
- What is the evidence of effectiveness (will they work)?

Scriven (2017) details a number of resources that might be available and it is important during the planning process to identify what exactly you are going to need to achieve your aim as well as what is already available. This might include professional input, existing policies and public health strategies, existing facilities and services, material resources, media resources and, most importantly, the target group or community themselves. The design, development and delivery of health promotion programmes is often practitioner-led; however, in this book we have highlighted the importance of participation and empowerment as key principles for health promotion. Thompson et al. (2014) also highlight the importance of community involvement at each stage of the planning process from the initial needs assessment to evaluating the effectiveness of the intervention. Laverack (2007) suggests four questions that can be asked of a programme to determine if it is 'top-down' (expert-led) or 'bottom-up' (community-led) in nature:

- Does the programme have a fixed timeframe or flexible timeframe?
- Is it the outside agent or the community who identifies the concerns to be addressed?
- Is it the outside agent or the community who has control over the management of the programme?
- How will the programme be evaluated?

EVALUATION AND EVIDENCE

The use of evidence is important at different stages of the planning process; for example, evidence of health need, evidence of what works (which will determine the methods that are used) and evidence of effectiveness (evaluation). Chapter 19, 'Health Promotion Research and Evaluation', discusses evidence in more detail, but the critical point to make here is about evidence-based practice. Evidence-based practice is another underpinning principle of health promotion, yet this is not always consistently applied in practice due to various challenges (Mabuza, 2018). These include a lack of knowledge about what constitutes evidence and how to actually use it (Owusu-Addo et al., 2017) as well as how evidence is translated into practice (Baldwin, 2020). In reality there are many different, and sometimes difficult, decisions to be made about how to apply and use evidence (Mabuza, 2018). These issues are discussed in more detail in the next chapter.

Evaluation is also a complex part of planning health promotion interventions. Again, Chapter 19 will expand more on this aspect of programme planning; however, it should be noted here that evaluation is an integral and essential part of a systematic approach to planning health promotion activities and should not be neglected. Typically, the complexity of health promotion interventions necessitates a 'multipronged', or triangulated, approach to evaluation (Mabuza, 2018: 94) but you will have noticed that all of the planning models we have looked at in this chapter have an evaluation phase or stage, even the simplest.

LOG FRAMES (LOGICAL FRAMEWORKS)

Logical frameworks (logframes) are a very useful evaluation tool and are frequently used to support evaluation, particularly in international contexts. They provide a clear structure for planning health promotion interventions including the activities of the programme, the intended impact of these and the intended outputs (Baldwin, 2020).

Table 18.1 A logical framework 4 x 4 matrix

	Narrative Summary	Verifiable Indicators	Means of Verification	Assumption
Goal				
Purpose				
Outputs				
Activities				

Source: Green et al. (2019: 189)

As you will see from Table 18.1 there are four key elements to a logframe represented in the left-hand column – Goal, Purpose, Outputs and Activities. Bell (2001) provides a useful explanation of each of these. Each logframe will typically have one *Goal* that is usually expressed in very broad terms (i.e. reducing unplanned teenage pregnancy or reducing childhood obesity). This is in order to address the question: 'Why do it?' The *Purpose* is the statement of the desired achievement of the intervention: 'What are you doing it for?' (i.e. increased physical activity; healthier eating). The *Outputs* are the outcomes you are hoping for such as immediate or longer-term results (i.e. material factors, organisation or behavioural change, i.e. one less unhealthy snack per day): 'What are you hoping to achieve?' Finally, the *Activities* are what will actually be done and address the question: 'How are you going to do it?' These need to be specified (i.e. working with parents to educate about healthier food choices). Each logframe should only have one goal so for a multipurpose intervention that has several goals you might need a few different logframes,

Table 18.2 An example logframe

	Narrative Summary	Verifiable Indicators	Means of Verification	Assumption
Goal	To reduce infant mortality	Number of deaths	Local clinic/hospital records	Infant mortality rates will go down
Purpose	Reduce the number of waterborne illness in young infants and children	Number of infections	Local epidemiological data about incidence and prevalence of water-borne illnesses	The number of waterborne illnesses will decrease
Outputs	90% of the community will have access to clean running water	Number of standpipes	Number of people with access to clean water	Improved awareness in the community and access to clean water will lead to changes in behaviour
	100% of the community will have increased awareness of good hygiene practices	Number of people with increased knowledge and awareness	Community surveys	
Activities	Install a minimum of ten new standing water pipes in the neighbourhood	Number of standing water pipes installed	Site (community) visits	Providing better access to water and sanitation facilities and information will improve hygiene practices in the community
	Deliver a local radio information campaign about water, sanitation and hygiene	Number of people educated on the issue	Community survey	

Table 18.3 A simple Gantt chart

	Months 1 & 2	Months 3 & 4	Months 5 & 6	Months 7 & 8	Months 9 & 10	Months 11 & 12
Needs assessment	▨					
Gathering baseline information and data		▨				
Recruiting key stakeholders involved in implementation			▨			
Training key stakeholders involved in implementation				▨		
Implementing the programme					▨	
Evaluating the programme						▨

although some of the content (i.e. methods) might overlap. Logframes, when done well, can provide a clear and concise summary of the whole health promotion intervention. This left-hand column represents what is called 'vertical logic', the assumption being that when one thing happens another will follow (Green et al., 2019). There will be a number of assumptions that underpin decision-making at different stages using a logframe that can be verified using vertical logic which is applied from the bottom of the column upwards. For example, if parents are educated about healthier eating using small group work (Activity), their children will choose healthier options (Output), healthier eating will result (Purpose) and childhood obesity will decrease (Goal). Clearly this is a simplified explanation however Table 18.2 provides a more detailed example of a logframe.

A logframe is also important for evaluation and how it happens. It should be used to assess whether or not you have achieved what you set out to. Along the top of a logframe matrix there are columns representing 'verifiable indicators' and 'means of verification'. Using a logframe enables a number of questions to be answered such as How should information be collected? What methods will you use to evaluate the intervention? How will you verify that something has taken place? These aspects of the logframe relate to evaluation and the specific objectives of the intervention. See Table 18.2 for examples.

GANTT CHARTS

Planning health promotion programmes is essentially about project management and will involve many of the same skill sets that are required to initiate, implement and bring a programme to completion (Cragg, 2006). Gantt charts provide a useful tool with which to manage your programme plan. They can provide a timeline for key activities and are very valuable for time management as well as mapping out what should happen when (Evans et al., 2017). Gantt charts set out what will be done and when, and can be used to guide the programme as well as to keep things on track, or highlight if things are falling behind.

CASE STUDY 18.1: NON-COMMUNICABLE DISEASE PREVENTION IN A SOUTHERN AFRICAN MARITIME PORT

Mabuza (2018) reports on an intervention that was intended to help prevent non-communicable diseases (NCDs) in a workplace setting that became beset by many challenges. The intervention was a self-care and employee wellness programme instigated by management without consultation with the workforce. Management had identified an increasing 'epidemic' of NCDs within the staff (over 3000 employees) at the port and the surrounding community and had decided to instigate a top-down, biomedically based approach to tackling it. The intervention was designed to improve health outcomes in relation to weight management, blood sugar control and high blood pressure. It was estimated that at least 50 per cent of the workforce had been diagnosed with one or more non-communicable diseases (diabetes Type 2, heart disease, hypertension, etc.) against the backdrop of an upwards trend in NCDs in the wider region. The intervention was a self-care programme aimed to educate staff about a range of 'risky' lifestyle factors such as poor diet, alcohol use, lack of physical activity, coping with stress and sleep hygiene. Two external providers were appointed to manage the intervention which was also extended to the staff's immediate family members. In addition, the on-site occupational health nurse conducted daily and weekly education sessions for the staff. The intervention was evaluated using quantitative means (a survey with the staff). Mabuza (2018) points out a number of difficulties with the intervention including the lack of attention given to the social determinants of health (for example, the disadvantaged circumstances that the staff lived in) and issues of cultural insensitivity (for example, the focus on weight loss in a culture where carrying extra weight symbolises status and wellness).

Source: Adapted and summarised from Mabuza (2018)

GO FURTHER 18.2

Consider the case study above and the challenges that arise within it. How would you design a more effective health promotion intervention to address non-communicable disease within this setting? Who would you involve and how? What methods would likely be most effective? How would you know that you had been successful? How could the intervention have been designed in order to increase acceptability for the staff, and to maximise effectiveness?

SUMMARY

Using a planning model in health promotion programme planning is highly recommended and can be very helpful in achieving success (Thompson et al., 2014). This chapter has presented a number of different planning models and outlined in some detail the common stages of these. The planning models discussed here are not exhaustive, there are other planning models that might appeal more or be more suitable and readers are encouraged to explore these. Planning health promotion interventions requires a strategic approach (Green et al., 2019). Having a strategy at the outset will greatly increase the likelihood of effectiveness. The discussion in this chapter has simplified the planning process in many ways but, as Whitehead (2010) points out, in real life promoting health is a complex, dynamic process. This is why strategic planning is so important.

SUGGESTED READING

Green, J., Cross, R., Woodall, J. and Tones, K. (2019) Health promotion planning – a systematic approach. *Health promotion: planning and strategies*. 4th edn. London, Sage. pp. 180–236.

Hubley, J., Copeman, J. and Woodall, J. (2021) Planning and management of health promotion. In *Practical health promotion*. 3rd edn. Cambridge, Polity. pp. 297–316.

Scriven, A. (2017) Planning and evaluating health promotion and public health interventions. In *Ewles and Simnett's promoting health: a practical guide*. 7th edn. London, Elsevier. pp. 71–98.

HEALTH PROMOTION RESEARCH AND EVALUATION

19

INTRODUCTION

Health promotion is a discipline with its own ideology and ordered field of study (Davies, 2013); in order to retain this it requires research to progress the development of theory and practice. Research informs the development of policy and practice and the evolution of theory. There is a long-standing tradition of research and evaluation activity in health promotion and now a suite of academic publications with the sole aim to publish health promotion research and scholarship. It is our view that health promoters should have a firm understanding of research and evaluation in their practice. This enables practitioners both to interpret and assess the quality of existing studies and also to conduct their own research and evaluation to answer practical challenges.

This chapter seeks to outline some key principles of health promotion research and evaluation. Given the space permitted it cannot be extensive, but instead it focuses on the key issues that may arise in health promotion research and evaluation specifically. The chapter begins by outlining what makes health promotion research distinct and then explains the recognised steps in the research process. The latter part of the chapter focuses on evaluation – an important component of practice – and illustrates the range of evaluation techniques and approaches.

DOING RESEARCH AND EVALUATION

Often the terms 'research' and 'evaluation' are bound together to suggest that these terms are similar and interchangeable. They are not. Evaluation, as will be explained later, aims to explore what is working or not working in a particular programme or intervention. Research, on the other hand, tries to develop new evidence or advance new knowledge. Not everyone who works in health promotion roles feels able to do research and evaluation – this is a very common scenario. Generally, concerns fall into four categories: competence, time and resources, quality and implementation of findings (Wright, 1999), and these are expanded in Box 19.1.

BOX 19.1 PRACTITIONER BARRIERS TO RESEARCH AND EVALUATION (WRIGHT, 1999)

Concerns about competence:

'I am not an academic'

'I don't know the language'

'I don't know statistics'

Concerns about quality:

'What is good enough research?'

'What level should I be working at?'

Concerns about time and resources:

'How can I fit this in?'

'I don't have time.'

'I have to get on with doing health promotion.'

Concerns and dissemination and implementation:

'If I do this research, will anyone care?'

'I can't produce anything worth publishing'

'Will the research be useful?'

There are some solutions to some of the issues raised in Box 19.1. Some of these solutions may facilitate or make the research and evaluation process easy for practitioners:

- Consider some research and evaluation training.
- Work with people who are more experienced and learn from them.
- Negotiate some time and support from your manager.
- Read a book.
- Develop a support network of other practitioners facing similar challenges (maybe a virtual group).

REFLECTIVE EXERCISE 19.1

Imagine that you are managing a health promotion team and your staff raise issues in relation to their ability to do research as part of their role (see Box 19.1). What additional strategies could you put in place to enable your team to integrate research activity as part of their working role?

WHAT MAKES HEALTH PROMOTION RESEARCH DISTINCT?

The primary question concerns what, if anything, makes health promotion distinctive from any other social science based or related discipline. Some have argued that there are a number of key characteristics that makes health promotion distinct (Woodall et al., 2018). These are:

1. Application to real-world contexts

The first element of distinctiveness is that health promotion research should be on the development of practice and on developing appropriate strategies for action on health (Koelen et al., 2001; Lahtinen et al., 2005). Health promotion research has direct applications to solving 'real world' issues and tends to avoid 'blue sky' research which focuses more on theoretical rather than applied issues. Indeed, Whitehead et al. (2003) have suggested how the tenets of action research, i.e. research designed explicitly to feed into and inform practice, resonates strongly with health promotion research.

2. Research values

As discussed more extensively in Chapter 6, health promotion is a values-driven discipline heavily informed by core principles to inform practice. These values extend further to health promotion research philosophy and practice. Health promotion's value base, derived from the Ottawa Charter (WHO, 1986), is clear in espousing ways of working that are enabling and empowering and which support individuals and communities to gain control over their own health. Some claim that health promotion research should reflect this and have an emphasis on control-enhancing action with values related to inclusion and participation explicitly woven into the research design (Lahtinen et al., 2005). Community participation, as an example, is regarded as a basic principle of health promotion and, by extension, should be a core value of health promotion research (Allison and Rootman, 1996). Practitioners of health promotion too have challenged the research community to ensure that their research design and method takes care 'to ensure that there is an adequate fit with health promotion principles and practice' (Watson and Platt, 2000: 12–13).

3. Relinquishing professional control

Given the privileging of lay perspectives in Chapter 1, it should come as no surprise that health promotion research reflects the importance and prominence of non-professional views.

The process of health promotion researchers as 'co-researchers with the participants in the co-production of knowledge' (Cross and Warwick-Booth, 2016: 9) is a distinctive feature of health promotion research. Such participatory approaches in health promotion research and the evidence that they derive asks people to adopt different attitudes to knowledge production and to reject traditional models of evidence or evidence hierarchy which may inadvertently favour experimental approaches or positivist ideas (Whitehead et al., 2003).

4.   Expansive methodological toolkit

The fourth area of distinctiveness is the expansive methodological toolkit that health promotion researchers can and should draw upon in their practice. Inherently interdisciplinary and not dogmatically tied to research paradigms, views or perspectives, health promotion research should be flexible and diverse to address the issue being explored or investigated. It is our view that such a position is upheld, especially given the range and types of work carried out under the health promotion banner. Ecological models of health promotion, for example, operate on the premise that health and determinants of health are produced by intrapersonal factors, interpersonal processes and primary groups, institutional factors, community factors and public policy (McLeroy et al., 1988).

THE RESEARCH PROCESS

This section outlines crucial steps in the research process. While many studies will vary, contingent on their design or methodological underpinning, there is generally some sequencing of considerations to ensure an effective research study. These broad principles are outlined here.

Understanding the research area and identifying the issue

One of the first stages in the research process is a broad understanding of the topic area itself. Without this understanding it is difficult to fully know what, if anything, your research is contributing. It could be, for instance, that the general issue you wish to examine is already adequately researched and therefore requires no further exploration at this time; or it could be that you identify a specific area that has not been adequately investigated. Ideally, this process is done through reading and identifying key journal articles from peer-reviewed sources – often deemed as 'high quality' – although this stage can also be undertaken through talking to people in the field you are interested to research.

Defining your research questions

The development of well-defined research questions is crucial to the foundation of a good research study and follows on from the first stage which concerns understanding the broad field of study. Once this has been done, it is crucial to begin to home in and identify specific research questions that your study seeks to address. Without clear research questions it is very difficult to undertake good-quality research. Good research questions, if answered, shed important or new insights into a research challenge or issue.

Choosing an appropriate methodology and method

The research questions that are developed will suggest an appropriate methodology and method to inform your research. So, if your research questions seek to explore and understand a given area then it is likely that a qualitative methodology may be best suited. If, however, your research questions are looking to find associations between variables, or to establish the prevalence of a given health issue, then a quantitative methodology may be better suited.

The methodology of a research study is the broad principles and framework for conducting research – a methodology provides an overarching view of how the research should be undertaken. As noted, this broadly relates to qualitative and quantitative methodology (see Box 19.2).

BOX 19.2 QUANTITATIVE AND QUALITATIVE METHODOLOGY

A methodology is a general approach to studying a research topic. While discussion varies, there are broadly qualitative or quantitative methodologies.

Qualitative research tends to study ideas in naturally occurring settings and is often driven by inductive processes - that being theory or issues grounded in empirical data rather than preconceived theories. Qualitative research is often characterised by being subjective in that it draws heavily on the researchers' interpretations. Qualitative methodology accepts that there can be multiple versions of reality to be discovered through the research process.

Quantitative research methodology seeks to discover single, identifiable truths through objective processes of investigation and testing. This approach takes place in controlled environments, often outside of natural settings. This methodology is premised on that things can be measured reliably and accurately and that these findings can be potentially generalised to wider populations and groups.

Methods, on the other hand, are seen as 'the nuts and bolts of research practice' (Carter and Little, 2007: 1325). There are no 'right' or 'wrong' methods for collecting data (Willig, 2001), although the procedures often adopted will use techniques such as interviews, focus groups, observations or surveys. Choosing appropriate methods for a research study should not be undertaken based on the researcher's familiarity with the approach or because some methods are easier or quicker to implement. Willig (2001: 8), for example, cautions that 'not all research methods are compatible with all methodologies'. Methods should be selected because they have the potential to answer the research aims and objectives and because they are consistent with the methodological position of the researcher (Carter and Little, 2007). There has been a tradition in health promotion to undertake mixed-methods research – this sees the combination of methods in order to gain a fuller picture of a research area (see Case Study 19.1).

CASE STUDY 19.1: MIXED-METHODS RESEARCH IN HEALTH PROMOTION

Taxi driving has the adverse effect of having several occupational risks, including muscle and back pain and stress related to the job (e.g. low income, safety threats). A study by Murray et al. (2019) used a mixed-methods approach to explore occupational health risks and opportunities for health interventions with taxi drivers. Qualitative and quantitative methods were used to explore the risks and opportunities. First, 19 taxi drivers took part in a focus group discussion – a semi-structured interview guide was followed and the primary questions included items such as 'What changes in your health have you noticed since becoming a taxi driver?', 'What are the challenges that make it difficult to stay healthy on the job?' and 'What are some ways that you currently try to stay healthy?' In addition, 75 taxi drivers completed a self-report questionnaire on their health status. Demographic information, work history (e.g. years as a driver, average hours worked, shift worked), health behaviours (e.g. physical activity, smoking) and self-reported health (e.g. musculoskeletal pain, fatigue, diabetes and stress) were gathered through the questionnaire. Height, weight and blood pressure were measured objectively by the research team. The research provided both quantitative and qualitative information to provide objective views of health and also strategies to promote and protect good health. The research offered implications to inform targeted health interventions that support the health and safety of taxi drivers.

Ethical approval and research governance

Almost all research comes with ethical risks and challenges that must be minimised to protect participants and the researchers themselves. Space does not permit a full review of all of the potential ethical considerations that arise in health promotion research, but given that health promotion research often focuses on the experiences of vulnerable groups there is an argument that particular sensitivities occur more frequently. Box 19.3 is not exhaustive, but highlights some of the common ethical issues.

BOX 19.3 COMMON ETHICAL ISSUES IN RESEARCH

- Informed consent – achieving informed consent is a paramount principle which is fundamental when conducting research. The failure to provide culturally sensitive and accessible study information to participants is unethical and can result in individuals agreeing to contribute to research studies without being fully aware of the implications.
- Confidentiality – the notion of confidentiality is grounded by the principle of respect for autonomy. This means that identifiable information about research participants collected during data collection must not be disclosed without permission (Wiles et al., 2008).
- Protecting participants – the ethical principles of beneficence and non-maleficence, i.e. do good while minimising potential harm (Noble-Adams, 1999), is also a critical research concern.
- Protecting the researcher – it is of paramount concern that the researchers themselves are fully protected in the research process.

Recognising participants' time and effort – whether research participants should be provided with incentives or payments is frequently debated and is of ethical concern as it can lead to coercion in research studies.

REFLECTIVE EXERCISE 19.2

Providing individuals with sufficient information about research and evaluation studies that they are participating in is fundamental. How would you ensure that the information was communicated effectively to all groups – consider, for example, people with poor literacy or those who cannot read at all. How would you overcome this to ensure that people could still fully participate?

Data gathering

It is surprising just how little is published or written on the actual process of data gathering. However, it is a critical period in the research study and often requires flexibility and the ability to be responsive to issues that occur in the field. The negotiation of gatekeepers and gaining access to sites does require negotiation skills and diplomacy – often which are not discussed or described that well in the literature. It is very likely that research is set in a context – maybe a setting, like a school, workplace, community or in primary care. It is important to remember that data gathering will be a priority for you and your research, but not always a priority in that particular setting. This awareness is often critical in order for the research to be non-intrusive and for the process to go smoothly.

Depending on the type of method you have chosen, this may result in many logistical challenges being considered and addressed. It may be that rooms require booking for private interviews or for focus groups, or it may mean being present to administer a questionnaire. Such logistics need careful consideration in advance to maximise the opportunities in the field – remembering to take a digital recorder, batteries, spare copies of information sheets and consent forms is a crucial part of being a prepared and effective researcher.

Data analysis

Data analysis is a crucial aspect of the research process as it moves the collected data (often referred to as raw data) into something far more meaningful and refined. In effect it is the process of moving between raw data to evidence-based interpretations (Rubin and Rubin, 2005). The data analysis strategy will vary depending on the methodology adopted.

In qualitative studies, data is generally in the form of text and words. Thematic analysis is commonly used in qualitative research – although there are many other approaches – and broadly follows a process of:

- Transcription – often producing a verbatim account of all verbal utterances, say in a focus group, in a way which was true to the original meaning (Poland, 2002).
- Immersion – a process of 'repeated reading' (Braun and Clarke, 2006: 87) and examining the data for patterns and areas of interest.
- Coding – the initial coding process reduces the raw data into more discrete elements and allows further reflection on the overall data set.
- Theme development (see Box 19.4) – 'A theme is a pattern found in the information that at the minimum describes and organizes the possible observations or at the maximum interprets aspects of the phenomenon. A theme may be identified at the manifest level (directly observable in the information) or at the latent level (categorizing issues underlying the phenomenon)' (Boyatzis, 1998: 161).

BOX 19.4 TECHNIQUES TO ARRIVE AT A THEME

Themes may emerge from the data itself (inductive) or from prior theoretical understandings of the area under study (deductive) (Boyatzis, 1998). Although researcher judgement is crucial to determining thematic categories (Braun and Clarke, 2006), Ryan and Bernard (2003) have proposed techniques for arriving at a theme.

Technique	Description
Repetitions	Repetition is one of the simplest forms of theme identification. The more the same concept or idea reoccurs in the raw data the more likely it is to be a theme.
Indigenous typologies	The use of terms or language that may sound unfamiliar or are used in unfamiliar ways.
Metaphors and analogies	Thoughts, behaviours and experiences are often represented through the form of metaphors and analogies. Analysis may, therefore, include searching for these linguistic tools.
Similarities and differences	This is similar to what has been termed the 'constant comparison method' which involves looking for similarities and differences across units of data.
Linguistic connectors	Examining texts for linguistic connectors can prove fruitful when identifying thematic areas of interest.
Theory-related material	Themes that may arise as a result of understanding of pre-existing theory or research.

In quantitative analysis, data usually comes in the form of numbers – collected in many ways, but often in the form of questionnaire responses. 'Descriptive analysis' covers a range of approaches to highlight patterns in the data. Tables and graphs are often used to present descriptive data – often information such as age of participants, gender, ethnicity or lifestyle issues such as smoking or alcohol intake. Descriptive statistics often report averages and standard deviations (the extent the data varies from the mean).

Inferential statistics enable researchers to try and infer that the data has transferability beyond the immediate data. Statistical tests are often used to determine whether the data is 'significant' which determines whether any pattern in the data is due to chance or fluke or actually due to an intervention or programme for instance. This process is based on developing a hypothesis and interpreting p-values (see Box 19.5) to accept or reject the hypotheses.

BOX 19.5 PROBABILITY VALUE (P-VALUE)

A p-value is the probability of obtaining a result due to chance or random errors. The smaller the value the less chance there is that the result was due to chance. If the p-value is less than 0.05 it is unlikely to be due to chance.

Take, for example, a study looking at the resting pulse rate (beats per minute) in a sample of smokers and non-smokers. The average pulse rate for the smokers is 75 and for the non-smokers 71.94. The p-value is calculated as 0.285. Are these differences in the sample statistically significantly different?

Using secondary data sources

We have described the process of gathering data using quantitative and qualitative approaches. Gathering this information to answer specific research questions is called 'empirical data' and is gathered through observations, interviews, questionnaires, and so on. However, there are data that have already been collected by other people, perhaps not specifically for research purposes, that could be of interest to health promotion researchers. This may be information already in the public domain that can be used by researchers to address evidence-based questions.

There are several ways in which existing data can be accessed; it is worth exploring some of these datasets to see if there is information already being held that can address particular evidence-based questions (see Box 19.6). Some of this is known as 'big data'.

BOX 19.6 EXAMPLES OF SECONDARY DATA SETS

- Open data: http://opendata.esriuk.com/
- UK Data Service: https://ukdataservice.ac.uk/
- ResearchOne: www.researchone.org/
- Office for National Statistics: www.ons.gov.uk/peoplepopulationandcommunity/ wellbeing
- National surveys, e.g. Community Life Survey: www.gov.uk/government/statistics/ community-life-survey-2017-18

Documentary analysis is one form of secondary data analysis. This can take myriad forms, but includes the systematic analysis of organisational and institutional reports and policies (Bowen 2009). This approach has been used to great effect in health promotion where accessing empirical evidence may be difficult or challenging for ethical or practical reasons (see Case Study 19.2).

CASE STUDY 19.2: PROMOTING HEALTH AND WELL-BEING IN PRISONS: AN ANALYSIS OF ONE YEAR'S PRISON INSPECTION REPORTS

This study used independent prison inspections, conducted by Her Majesty's Inspectorate of Prisons for England and Wales (HMIP), to explore ways of promoting health in prison. The research analysed one year (2018) of inspection reports in 38 male prisons. Reports were identified through the HMIP website (www.justiceinspectorates. gov.uk/hmiprisons/), a free to access resource in the public domain. For further details, see Woodall and Freeman (2019).

Writing up and dissemination

Writing up research can be a challenging undertaking. It frequently requires skills in effective communication and distilling complex ideas into things that are meaningful for people. Knowing the audience you are writing for is crucial and without being clear on this, it is likely that your write-up will not resonate appropriately.

REFLECTIVE EXERCISE 19.3

Researchers must often communicate their findings to a range of audiences and the style and communication mode needs to reflect these varying stakeholder groups. Imagine that you have completed your research and now need to communicate the key findings. What strategies or methods would you use for the following audiences? What would the focus of the message be on? What would the format of the communication be and what considerations would you give to the language and layout?

- Academics
- Policy-makers
- Health promotion practitioners
- Community members

Dissemination – the art of spreading information widely – is a crucial aspect of the research process as it is the way in which practice and policy can be shaped. It is the way in which ideas are taken up and applied, and practice and policy are refined. The writing up and dissemination strategy employed will be largely dependent on the purpose of the research. Research outputs can look quite different – most traditionally, though, in the form of a peer-reviewed journal article. However, most practitioners do not have the time or motivation to do this and so often research for practice can be presented in reports, posters and presentations at conferences. The peer-reviewed academic article, while not perfect, is often deemed as a gold standard as the work will be assessed by experts in the field before it is published or disseminated widely. This offers *some* assurance that the research you are reading is of good quality, but not always! The process of getting research published is often lengthy and requires some resilience, as your research is scrutinised carefully and thoroughly often demanding multiple drafts before it is accepted.

There are, however, other ways in which research can be written and disseminated. Blogs are now becoming a useful way to share research findings quickly and at scale. While blogs do not come with a peer-reviewed assurance, they are often effective ways to reach larger audiences and to communicate key issues in a simple and succinct way. Social media also open up opportunities to share research findings and is often a good way to highlight or signpost people to the full research study.

EVALUATION

Evaluation is a crucial skill for any health promoter and moreover is seen as being a critical competency for professional practice (Barry et al., 2009). The reason for this is that evaluation of interventions and of practice directly informs evidence-based practice and decision-making. Evaluation is a key stage of the planning cycle as it provides an assessment of a programme and its impact (South and Woodall, 2012). A credible discipline requires an evidence base on which practitioners and decision-makers can base their practices (Deehan and Wylie, 2010).

In its simplest form, an evaluation is to assess the extent to which interventions have achieved their goals (Green et al., 2019). Evaluations can be flexible in what they seek to achieve, but broadly speaking can provide four functions:

- evaluation for accountability
- evaluation for programme management and development
- evaluation for learning
- evaluation as an ethical obligation (Green and South, 2006)

Health promotion evaluation does pose significant challenges, including the existence of profound debates, and indeed methodological divisions, about appropriate approaches to evaluation (South and Woodall, 2012). Indeed, there are lots of challenges and pitfalls when evaluating (see Box 19.7).

BOX 19.7 COMMON EVALUATION PROBLEMS (FROM HUBLEY ET AL., 2013)

- No objectives/targets were set at the beginning, so it was not clear what the purpose of the programme was.
- The objectives/targets are not measurable because they were set out in terms that were too general (e.g. increase exercise, increase awareness, empower people).
- No baseline study was carried out, so it is not possible to demonstrate any improvement as a result of the health promotion activity.

- Unanticipated benefits or negative outcomes are not picked up. The evaluation was focused only on the achievement or non-achievement of the objectives, so other changes were not noticed.
- A lack of impact is demonstrated, but reasons for failure are not known because insufficient supporting information was collected.
- An impact is demonstrated, but it could be for reasons other than the programme. A lack of controls or supporting information make it difficult to prove that the change observed was a result of the health promotion.
- The benefits of the health promotion are seen only after the end of the programme and are not noticed in the evaluation (sleeper effect).
- Improvements in the community are not sustained and the situation reverts back to the original state (backsliding).

Most evaluations are comprised of two components. First, the assessment of outcomes – that is the changes that result from an intervention. The intervention could be a programme or a policy, for example, and the purpose is to determine what, if anything, has changed as a result of that intervention. In contrast, the assessment of process is looking at the mechanisms operating within interventions and the influence of contextual factors (South and Woodall, 2012). Saunders et al. (2005) suggest seven elements to be included in a process evaluation plan: fidelity (whether the programme was implemented as planned); completeness (whether all elements were delivered to participants); exposure, satisfaction, reach, recruitment and context (whether environmental aspects have influenced the programme).

GO FURTHER 19.1

Combining the evaluation of intervention outcomes and process is a valuable approach in health promotion. What strengths do each of these approaches bring and why would that be important for understanding how health promotion interventions work?

Outcomes from interventions can be evaluated using indicators of success. Indicators measure different types of health promotion outcomes and can be behavioural, educational, social, policy, environmental or even physiological and will relate to different levels of programme outcomes (South and Woodall, 2012):

- individual – for example, measuring changes such as knowledge, beliefs or behaviour;
- organisational – for example, measuring changes in staff skills or service improvements;

Table 19.1 Indicators for evaluation – strengths and weaknesses

Type of change	Indicators	Strengths and weaknesses as an indicator for evaluation
Changes in health	Mortality – death rates Morbidity – (sickness rates, workplace absenteeism through ill health) Injury rates Notifiable diseases Quality of life indicators	Mortality rates are good for convincing policy makers of the benefits of health promotion. However, it is difficult to achieve changes in health within a period of less than five years. Mortality is unsuitable for small-scale programmes because numbers are too small to make statistical comparisons with control communities.
Changes in behaviour	Lifestyle changes – diet, exercise, alcohol consumption Uptake of services, e.g. immunisation, screening, Adherence to prescribed courses of medicines.	Behaviour changes are more suitable than changes in health/disease status for evaluation of health promotion because improvements in health can take a long time. However, changes in behaviours are more appropriate to programmes based on persuasion models rather than empowerment.
Health Empowerment	Self-efficacy scales Health literacy	This would be more suitable for community development and empowerment approaches.
Knowledge/ awareness/ attitudes	Knowledge of symptoms, causes, preventive measures for particular health conditions. Perceived importance and susceptibility	Knowledge and attitudes can be measured using scales and are good indicators for measuring short-term impact. But change in knowledge or attitude does not necessarily imply changing behaviour so these indicators are insufficient on their own.
Skills	Ability to perform specific skills, e.g. communication, decision-making.	For some programmes this is a useful indicator but it is important to measure not only whether people have acquired the skills but also whether they are actually using them in their own lives.
Advocacy	Enactment of legislation/policy. Implementation of policies. Media coverage of issues.	These kinds of objectives are appropriate for advocacy components of programmes.
Service Improvement	Training of staff. Numbers of health promotion sessions delivered. Uptake of new services. Contacts between service providers and service users. Quality/satisfaction indicators.	Improving services are an important goal of health promotion. It is also important to establish that those services are being used by those in greatest need.

Source: Hubley et al. (2013) reproduced by kind permission of Polity Press

- community – for example, measuring changes in social capital or increased community mobilisation.
- policy – for example, measuring changes in policy to support health or increased participation in policy processes.

Hubley et al. (2013) has usefully offered a series of common indicators used to measure changes in health or health-related behaviours. These have been presented in Table 19.1 with an additional commentary indicating the relative strengths and weaknesses of adopting these measures of success.

In terms of how outcomes are measured, experimental designs, most notably randomised control trials, are often used in evaluations as a useful way to assess changes caused by an intervention. Using this evaluation design makes sense, given that change can often be attributable to the intervention – especially when randomised controlled trials are used (see Box 19.8).

BOX 19.8 THE RANDOMISED CONTROLLED TRIAL (RCT)

The randomised control trial (RCT) is a study in which a number of people or communities are randomly assigned to two (or more) groups. One group (the experimental group) receives the intervention being tested, the other (the comparison group or control group) has either an alternative intervention, a dummy intervention (placebo), or no intervention at all. The groups are assessed to see if there are differences between them, thus demonstrating the effectiveness of the intervention.

Source: Adapted from (Kendall, 2003)

Within health promotion, though, the randomised controlled trial and similar experimental approaches have often been criticised as being inappropriate (Green and Tones, 1999), although there are some exceptions (see Case Study 19.3). Green et al. (2019) have summarised these limitations as follows:

- inability to cope with the complexity of health promotion programmes;
- do not pay sufficient attention to process and the quality of interventions;
- practical difficulties in relation to randomisation;

- contamination of control or reference groups;
- are ideologically incompatible with health promotion in relation to:
  - o commitment to 'active' individual and community participation in the research process;
  - o contributing to its empowering and 'emancipatory' role;
  - o the use of research as a tool for achieving political and social change.

CASE STUDY 19.3: EVALUATION OF THE IMPACT OF A SCHOOL GARDENING INTERVENTION ON CHILDREN'S FRUIT AND VEGETABLE INTAKE: A RANDOMISED CONTROLLED TRIAL

The RCT is often criticised for being incompatible with the values and philosophy of health promotion, but the RCT has been used to good effect in some cases. Christian et al. (2014) demonstrated, using a cluster randomisation of schools, the effectiveness of a school gardening programme on children's fruit and vegetable intake. The study evaluated the impact of a Royal Horticultural Society (RHS) led intervention against a less involved teacher-led intervention.

Ten schools in London were randomly allocated to receive the Royal Horticultural Society (RHS) led intervention and 13 schools were allocated to receive the teacher-led intervention. The results have found very little evidence to support the claims that school gardening alone can improve children's daily fruit and vegetable intake. Nonetheless, when a gardening intervention is implemented at a high level within the school it may improve children's daily fruit and vegetable intake by a portion.

Participatory evaluation approaches are often favoured in health promotion – this is for a range of reasons, but essentially because they resonate so well with health promotion's core values (see Chapter 6) and can potentially offer greater illumination of issues with findings more likely to be considered and implemented. The meaning of participatory research varies, but Mantoura and Potvin (2013) usefully suggest that it should be defined in relational terms exemplified by the interaction between those conducting research and those whose lives are the focus of the research (Wright et al., 2010).

As an example, the use of storyboards, as a creative participatory evaluative method, can be used to neutralise power relations. Research has shown that the storyboard approach can be used with young, vulnerable women to understand their social context and to reflect on their engagement with a service designed to support their health and social needs. The approach was contingent on building rapport and relationships with the young women in order to increase trust and eradicate any perceived power relationships. Participants were supported to develop a storyboard of their lives before and during their engagement with the service and to envisage what life may be like in the future. Participants were encouraged to use creative and artistic ways to do this and this formed the basis of further discussion – such an approach was designed to put participants at ease. While not without challenges, the participatory evaluation approach used was concluded to have provided rich data, promoted engagement and empowerment and enabled individuals to have more power over the research process (Cross and Warwick-Booth, 2016). As demonstrated here, participatory approaches can be used both to explore outcomes as a result of an intervention and processes in the conception and implementation of the intervention.

There has been growth in the use of theory-based evaluation in health promotion, particularly realistic evaluation approaches. Theory of change is one such approach which is useful when evaluating complex interventions (which most health promotion interventions are). Theory of change approaches involve a participatory process whereby the long-term aims of a programme, policy or intervention are identified and then a process of 'backwards-mapping' seeks to identify the steps along the change pathway. This is useful both for practitioners in understanding the 'logic' of their interventions and also for evaluators in identifying useful indicators of success.

SUMMARY

Research and evaluation are important elements of health promotion both to extend understanding of theory and also to inform policy and practice. The delivery of research and evaluation should recognise the unique disciplinary context and complement, rather than compromise, the core values and philosophy of inclusion, empowerment and enablement. The chapter has illustrated some of the key considerations and processes in the research process – ranging from conception of idea, to developing research questions, to analysis and dissemination. This shouldn't be seen as being prescriptive, but as a framework to work with and modify. The latter part of the chapter has focused on evaluation as a core component to understand both the effectiveness of interventions (i.e. do they work?) and issues relating to processes (i.e. how/why do they work?). Evaluation designs can take a range of forms and should be selected carefully to ensure appropriate fit – in some cases, such designs can align coherently to the core function of health promotion, through inclusive activities and in other cases may actively contradict this.

SUGGESTED READING

Green, J., Cross, R., Woodall, J. et al. (2019) *Health promotion: planning and strategies.* 4th edn. London, Sage.

Green, J. and South, J. (2006) *Evaluation.* Maidenhead, Open University Press.

Woodall, J., Warwick-Booth, L., South, J. et al. (2018) What makes health promotion distinct? *Scandinavian Journal of Public Health*, 46: 118–122.

COMMUNICATING EFFECTIVELY

20

INTRODUCTION

This final chapter considers communication, a vital component of health promotion. It is nearly impossible to promote health without communicating in some way. Being able to communicate effectively is therefore vital and is a core domain of health promotion practice. This chapter explores communication strategies, considers different types of audiences and how communication strategies should be tailored appropriately. We discuss the practicalities of communication and persuasion looking specifically at using written, oral and electronic strategies so each of these are discussed in turn. Finally, some practical advice is offered about how to use social media to disseminate information for health promotion.

THE IMPORTANCE OF COMMUNICATION

As stated in the introduction, communication is a vital component of health promotion. Chapter 16, 'Professional Competencies and Core Skills', highlighted the importance of good communication skills for the health promotion practitioner. All public health/health promotion professional competency frameworks have a communication component in them because effective communication is crucial in order to improve health outcomes and achieve health gain. In order for health promotion efforts to be successful we need to communicate effectively (Scriven, 2017).

There are several different models of communication in the wider literature; however, one of the most comprehensive is Green et al.'s (2019) communication model which derives from telecommunications (see Figure 20.1). This model takes into account the characteristics of the source of the communication (which may be a person in interpersonal communication or some other kind of source such as a leaflet or TV campaign) and the characteristics of those who are receiving the message (such as the recipients' beliefs or culture, for example). It acknowledges the reciprocal relationship between the sender (or source) and the receiver (Cross et al., 2017). It also accounts for the *process* of communication and how messages are encoded by the sender and decoded by the receiver.

According to this model, the message may be coded in several different ways. If the source is a person then non-verbal communication (NVC) will accompany the verbal communication if the person is actually visible. A *symbolic* message will use written language or symbols; an *iconic* message will use pictures or diagrams; and an *enactive* message will have people involved in some kind of activity. Crucially, this model contains a *feedback loop* which is an important feature in communication although note that sometimes communication for health promotion is one-way and does not involve any feedback at all (for example, think about the use of billboards or radio to convey health information).

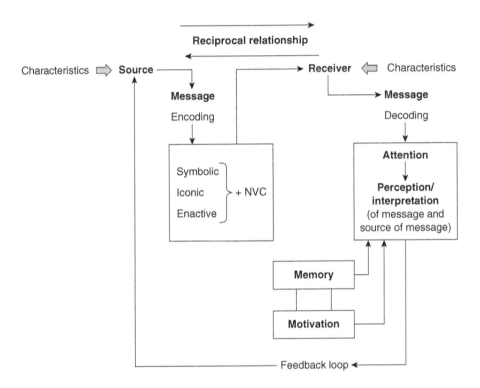

Figure 20.1 A communication model

Source: Green et al. (2019: 345)

Communication in health promotion can take place at different levels from the individual to the institutional to the community (Corcoran, 2013). Corcoran (2013: 9) has identified five categories of communication methods as follows:

Intrapersonal: Internal communication (for example, what we think)

Interpersonal: One-to-one, small groups, email, telephone calls, etc.

Organisational: Lectures, seminars, meetings, newsletters, intranets, etc.

Community: Local radio, debates, local newspapers, bus wraps, health fairs, etc.

Public/Mass communication: Newspapers, television, Internet, mobile phones, etc.

The methods and strategies we use will depend on which category of communication we are working in and what we are trying to achieve but one of the first steps to effective communication is knowing your audience.

KNOWING YOUR AUDIENCE

One of the most important aspects of communication is the intended recipients of it, or the 'audience'. Knowing who you are communicating with (or to) is vital in order that the message is framed and delivered in the most appropriate, accessible way. In social marketing identifying who your audience is and determining what their characteristics, behaviours, values and desires are is referred to as *audience segmentation* (Nutland, 2015). Different types of communication will be appropriate to different audiences and this will depend on what the intended outcome of the communication is. The premise of audience segmentation is that populations can be segmented or broken up into smaller 'units' depending on factors such as demographics, lifestyle, geography, and so on (Brocklehurst et al., 2012), and the purpose is to establish some degree of heterogeneity whereby people with similar wants and needs can be identified and therefore grouped together. For example, an audience might be male students in a high school or pregnant women aged 18–24 years. The size of the audience will vary from a single person to whole populations. The method of communication will have to be adapted depending on this. The nature of the audience will also have an impact; for example, how old people are, how much formal education they have received and what their socio-cultural background is.

An important aspect of communication for health promotion takes place at the one-to-one level through interpersonal communication. This can take many forms. Bandura's Social Learning Theory (David, 2019) proposes that we are more likely to pay attention to, and learn from, people that we know and trust and so it stands to reason that our social networks (interpersonal relationships) have a large influence in terms of health communication. Thus, peer-to-peer strategies for promoting health are often effective since they use existing social and peer networks as a means to promote health (Forrest, 2015). Peer education comprises teaching and the communication of health information, values and behaviours between people who have something in common be that age, social status or other characteristics (South, Bagnall and Woodall, 2017). Peer education is a popular method of interpersonal communication especially for certain public health issues such as teenage sexual health, or with groups of people who are traditionally viewed as difficult to connect with (Cross et al., 2017). A systematic review by Wong et al. (2019: 652) found that 'peer education was beneficial for increasing knowledge of sexual health topics and creating some behaviour change such as increased condom use and HIV testing' in college (university) students. Similarly, another systematic review by Vujcich et al. (2018), which aimed to determine the range, nature and success of Indigenous youth peer-led health promotion in Canada, New Zealand, Australia and the United States, found that such interventions improved knowledge, attitudes and behaviours in Indigenous young people. Having a good relationship with your audience (or being perceived as having a good image) makes a difference to the effectiveness of health communication efforts (Rodham, 2019).

THE ART OF PERSUASION

Giving information or advice is often not enough to effect behaviour change, people may also need to be persuaded in some way to take action or change what they are doing (Abraham et al., 2008). Successful persuasion can lead to changes in attitudes, intentions and behaviours resulting in improved health experience. Persuasion is distinguishable from coercion because coercion is typically punitive; that is, it uses threat or 'punishment' (Cross et al., 2017). Persuasive techniques in health promotion are subject to critique on ethical grounds because they are arguably not in line with empowering ways of working (Hubley et al., 2021). However, we do use persuasion as well as coercion and manipulation as means of promoting health. Persuasive techniques include trying to influence people to change their behaviour through 'explanations, advice and argument' (Hubley et al., 2013: 25). The purpose is to try to convince people to do something different or even to give something up. Different methods can be used to persuade people to change their behaviour. Here we discuss two techniques – message framing and social influence.

Message framing is based on prospect theory which is actually located in economics; however, it has utility in communication for health promotion as you'll see. Prospect theory was first devised in the late 1970s by Kahneman and Tversky and it theorises that people make decisions based on what they hope to gain rather than what they think they will lose. For this reason, the theory is also sometimes referred to as the 'loss-aversion' theory (Abraham et al., 2008). So, the assumption is that, faced with a choice, people will choose the option that provides a potential gain or benefit over the option that will result in a possible loss or cost (Rodham, 2019). Many health promotion messages can be communicated in these two different ways. A negatively framed anti-smoking message would emphasise potential losses; for example, 'Give up smoking or you are much more likely to get lung cancer'. A positively framed anti-smoking message would emphasise the benefits of giving up smoking such as saving money or having a better complexion/fresher breath.

Social influence is important because it affects our motivation and behaviour. People can influence us in different ways. *Informational influence* refers to the influence that other people have when we perceive them to have more knowledge than we do (they might be an expert or better informed; for example, a healthcare professional) (Rodham, 2019). *Normative influence* refers to our desire to fit in with our peers. This desire can motivate us to do things that we would not necessarily choose to do if we were left to our own devices. Normative influence is very relevant to peer-education strategies which are discussed in more detail later in this chapter.

GO FURTHER 20.1

Choose a public health issue and a method of communication discussed in this chapter and then see if you can find a systematic review or meta-analysis which examines the effectiveness of that method. For example, you could look for research that has been done on the effectiveness of motivational interviewing for reducing alcohol consumption or the effectiveness of group participation for weight loss. Use the internet or your university library search engine. See if you can determine what the consistent elements of success are.

ORAL STRATEGIES

Oral strategies for communicating health take many forms and often involve one-to-one interventions including giving advice and counselling. Such approaches are widely used in many different settings including clinical and community contexts (Hubley et al., 2021). This type of intervention typically takes place in person face-to-face but can also be via the telephone or electronic means such as asynchronous online web or live text-chats. Interpersonal communication comes into play here primarily verbal and non-verbal communication. Verbal communication is, of course, what we *say*. However, we also communicate with each other through non-verbal communication which includes body language and contact, direct gaze and eye contact, voice tone/volume, posture, physical appearance, body movement and facial expressions (Scriven, 2017). Active listening and effective interpersonal communication are very important in health promotion. See Boxes 20.1 and 20.2 for more information on this.

BOX 20.1 ACTIVE LISTENING

Active listening involves:

- inviting the person to talk;
- giving the person attention;
- allowing the person time to explain themselves;
- not interrupting;
- encouraging the person to talk by using non-verbal communication strategies such as nods and smiles, and verbal remarks such as 'Umm', 'That's interesting', 'Can you say more about that?';
- clarifying what is being said by asking questions, paraphrasing and reflecting things back to the person;
- showing empathy and understanding;
- looking interested and making appropriate eye contact;
- asking open-ended questions (those that cannot be answered with a 'yes' or 'no');
- summarising what has been said and reflecting it back to the person.

Sources: Hubley et al. (2021); Scriven (2017)

BOX 20.2 TOP TIPS FOR EFFECTIVE INTERPERSONAL COMMUNICATION

- Engage in active listening (see Box 20.1)
- Avoid using health or medical jargon
- Treat each person as an individual
- Respect people's differences
- Adopt a non-judgemental attitude
- Practise self-awareness and reflection (how are you coming across?)

There are different types of one-to-one interventions in health promotion. These include health coaching and motivational interviewing, each of which will now be discussed in turn.

Health coaching is becoming more common in recent years as a means for addressing health behaviour 'positioning people to become powerful drivers of change in their own lives' (Root, 2019: 53). Research into health coaching for weight loss suggests that the nature of the relationship between the coach and client is key and that developing a therapeutic alliance is important (Nagy et al., 2018). Not surprisingly perhaps, there is a better likelihood of bonding between coach and client when more time is given to the coaching session. Health coaching clearly has positive impacts on behaviour change even though it takes different forms and there is no agreed understanding in the literature about what it actually is (Finn and Watson, 2017). It typically involves strategies such as goal-setting, self-management and individual feedback. The 'health champions' model in England provides a similar framework of support. A health champion is a trained member of staff who helps people adopt healthier behaviours (for example, smoking cessation, reduced alcohol consumption, weight management, etc.) as well as signposting them to more specialised services (Micallef et al., 2019).

Motivational interviewing is a method of enabling behaviour change that was originally devised by Miller and Rollnick in the 1980s to help people with addictive behaviours. It has since been adapted for use in a range of lifestyle issues such as healthy eating and physical activity. It is a one-to-one method tailored to the individual and where they are at and is designed to help people work through any ambivalence they might have towards changing their behaviour through setting goals (Green et al., 2019). Through the process of motivational interviewing (or 'change talk' – Szczekala et al., 2018: 128) the 'interviewer' determines the person's readiness to change and structures their responses/interactions accordingly. A review of the literature on motivational interviewing concluded that it can result in improved health behaviours as well as better self-esteem and self-efficacy, internal motivation and increased willingness to change habits (Szczekala et al., 2018).

Health education techniques with communities who cannot read and write also involve verbal and non-verbal communication and can include a range of strategies such as drama, pictorial storyboards, poetry, mime, role play and song. This often takes place in some kind of group.

Working with groups. Health promotion also takes place in groups and will necessarily involve oral strategies, often alongside other types of strategy. Groups can take different forms such as teaching/learning groups, self-help groups, problem-solving groups and community-based groups (Hubley et al., 2021). Groups vary enormously and the purpose of them will differ; however, the challenges of working in groups are fairly universal, as are the keys to success. See Box 20.3 for further information.

BOX 20.3 WORKING WITH GROUPS TO PROMOTE HEALTH

SOME POTENTIAL CHALLENGES:

- Lack of common purpose
- Unequal contribution by group members (for example, someone may dominate)
- Disagreement and lack of cohesion
- Poor or irregular attendance
- Lack of decision-making or task fulfilment
- Group is too big (or too small)

SOME KEYS TO SUCCESS:

- Group size around 8-12 people
- Clear, defined purpose
- Effective facilitation (or leadership)
- Group consensus (going with the majority view)
- Meaningful participation

Source: Adapted from Hubley et al. (2021)

WRITTEN STRATEGIES

Health communication often takes written form, from posters to leaflets to all manner of printed material designed to relay information to improve health. Of course, such communication relies on people's ability to read and also on their ability to make sense of information and act on it. This is where the concept of 'health literacy' comes in. There are many different definitions of health literacy in the literature; however, it generally refers to people's understandings of health information and their ability/capacity to act on it (Cross et al., 2017). The higher the level of someone's health literacy, the better their health is likely to be, and the more they are likely to be able to engage with, and act upon, health information. See Box 20.4 for further details about the different types of health literacy.

BOX 20.4 TYPES OF HEALTH LITERACY

Functional health literacy – concerned with improved knowledge of health risks and health services, and compliance with prescribed actions. It requires a level of basic reading and writing skills to be able to function effectively in everyday situations.

Interactive health literacy – developing personal and social skills to act independently on knowledge and to improve motivation and self-confidence to act on advice received. It requires more advanced cognitive and literacy skills so that people can participate in everyday activities and apply new information in changing circumstances.

Critical health literacy – 'reflects the cognitive and skills development outcomes which are oriented towards supporting effective social and political action, as well as individual action'. It requires even more advanced skills, together with social skills, which can be applied to analyse information and use it to exert greater control over life events and situations.

Source: Cross et al. (2017); Nutbeam and Kickbusch (2000: 265)

Readability is another important factor for written communication strategies. It is vital that the message is accessible and understandable (Cross et al., 2017). However, there is evidence that many health education materials are beyond the average person's reading skills (Rudd, 2015). One way of testing the readability of written material is to carry out a SMOG test. 'SMOG' stands for 'Simple Measure of Gobbledygook'. See Box 20.5 for how to carry out a SMOG test on written material.

BOX 20.5 SIMPLE MEASURE OF GOBBLEDYGOOK (SMOG)

How to carry out a SMOG test of text readability:

1. Take the entire text to be assessed.
2. Count 10 sentences in a row near the beginning, 10 in the middle and 10 near the end to get a total of 30 sentences.
3. Count every word with three or more syllables in the 30 sentences, even if the same word appears more than once.
4. Calculate the square root of the number arrived at in step 3 and round it off to the nearest 10.
5. Add 3 to the figure you arrived at in step 4 to get the SMOG score.
6. The higher the SMOG score, the lower the readability of the text.

Source: Adapted from McLaughlin (1969)

REFLECTIVE EXERCISE 20.1: SMOG TEST

Find an example of written health promotion; a leaflet or website would be ideal. Carry out a SMOG test on the material and see what the final score is. It is likely that the reading age will be higher than it should be. Consider the material. How could it be improved? Can you re-word the content to make it more accessible and reduce the overall score? Would another method of communication be more effective? If so, what would you suggest and why? Compare two or three different examples and see which comes out as most readable.

Communicating messages in writing is not easy but there are strategies that can be adopted to enhance effectiveness. Hubley et al. (2013: 145) offer a practical checklist to ensure that written information is provided in plain English as follows:

1. Have the intended reader clearly in mind when you are writing.
2. Use words that are likely to be familiar to the reader.
3. Avoid jargon – if you really need to use a technical word it needs to be defined.
4. Keep acronyms to a minimum.
5. If there is a choice between a long word and a short word, use the short word!
6. Use concrete language rather than general phrases – e.g. instead of 'interact with your children', say 'talk with your children'.
7. Try reading it aloud. If it is difficult to read aloud you need to rewrite it.
8. Use short sentences and paragraphs. Commas and full stops are your friends!
9. Use lists and bullet points.
10. Pre-test what you have written by giving it to someone and asking if they understand it.

ELECTRONIC STRATEGIES

There has been a significant shift in the way that people access information about health over the past two decades with more and more people relying on electronic media such as internet sources; information about health is rife (Palfrey, 2018). One reason for this is the increasing relative ease of access since information can be found at the click of a button or simply by asking 'Alexa' (or any other kind of smart speaker). Never has it been so accessible to find out things and the existence of Wi-Fi makes it even easier (Rodham, 2019). However, the quality of online (or electronic) information cannot always be determined and, coupled with the overwhelming amount of information that is available, it can be hard to discern what to pay attention to. In addition, there is a lot of unreliable and contradictory health advice available online which can be confusing. Nevertheless, technology is changing all the time and health promotion can embrace it to increase efforts to improve health experience and health outcomes in many areas. Chapter 15, 'Virtual Settings for Health', provides a more detailed discussion of the issues related to this but see Case Study 20.1 for an example of the use of mHealth to improve postnatal care in rural areas in low- and middle-income countries.

CASE STUDY 20.1: HEALTH COMMUNICATION AND POSTNATAL CARE IN RURAL AREAS

Women living in rural areas typically access postnatal care less than their urban counterparts which has potentially negative implications for maternal and infant morbidity and mortality. mHealth strategies have been employed as a means to improve postnatal care in urban settings. Mbuthia et al. (2019) carried out a systematic review that aimed to determine the best means of using mHealth communication strategies to enhance post-natal care in rural settings in low- and middle-income countries such as Kenya, Tanzania and Nigeria. Seven types of mHealth communication were used with the mothers in the studies selected. These included phone calls, one-way messaging, interactive messaging, audiovisual material and videos, voice messages, and combined messaging and phone calls. The review concluded that a variety of mHealth communication can be used to strengthen post-natal care in rural settings, particularly one-way mobile messaging which appears to be the mHealth communication method of choice for many, and results in the best outcomes. Mbuthia et al. (2019) concluded that mHealth interventions can improve the uptake of post-natal care by influencing intention and skills, and because they reduce environmental constraints (i.e. access to skilled support). Advice can be given in this way about several aspects of post-natal care such as breastfeeding and safer sleep practices. Such approaches therefore have the potential to reduce health inequalities.

Source: Mbuthia et al. (2019)

BOX 20.6 ASSESSING THE QUALITY OF HEALTH INFORMATION ON THE INTERNET

1. Who has written the information? Who is the author? Is it an organization or an individual person? Is there a way to contact them?
2. Are the aims of the site clear? What are the aims of the site? What is it for? Who is it for?
3. Does the site achieve its aims? Does the site do what it says it will?
4. Is the site relevant to me? List five things you want to find out from the site.
5. Can the information be checked? Is the author qualified to write the site? Has anyone else said the same things anywhere else? Is there any way of checking this out? If the information is new, is there any proof?
6. When was the site produced and last updated? Is it up to date? Can you check to see if the information is up to date, and not just the site?
7. Is the information biased in any way? Has the site got a particular reason for wanting you to think in a particular way? Is it a balanced view?
8. Does the site tell you about choices open to you? Does the site give you advice? Does it tell you about other ideas?

Source: Scriven (2017:160)

CASE STUDY 20.2: LESSONS FOR PUBLIC HEALTH FROM A PRESIDENTIAL ELECTION CAMPAIGN

Barack Obama's election campaign strategy reached millions of people in a previously unprecedented manner. Central to the campaign was the use of electronic media, namely the internet, digital video and mobile devices, which can be grouped into five types as follows: 1) the campaign website, 2) the campaign TV channel, 3) social network sites, 4) mobile phones and 5) unofficial campaign materials created by Obama's supporters using electronic media. History testifies the success of the campaign. Abroms and Lefebvre (2009: 402) argue that health communication can learn from how the campaign operated and point out the following key lessons for public health efforts:

- Consider new media – social network sites, uploaded videos, mobile text messages, and blogs – as part of a comprehensive media mix
- Encourage horizontal (i.e. peer-to-peer and social network) communication of the campaign message as social influence and modelling are important drivers of behaviour. Embrace user-generated messages and content, especially in the case where top-down campaign messages are straightforward and translatable by the public.
- Use new media to encourage small acts of engagement. Small acts of engagement are important for relationship building and can lead to larger acts of engagement in the future. Additionally, small acts of engagement can have effects that ripple throughout a social network.
- Use social media to facilitate in-person grassroots activities, not to substitute for them.

Source: Abroms and Lefebvre (2009)

REFLECTIVE EXERCISE 20.2

Following on from Case Study 20.2 and the implications of the success of the methods used in the presidential campaign for health communication, can you think of any other ways in which communication strategies can be extended to include more recent advances in electronic media and technology? Use the internet to find out what is at the cutting edge of technological advances and your own creativity to imagine how technology might be harnessed to promote health at an individual or population level.

SOCIAL MEDIA AND HEALTH PROMOTION

Social media is becoming more and more vital as a method for health promotion. As Nutland (2015) points out, in contrast to mass media which tends to be a one-way form of communication, social media has the potential for interaction (two-way communication) which distinguishes it from more traditional methods of media such as TV and radio.

Types of social media vary and include platforms such as Facebook, Twitter, Instagram and YouTube as well as mobile apps. For more discussion on the use of social media to promote health see Chapter 15, 'Virtual Settings for Health'. See Box 20.7 for tips on how to use social media to promote health.

BOX 20.7 TEN TIPS FOR USING SOCIAL MEDIA TO PROMOTE HEALTH

1. *Position your campaign as a cause.* Social media provides a platform to generate or gain people's interest and to engage them in something they feel strongly about.
2. *Know your social media platform and tailor accordingly.* For example, Facebook is used primarily for personal use whilst Twitter is mostly professional.
3. *Use a hashtag (#).* These will help you (and others) monitor and track campaign activity.
4. *Shareability.* Shareability is important so make it something that people will want to share. The more sharing, the greater the reach of the campaign.
5. *Use images.* Posts accompanied by photos or images are more successful.
6. *Use humour.* Use humour as appropriate - people use social media to converse, engage and have fun.
7. *Know your audience and post when they are most likely to engage.* For example, posting at a similar time each week can be a good strategy. Weekday evenings might be better if you're trying to reach parents whilst it's probably best to avoid before midday if you're trying to reach teenagers!
8. *Maintain a minimum level of activity.* It is useful to have a daily or weekly target to work to.
9. *Get others involved.* This can amplify your campaign. For example, other people can join in the conversation - tag them!
10. *Social media is just one branch of a tree.* It is best used as part of a comprehensive programme of activity, not as a standalone method.

Source: Zosel (2014), https://www.phaa.net.au/documents/item/430 reproduced by kind permission of Rebecca Zosel, Public Health Consultant, Melbourne, Australia

---

GO FURTHER 20.2

This chapter has provided an introduction to communication for health promotion. If you want to read something that is more critical and which provides a more in-depth discussion about the challenges of communicating for health, see R. Cross, S. Davis and I. O'Neil (2017) *Health communication: theoretical and critical perspectives.* Cambridge, Polity.

SUMMARY

This chapter has considered effective communication in health promotion. At the outset the point was made that communication is integral to promoting health. Indeed, it is very difficult to think of how health can be promoted without involving some element of communication. Communication happens at different levels and in different contexts and, in order to be effective, it needs to be tailored to the circumstances in which it is taking place. The role of the health promoter is therefore central, as is a clear notion of what is trying to be achieved. This chapter provides an overview of some of the key aspects of communication and some strategies for effectiveness. For more in-depth information see the suggestions for further reading that follow.

SUGGESTED READING

Corcoran, N. (ed.) (2013) *Communicating health: strategies for health promotion.* 2nd edn. London, Sage.

Cross, R., Davis, S. and O'Neil, I. (2017) *Health communication: theoretical and critical perspectives.* Cambridge, Polity.

O'Neil, I. (2019) *Digital health promotion: a critical introduction.* Cambridge, Polity.

REFERENCES

Abel, T. & McQueen, D. (2020) Critical health literacy and the COVID-19 crisis. *Health Promotion International*, https://doi.org/10.1093/heapro/daaa040.

Abelson, J., Forest, P.G., Eyles, J., Smith, P., Martin, E. & Gauvin, F.P. (2003) Deliberations about deliberative methods: issues in the design and evaluation of public participation processes. *Social Science & Medicine*, 57, 239–251.

Abdulmalik, J., Nwefoh, E., Obindo, J., Dakwak, S., Ayobola, M., Umaru, J., Samuel, E., Ogoshi, C. and Eaton, J. (2018) Emotional difficulties and experiences of stigma among persons with lymphatic filariasis in Plateau State, Nigeria. *Health & Human Rights*, 20, 27–40.

Abraham, C., Conner, M., Jones, F. and O'Connor, D. (2008) *Health Psychology*. London, Hodder Education.

Abrahams, N. and Gevers, A. (2017) A rapid appraisal of the status of mental health support in post-rape care services in the Western Cape. *South African Journal of Psychiatry*, 23, 959–968.

Abroms, L.C. and Lefebvre, R.C. (2009) Obama's wired campaign: lessons for public health communication. *Journal of Health Communication*, 14, 415–423.

Adams, C., Harder, B.M., Chatterjee, A. and Mathias, L.H. (2019) Healthworlds, cultural health toolkits, and choice: how acculturation affects patients' views of prescription drugs and prescription drug advertising. *Qualitative Health Research*, https://doi.org/10.1177.1049732319827282.

Adeloye, D., Thompson, J., Akanbi, M.A., Azuh, D., Samuel, V., Omoregbe, N. and Ayo, C.K. (2016) The burden of road traffic crashes, injuries and deaths in Africa: a systematic review and meta-analysis. *Bulletin of the World Health Organization*, 94, 510–521.

Age UK (n.d.) Healthy ageing evidence review. London, Age UK.

Ahn, J., Bivona, L. K. and DiScala, J. (2011) Social media access in K-12 schools: Intractable policy controversies in an evolving world. *Proceedings of the American Society for Information Science and Technology*, 48, 1–10.

Ajzen, I. (1988) The theory of planned behaviour. *Organizational Behavior and Human Decision Processes*, 50, 179–211.

Akter, S.F.U., Rani, M.F.A., Nordin, M.S., Ab Rahman, J., Aris, M. and Rathor, M.Y. (2012) Dementia: prevalence and risk factors. *International Review of Social Sciences and Humanities*, 2, 176–184.

Al-Qdah, T.A.K. and Lacroix, M. (2017) Syrian refugees in Jordan: Social workers use a Participatory Rapid Appraisal (PRA) methodology for needs assessment, human rights and community development. *International Social Work*, 60 (3), 614–627.

Allegrante, J.P. and Auld, M.E. (2019) Advancing the Promise of Digital Technology and Social Media to Promote Population Health. *Health Education and Behavior*, 46 (2), 5S–8S.

Allison, K.R. and Rootman, I. (1996) Scientific rigor and community participation in health promotion research: are they compatible? *Health Promotion International*, 11, 333–340.

Allmark, P. and Tod, A. (2006) How should public health professionals engage with lay epidemiology? *Journal of Medical Ethics*, 32 (8), 460–463.

Amuyunzu-Nyamongo, M., Jones, C. and McQueen, D. (2009) Repositioning health promotion in Africa. In M. Amuyunzu-Nyamongo and D. Nyamwaya (eds) *Evidence of health promotion effectiveness in Africa*. Nairobi, African Institute for Health.

Anderson, R.S., Nichter, M. and Risør, M.B. (2017) Introduction: sensations, symptoms and healthcare seeking. *Anthropology in Action*, 24 (1), 1–5.

Angner, E., Midge, N.R., Saag, K.G. and Allison, J.J. (2009) Health and happiness among older adults: a community-based study. *Journal of Health Psychology*, https://doi/org/10/1177/1359105309103570

Ansett, S. (2010) *Boundary spanner: the gatekeeper of innovation in partnerships* [Online]. Available: www.greenleaf-publishing.com/content/pdfs/af06anse.pdf [Accessed 27 May 2020].

Antonovsky, A. (1996) The salutogenic model as a theory to guide health promotion. *Health Promotion International*, 11, 11–18.

Arnstein, S. (1969) A ladder of citizen participation. *American Institute of Planners Journal*, 35, 216–224.

ASA (2013) Children and advertising on social media websites. London, Advertising Standards Authority.

Assefa, Y., Van Damme, W., Williams, O.D. and Hill, P.S. (2017) Successes and challenges of the millennium development goals in Ethiopia: lessons for the sustainable development goals. *BMJ Global Health*, 2 (2), doi: 10.1136/bmjgh-2017-000318

Australian Health Promotion Association (2009) *Core Competencies for Health Promotion Practitioners*. Australia, Queensland, Australian Health Promotion Association.

Aveyard, H. and Sharp, P. (2009) *A beginner's guide to evidence-based practice in health and social care*. London, McGraw-Hill Education.

Ayo, N. (2012) Understanding health promotion in a neoliberal climate and the making of health conscious citizens. *Critical Public Health*, 22, 99–105.

Babu, B.V., Hazra, R.K., Chhotary, G.P. and Satyanarayana, K. (2004) Knowledge and beliefs about elephantiasis and hydrocele of lymphatic filariasis and some socio-demographic determinants in an endemic community of Eastern India. *Public Health*, 118 (2), 121–127.

Bagnall, A.-M., Radley, D., Jones, R., Gately, P., Nobles, J., Van Dijk, M., Blackshaw, J., Montel, S. and Sahota, P. (2019) Whole systems approaches to obesity and other complex public health challenges: a systematic review. *BMC Public Health*, 19, 1–4.

Bagnall, A., Jones, R., Akhter, H. and Woodall, J. (2016) Report on evidence for interventions to prevent burnout in high risk individuals. London, Public Health England.

Baker, S.A. and Rojeck, C. (2019) The scandal that should force us to reconsider wellness advice from influencers. *The Conversation*. [Online] Available: https://theconversation. com/the-scandal-that-should-force-us-to-reconsider-wellness-advice-from-influencers-117041 [Accessed 22 July 2019].

Baldwin, L. (2020) Planning and implementing health promotion programs. In M. Fleming and L. Baldwin (eds) *Health promotion in the 21st century: new approaches for achieving health for all*. London, Allen & Unwin.

Barić, L. (1998) *People in settings*. Altrincham, Barns Publications.

Barić, L. (2000) Keynote speech: health education and promotion programmes – the accountability aspect. *Vaccine*, 18, S6–S9.

Barry, H. (2018) *Emotional resilience: how to safeguard your mental health*. London, Orion Spring.

Barry, M.M., Allegrante, J.P., Lamarre, M.-C., Auld, M.E. and Taub, A. (2009) The Galway Consensus Conference: international collaboration on the development of core competencies for health promotion and health education. *Global Health Promotion*, 16, 5–11.

Barry, M.M., Clarke, A.M., Jenkins, R. and Patel, V. (2013) A systematic review of the effectiveness of mental health promotion interventions for young people in low and middle income countries. *BMC Public Health*, 13, 835, 1–19.

Bartley, M. (2017) *Health inequality: an introduction to concepts, theories and methods*. Cambridge, Polity Press.

Battel-Kirk, B. and Barry, M.M. (2019) Implementation of health promotion competencies in Ireland and Italy – a case study. *International Journal of Environmental Research and Public Health*, 16 (24): 4992, 1–21. doi: 10.3390/ijerph16244992

Baum, F. (2003) *The new public health*. Melbourne, Oxford University Press.

Baum, F. and Fisher, M. (2014) Why behavioural health promotion endures despite its failure to reduce health inequities. *Sociology of Health & Illness*, 36, 213–225.

Baybutt, M., Hayton, P. and Dooris, M. (2010) Prisons in England and Wales: an important public health opportunity? In J. Douglas, S. Eearle, S. Handsley, L. Jones, C. Lloyd and S. Spurr (eds) *A reader in promoting public health: challenge and controversy*, 2nd edn. Milton Keynes: Open University Press.

Beattie, A. (1991) Knowledge and control in health promotion: a test case for social policy and social theory. In J. Gabe, M. Calnan and M. Bury (eds) *The sociology of the health service*. London, Routledge.

Belcher, J.M., Butler, T., Richmond, R.L., Wodak, A.D. and Wilhelm, K. (2006) Smoking and its correlates in an Australian prisoner population. *Drug and Alcohol Review*, 25, 343–348.

Bell, S. (2001) *LogFrames: Improved NRSP Research Project Planning and Monitoring*. Hemel Hampstead, DFID, NRSP.

Bell, K., Salmon, A. and McNaughton, D. (2011) Editorial: Alcohol, tobacco, obesity and the new public health. *Critical Public Health*, 21, 1–8.

Bellis, M.A., Hughes, K. and Lowey, H. (2002) Healthy nightclubs and recreational substance use: from a harm minimisation to a healthy settings approach. *Addictive Behaviors*, 27, 1025–1035.

Bennett, B.L., Goldstein, C.M., Gathright, E.C., Hughes, J.W. and Latner, J.D. (2017) Internal health locus of control predicts willingness to track health behaviors online and with smartphone applications. *Psychology, Health & Medicine*, 22 (10), 1224–1229.

Berkley-Patton, J., Thompson, C.B., Bradley-Ewing, A., Berman, M., Bauer, A., Catley, D., Goggin, K., Williams, E., Wainwright, C., Petty, T. and Aduloju-Ajijola, N. (2018) Identifying health conditions, priorities, and relevant multilevel health promotion strategies in African American churches: a faith community health needs assessment. *Evaluation and Program Planning*, 67, 19–28.

Bertotti, M., Frostick, C., Hutt, P., Sohanpal, R. and Carnes, D. (2018) A realist evaluation of social prescribing: an exploration into the context and mechanisms underpinning a pathway linking primary care with the voluntary sector. *Primary Health Care Research & Development*, 19 (3), 232–245.

Bhutta, Z.A., Atun, R., Ladher, N. and Abbasi, K. (2018) Alma Ata and primary healthcare: back to the future. *BMJ*, 363: k4433. doi: 10.1136/bmj.k4433

Bickerdike, L., Booth, A., Wilson, P.M., Farley, K. and Wright, K. (2017) Social prescribing: less rhetoric and more reality. A systematic review of the evidence. *BMJ Open*, 7, e013384.

Biddle, S. and Seymour, M. (2012) Healthy neighbourhoods and communities: policy and practice. In A. Scriven and M. Hodgins (eds) *Health promotion settings: principles and practice*. London, Sage.

Bird, Y., Lemstra, M. and Rogers, M. (2017) The effects of household income distribution on stroke prevalence and its risk factors of high blood pressure and smoking cross sectional study in Saskatchewan, Canada. *Perspectives in Public Health*, 137 (2), 114–121.

Birmingham, L., Wilson, S. and Adshead, G. (2006) Prison medicine: ethics and equivalence. *British Journal of Psychiatry*, 188, 4–6.

Bishop, F. and Yardley, L. (2010) The development and initial validation of a new measure of lay definitions of health: the wellness beliefs scale. *Psychology & Health*, 25 (3), 271–287.

Blaxter, M. (2004) *Health*. Cambridge, Polity Press.

Blaxter, M. (2010) *Health*, 2nd edn. Cambridge, Polity Press.

Bloch, P., Toft, U., Reinbach, H.C., Clausen, L.T., Mikkelsen, B.E., Poulsen, K. and Jensen, B.B. (2014) Revitalizing the setting approach – supersettings for sustainable impact in community health promotion. *International Journal of Behavioral Nutrition and Physical Activity*, 11, 118 1–15.

Bonita, R., Beaglehole, R. and Kjellström, T. (2006) *Basic Epidemiology*. 2nd edn. Geneva, WHO.

Bopp, M., Braun, J., Gutzwiller, F. and Faeh, D. (2012) Health risk or resource? Gradual and independent association between self-rated health and mortality persists over 30 years. *Plos ONE*, https://doi.org/10.1371/journal.pone.0030795

Bowden, J. (2017) Evaluation in health promotion. In J. Bowden and V. Manning (eds) *Health promotion in Midwifery: principles and practice*, 3rd edn. London, CRC Press.

Boyatzis, R. E. (1998) *Transforming qualitative information: thematic analysis and code development*. London, Sage.

Boydell, L. (2001) Partnership framework: a model for partnerships in health. Dublin: Institute of Public Health in Ireland.

Bradshaw, J. (1972) The concept of social need. *New Society*, 30 March.

Bramley, G., Fitzpatrick, S., Edwards, J., Ford, D., Johnsen, S., Sosenko, F. and Watkins, D. (2015) *Hard edges: mapping severe and multiple disadvantage*. London: Lankelly Chase.

Brandenburg, U. (2012) Volkswagen: a comprehensive approach to health promotion in the workplace. In A. Scriven and M. Hodgins (eds) *Health promotion settings: principles and practice*. London, Sage.

Braun, V. and Clarke, V. (2006) Using thematic analysis in psychology. *Qualitative Research in Psychology*, 3, 77–101.

Brende, B. and Hoie, B. (2015) Towards evidence-based, quantitative sustainable development goals for 2030. *The Lancet*, 385 (9964), 206–208.

Brine, S. (2019) Letter to Duncan Selbie, Chief Executive, Public Health England. 22 March. Available: https://assets/publishing.service.gov.uk/government [Accessed 7 July 2019].

Bringewatt, E.H. and Gershoff, E.T. (2010) Falling through the cracks: gaps and barriers in the mental health system for America's disadvantaged children. *Children and Youth Services Review*, 32, 1291–1299.

Brocklehurst, P.R., Morris, P. and Tickle, M. (2012) Social marketing: an appropriate strategy to reduce oral health inequalities? *International Journal of Health Promotion and Education*, 50 (2), 81–91.

Brownson, R.C., Fielding, J.E. and Maylahn, C.M. (2009) Evidence-based public health: a fundamental concept for public health practice. *Annual Review of Public Health*, 30, 175–201.

Buck, D. and Frosini, F. (2012) *Clustering of unhealthy behaviours over time: Implications for policy and practice*. London, The King's Fund.

Bunton, R. and Macdonald, G. (2004) *Health promotion: disciplines, diversity and developments*, 2nd edn. London, Routledge.

Burgess-Allen, J., Langlois, M. and Whittaker, P. (2006) The health needs of ex-prisoners, implications for successful resettlement: a qualitative study. *International Journal of Prisoner Health*, 2, 291–301.

Burns, D. (2014) How far we have come in the last 50 years in smoking attitudes and actions. *Annals of the American Thoracic Society*, 11 (2), doi:org/10.1513/AnnalsATS.201308-258PS

Caffrey, A., Pointer, C., Steward, D. and Vohra, S. (2018) The role of community health needs assessments in medicalizing poverty. *The Journal of Law, Medicine & Ethics*, 46, 615–621.

Calderwood, P.E. (2003) Toward a professional community for social justice. *Journal of Transformative Education*, 1, 301–320.

Caley, M.J., O'Leary, R.A., Fisher, R., Low-Choy, S., Johnson, S. and Mengersen, K. (2014) What is an expert? A systems perspective on expertise. *Ecology and Evolution*, 4, 231–242.

Callaghan, D. (2000) Promoting healthy behavior: how much freedom? Whose responsibility?, New York, Georgetown University Press.

Cameron, I. (2018) *Nobody left behind: good health and a strong economy. The annual report of the director of public health in Leeds 2017/18*. Leeds, Leeds City Council.

Capland, R. and Holland, R. (1990) Rethinking health education theory. *Health Education Journal*, 49 (1), 10–12.

Caraher, M., Dixon, P., Hayton, P., Carr-Hill, R., McGough, H. and Bird, L. (2002) Are health-promoting prisons an impossibility? Lessons from England and Wales. *Health Education*, 102, 219–229.

Carey, G., Malbon, E., Crammond, B., Pescud, M. and Baker, P. (2016) Can the sociology of social problems help us to understand and manage 'lifestyle drift'? *Health Promotion International*, doi: 10.1093/heapro/dav116, 1–7.

Carneiro, I. and Howard, N. (2011) *Introduction to epidemiology*, 2nd edn. Maidenhead, Open University Press.

Carstairs, C., Philpott, B. and Wilmshurst, S. (2019) *Be wise! Be healthy! Morality and citizenship in Canadian public health campaigns*. Toronto, UBC Press.

Carter, S., Cribb, A. and Allegrante, A. (2012) How to think about health promotion ethics. *Public Health Reviews*, 34 (1) doi: 10.1107/BF03391661

Carter, S.M. and Little, M. (2007) Justifying knowledge, justifying method, taking action: epistemologies, methodologies, and methods in qualitative research. *Qualitative Health Research*, 17, 1316–1328.

Catford, J. (2008) Food security, climate change and health promotion: opening up the streams not just helping out down stream. *Health Promotion International* 23, 105–108.

Catford, J. (2010) Implementing the Nairobi call to action: Africa's opportunity to light the way. *Health Promotion International*, 25 (1), 1–4.

Cattan, M., White, M., Bond, J. and Learmouth, A. (2002) Preventing social isolation and loneliness among older people: a systematic review of health promotion interventions. *Ageing & Society*, 25, 41–67.

Cattaruzza, M.S. and West, R. (2013) Why do doctors and medical students smoke when they know how harmful it is? *European Journal of Public Health*, 23 (2), 188–189.

Cavanagh, S. and Chadwick, K. (2005) Needs assessment. In W. Macdowell, C. Bonell and M. Davies (eds) *Health promotion practice*. Maidenhead, Open University Press.

Centre for Reviews and Dissemination (2009) Systematic reviews: CRD's guidance for undertaking reviews in healthcare. York, CRD.

Cheong, W.L., Mohan, D., Warren, N. and Reidpath, D.D. (2018) Multiple sclerosis in the Asia Pacific region: a systematic review of a neglected neurological disease. *Frontiers in Neurology*, 1–9.

Cherry, K. (2019) The five levels of Maslow's hierarchy of needs. [Online] Available: www.verywellmind.com [Accessed 29 June 2019].

Cheshire, J. (2012) Featured graphic. Lives on the line: mapping life expectancy along the London Tube network. *Environment and Planning A*, 44, 1525–1528.

Child, J. and Faulkner, D. (1998) *Strategies of cooperation: managing alliances, networks, and joint ventures*. Oxford, Oxford University Press.

Chirico, F. (2016) Spiritual well-being in the 21st century: it's time to revise the current WHO's health definition? *Journal of Health and Social Sciences*, 1 (1), 11–16.

Choi, Y. (2019) 'Are you a good female citizen?' Media discourses on self-governing represented in popular Korean weight-loss reality TV shows. *Sociological Research Online*, 24 (2), 154–166.

Chou, W.-Y.S., Prestin, A., Lyons, C. and Wen, K.-Y. (2013) Web 2.0 for health promotion: reviewing the current evidence. *American Journal of Public Health*, 103, e9–e18.

Christensen, K., Doblhammer, G., Rau, R. and Vaupel, J.W. (2009) Ageing populations: the challenges ahead. *The Lancet*, 374, 1196–1208.

Christensen, P. (2004) The health-promoting family: a conceptual framework for future research. *Social Science & Medicine*, 59, 377–387.

Christian, M.S., Evans, C.E.L., Nykjaer, C., Hancock, N. and Cade, J.E. (2014) Evaluation of the impact of a school gardening intervention on children's fruit and vegetable intake: a randomised controlled trial. *International Journal of Behavioral Nutrition and Physical Activity*, 11, 9, 1–15.

CLES (2016) Inspiring Change Manchester. Systems change report – phase 2. Manchester, CLES.

Cloninger, R.C. and Zohar, A.H. (2011) Personality and the perception of health and happiness. *Journal of Affective Disorders*, 128 (1–2), 24–32.

Cockerham, W.C. (2007) *Social causes of health and disease*. Cambridge, Polity Press.

Cockerham, W.C., Abel, T. and Luschen, G. (1993) Max Weber, formal rationality, and health lifestyles. *The Sociological Quarterly*, 34, 413–425.

Coffey, D., Gupta, A., Hathi, P., Khurana, N., Spears, D., Srivastav, N. and Vyas, S. (2014) Revealed preference for open defecation: evidence from a new survey in rural north India. *Economic & Political Weekly*, XLIX (38), 43–55.

Cohen, R.L., Bishai, D.M., Alfonso, Y.N., Kuruvilla, S. and Schweitzer, J. (2014) Post-2015 health goals: could country specific targets supplement global ones? *The Lancet, Global Health*, 2 (7), e373–e374.

Condon, L., Hek, G. and Harris, F. (2008) Choosing health in prison: prisoners' views on making healthy choices in English prisons. *Health Education Journal*, 67, 155–166.

Connor, M. and Norman, P. (2015) *Predicting and changing health behaviour: research and practice with social cognition models*, 3rd edn. Maidenhead, Open University Press.

Connor, M. and Norman, P. (2017) Health behaviour: Current issues and challenges. *Psychology & Health*, 32, 895–906.

Corcoran, N. (2011) *Working on health communication*. London, Sage.

Corcoran, N. (2013) *Communicating health: strategies for health promotion*, 2nd edn. London, Sage.

Cragg, L. (2006) Project planning and budgeting. In W. Macdowall, C. Bonell and M. Davies (eds) *Health promotion practice*. Maidenhead, Open University Press.

Crawford, R. (1980) Healthism and the medicalization of everyday life. *International Journal of Health Services*, 10, 365–388.

Cribb, A. and Duncan, P. (2002) *Health promotion and professional ethics*. London, Blackwell.

Crichton, N. and Mulhall, A. (2015) Epidemiology and health. In J. Naidoo and J. Wills (eds) *Health studies: an introduction*. London: Palgrave Macmillan.

Cross, R. (2010) Health promotion theory: models and approaches. In D. Whitehead and F. Irvine (eds) *Health promotion & education in Nursing*. Basingstoke, Palgrave Macmillan.

Cross, R. (2013) The social construction of risk: young women and health. PhD thesis. Leeds, Leeds Metropolitan University.

Cross, R. (2020) Understanding the importance of concepts of health. *Nursing Standard*, doi: 107748/ns.2020.e11539

Cross, R., Davis, S. and O'Neil, I. (2017) *Health communication: theoretical and critical perspectives*. Cambridge, Polity.

Cross, R., Rowlands, S. and Foster, S. (2021) Foundations of health promotion. In R. Cross, L. Warwick-Booth, S. Rowlands, J. Woodall, I. O'Neil and S. Foster (eds) *Health promotion: global principles and practice*, 2nd edn. London, CABI.

Cross, R. and Warwick-Booth, L. (2016) Using storyboards in participatory research. *Nurse Researcher*, 23, 8–12.

Cross, R., Warwick-Booth, L. and Foster, S. (2021) Towards the future of health promotion. In R. Cross, L. Warwick-Booth, S. Rowlands, J. Woodall, I. O'Neil and S. Foster (eds) *Health promotion: global principles and practice*, 2nd edn. London, CABI.

Cuartas Ricaurte, J., Karim, L.L., Martínez Botero, M.A. and Hessel, P. (2019) The invisible wounds of five decades of armed conflict: inequalities in mental health and their determinants in Colombia. *International Journal of Public Health*, 64, 703–711.

Dahlgren, G. and Whitehead, M. (1991) Policies and strategies to promote social equity in health. Stockholm: Institute for Futures Studies.

David, L. (2019) Social Learning Theory (Bandura). *Learning theories*. Available: www.learning-theories.com/social-learning-theory-bandura [Accessed 4 November 2019].

Davies, J.K. (2013) Health promotion: a unique discipline? Auckland, Health promotion forum of New Zealand.

Davison, C. and Davey Smith, G. (1995) The baby and the bath water: examining socio-cultural and free-market critiques of health promotion. In R. Bunton, S. Nettleton and R. Burrows (eds) *The sociology of health promotion*. London, Routledge.

De Jong, N., Collins, A. and Plüg, S. (2019) 'To be healthy to me is to be free': How discourses of freedom are used to construct healthiness among young South African Adults. *International Journal of Qualitative Studies on Health and Well-Being*, 14, 1603518 doi: 10.1080/17482631.2019.1602518

de Leeuw, E., Crimeen, A., Freestone, R., Jalaludin, B., Sainsbury, P., Hirono, K. and Reid, A. (2018) Healthy airports. Sydney: Centre for Health Equity Training, Research and Evaluation (CHETRE), University of New South Wales.

de Viggiani, N. (2006) A new approach to prison public health? Challenging and advancing the agenda for prison health. *Critical Public Health*, 16, 307–316.

Deehan, A. and Wylie, A. (2010) Health promotion: the challenges, the questions of definition, discipline status and evidence base. In A. Wylie, T. Holt and A. Howe (eds) *Health promotion in medical education: from rhetoric to action*. Oxford, Radcliffe Publishing.

Department of Health (2002) *Health promoting prisons: a shared approach*. London, Crown.

Deribe, K., Beng, A.A., Cano, J., Njouendo, A.J., Fur-Cho, J., Awah, A.R. (2018) Mapping the geographical distribution of podoconiosis in Cameroon using parasitological, serological, and clinical evidence to exclude other causes of lymphedema. *PLOS Neglected Tropical Diseases*, 12 (1) https://doi.org/10.1371/journal.pntd.0006126

Dewi, T.K., Massar, K., Ruiter, R.A.C. and Leonardi, T. (2019) Determinants of breast self-examination practice among women in Surabaya, Indonesia: an application of the health belief model. *BMC Public Health*, 19, 1581, 1 –8. https://doi.org/10.1186/s12889-019-7951-2

Diepeveen, S., Ling, T., Suhrcke, M., Roland, M. and Marteau, T. M. (2013) Public acceptability of government intervention to change health-related behaviours: a systematic review and narrative synthesis. *BMC Public Health*, 13, 756.1 –11.

Dignan, M.B. and Carr, P.A. (1992) *Program planning for health* (2nd edn). Malvern, PA, Lee & Febiger.

Dixey, R. (2013) Towards the future of health promotion. In R. Dixey (ed.) *Health promotion: global principles and practice*. London, CABI.

Dixey, R., Cross, R., Foster, S. and Woodall, J. (2013) Foundations of health promotion. In R. Dixey (ed.) *Health promotion: global principles and practice*. London: CABI.

Dixey, R., Nyambe, S., Foster, S., Woodall, J. and Baybutt, M. (2015) Health promoting prisons – An impossibility for women prisoners in Africa? *Agenda*, 29 (4) 1–8.

Dixey, R., Woodall, J. and Lowcock, D. (2013) Practising health promotion. In R. Dixey (ed.) *Health promotion: global principles and practice*. London, CABI.

Dobbinson, S.J., Hayman, J.A. and Livingston, P.M. (2006) Prevalence of health promotion policies in sports clubs in Victoria, Australia. *Health Promotion International*, 21, 121–129.

Dorling, H., Blervacq, J. and Gidron, Y. (2018) Effects of psychological inoculation versus health education on physical activity: two randomized controlled studies. *Journal of Physical Activity and Health*, 15, 295–302.

Donnelly, P. (2003) Sport and social theory. In B. Houlihan (ed.) *Sport and society*. London, Sage.

Dooris, M. (2001) The 'Health Promoting University': a critical exploration of theory and practice. *Health Education*, 101, 51–60.

Dooris, M. (2004) Joining up settings for health: a valuable investment for strategic partnerships? *Critical Public Health*, 14, 37–49.

Dooris, M. (2005) Healthy settings: challenges to generating evidence of effectiveness. *Health Promotion International*, 21, 55–65.

Dooris, M. (2006) Health promoting settings: future directions. *Promotion & Education*, 13, 4–6.

Dooris, M. (2007) Healthy settings: past, present and future. Unpublished PhD thesis. Deakin University, Geelong.

Dooris, M. (2013) Expert voices for change: Bridging the silos – towards healthy and sustainable settings for the 21st century. *Health & Place*, 20, 39–50.

Dooris, M. and Hunter, D.J. (2007) Organisations and settings for promoting public health. In C.E. Lloyd, S. Handsley, J. Douglas, S. Earle and S. Spurr (eds) *Policy and practice in promoting public health*. London, Sage.

Dooris, M., Poland, B., Kolbe, L., Leeuw, E.D., McCall, D. and Wharf-Higgins, J. (2007) Healthy settings. Building evidence for the effectiveness of whole system health promotion – challenges and future directions. In D.V. McQueen and C.M. Jones (eds) *Global perspectives on health promotion effectiveness*. New York, Springer.

Dooris, M. and Thompson, J. (2001) Health-promoting universities: an overview. In A. Scriven and J. Orme (eds) *Health promotion: professional perspectives*, 2nd edn. London, Palgrave.

Downie, R.S., Tannahill, C. and Tannahill, A. (1996) *Health promotion: models and values*. Oxford, Oxford University Press.

Dreyfus, S.E. (2004) The five-stage model of adult skill acquisition. *Bulletin of Science, Technology & Society*, 24: 177 doi: 10.1177/0270467604264992.

Duncan, P. (2004) Dispute, dissent and the place of health promotion in a 'disrupted tradition' of health improvement. *Public Understanding of Science*, 13, 177–190.

Duncan, P. (2013) Failing to professionalise, struggling to specialise: the rise and fall of health promotion as a putative specialism in England, 1980–2000. *Medical History*, 57 (3), 377–396.

El Achhab, Y., El Ammari, A., El Kazdouh, H., Najdi, A., Berraho, M., Tachfouti, N., Lamri, D., El Fakir, S. and Nejjari, C. (2016) Health risk behaviours amongst school adolescents: protocol for a mixed methods study. *BMC Public Health, 16*, doi: 10.1186/s12889-016-3873-4

Estacio, E., Oliver, M., Downing, B., Kurth, J. and Protheroe, J. (2017) Effective partnership in community-based health promotion: lessons from the health literacy partnership. *International Journal of Environmental Research and Public Health*, 14, 1550, 1–8.

EuroHealthNet (n.d.) Making the link: gender equality and health. Brussels, EC.

Evandrou, M., Falkingham, J., Feng, Z. and Vlachantoni, A. (2016) Ethnic inequalities in limiting health and self-reported health in later life revisited. *Journal of Epidemiology and Community Health*, 70, 653–662.

Evans, D., Coutsaftiki, D. and Fathers, C.P. (2017) *Health promotion and public health for nursing students*, 3rd edn. London, Sage.

Evans, J.M., Connelly, J., Jepson, R., Gray, C., Shepherd, A. and Mackison, D. (2018) A physical activity intervention in a Bingo club: significance of the setting. *Health Education Journal*, 77, 377–384.

Farrell, M. and Marsden, J. (2008) Acute risk of drug related death among newly released prisoners in England and Wales. *Addiction*, 103, 251–255.

Fawkes, S., Fudge, C. and Engelhardt, K. (2012) Healthy cities: comprehensive solutions to urban health improvement. In A. Scriven and M. Hodgins (eds) *Health promotion settings: principles and practice*. London, Sage.

Ferrer, R.A. and Mendes, W.B. (2018) Emotion, health decision-making, and health behaviour. *Psychology & Health*, 33 (1), 1–16.

Finn, H.E. and Watson, R.A. (2017) The use of health coaching to improve health outcomes: implications for applied behavior Analysis. *Psychological Record*, 67, 181–187.

Fisher, B. J. and Gosselink, C. A. (2008) Enhancing the Efficacy and Empowerment of Older Adults Through Group Formation. *Journal of Gerontological Social Work*, 51, 1–2.

Fisher, J.W., Francis, L.J. and Johnson, P. (2000) Assessing spiritual health via four domains of spiritual wellbeing: the SH4DI. *Pastoral Psychology*, 49 (2), 133–145.

Fitzgerald, F.T. (1994) The tyranny of health. *The New England Journal of Medicine*, 3, 196–198.

Fitzpatrick, M. (2001) *The tyranny of health*. London, Routledge.

Fletcher, D. and Mustafa, S. (2013) Psychological resilience: a review and critique of definitions, concepts, and theory. *European Psychological*, 18 (1), 12–23.

Fogle, B. and Fogle, M. (2018) *Up: my life's journey to the top of Everest*. London, William Collins.

Forrest, S. (2015) Peer education. In W. Nutland and L. Cragg (eds) *Health promotion practice*, 2nd edn. Maidenhead, Open University Press.

Freeman, B. and Chapman, S. (2007) Is 'YouTube' telling or selling you something? Tobacco content on the YouTube video-sharing website. *Tobacco Control*, 16, 207–210.

Fried, J., Harris, B., Eyles, J. and Moshabela, M. (2015) Acceptable care? Illness constructions, healthworlds, and accessible chronic treatment in South Africa. *Qualitative Health Research*, 25 (5), 622–635.

Gardner, B., Lally, P. and Wardle, J. (2012) Making health habitual: the psychology of 'habit-formation' and general practice. *British Journal of General Practice*, 62 (605), 664–666.

Garthwaite, K. and Bambra, C. (2017) 'How the other half live': lay perspectives on health inequality in an age of austerity. *Social Science and Medicine*, 187, 268–275.

Gately, C., Bowen, A., Kennedy, A., MacDonald, W. and Rogers, A. (2006) Prisoner perspectives on managing long term conditions: a qualitative study. *International Journal of Prisoner Health* 2, 91–99.

Gatherer, A. and Møller, L. (2009) Social justice, public health and the vulnerable: health in prisons raises key public health issues. *Public Health*, 123, 407–409.

Gatherer, A., Møller, L. and Hayton, P. (2005) The World Health Organization European health in prisons project after 10 years: persistent barriers and achievements. *American Journal of Public Health*, 95, 1696–700.

Gebremariam, B., Hagos, G. and Abay, M. (2018) Assessment of community led total sanitation and hygiene approach on improvement of latrine utilization in Laelay Maichew District, North Ethiopia. A comparative cross-sectional study. *PLOS ONE*, 13 (9): e0203458

Geeraert, N. (2018) How knowledge about different cultures is shaking the foundations of psychology. *The Conversation*. [Online] Available: https://theconversation.com [Accessed 22 July 2019].

Germond, P. and Cochrane, J. (2010) Healthworlds: conceptualising landscapes of health & healing. *Sociology*, 44, 307–324.

Gertler, P., Shah, M., Alzua, M.L., Cameron, L., Martinez, S. and Patil, S. (2015) How does health promotion work? Evidence from the dirty business of eliminating open defecation. NBER Working Paper No. 20997. JEL No. I12.I15.O15. Available: www.nber.org/papers/w20997.pdf [Accessed 7 March 2020].

Gill, R. (2008) Body talk: negotiating body image and masculinity. In S. Riley, M. Burns, H. Frith, S. Wiggins and P. Markula (eds) *Critical bodies: representations, identities and practices of body management*. Basingstoke, Palgrave Macmillan.

Gill, R. and Scharff, C. (2011) Introduction. In R. Gill and C. Scharff (eds) *New femininities: postfeminism, neoliberalism and subjectivity*. Basingstoke, Palgrave Macmillan.

Glouberman, S. and Millar, J. (2003) Evolution of the determinants of health, health policy, and health information systems in Canada. *American Journal of Public Health*, 93 (3), 388–392.

Glover, M. and Kira, A. (2011) Why Māori women continue to smoke while pregnant. *The New Zealand Medical Journal*, 124 (1339), 22–31.

Godderis, R. (2006) Food for thought: an analysis of power and identity in prison food narratives. *Berkeley Journal of Sociology*, 50, 61–75.

Gold, J., Pedrana, A.E., Sacks-Davis, R., Hellard, M.E., Chang, S., Howard, S., Keogh, L., Hocking, J.S. and Stoove, M.A. (2011) A systematic examination of the use of online social networking sites for sexual health promotion. *BMC Public Health*, 11, 583, 1–9.

Goldberg, D.P., Gater, R., Sartorius, N., Ustun, T.B., Piccinelli, M., Gureje, O. and Rutter, C. (1997) The validity of two versions of the GHQ in the WHO study of mental illness in general health care. *Psychological Medicine*. 27(1), 191–197.

Golden, S.D. and Earp, J.L. (2012) Socio ecological approaches to individuals and their contexts: twenty years of health education & behavior health promotion interventions. *Health Education & Behavior*, 39 (3), 364–372.

Golombok, S. (2015) *Modern families: parents and children in new family forms*. Cambridge, Cambridge University Press.

Good, M.J. and Hannah, S.D. (2015) 'Shattering culture': perspectives on cultural competence and evidence-based practice in mental health services. *Transcultural Psychiatry*, 52 (2), 198–221.

Goodman-Brown, J. (2012) Developing self-awareness. In M. Gottwald and J.A. Goodman-Brown, *A guide to practical health promotion*. Maidenhead, Open University Press, pp. 89–110.

Gopalkrishnan, N. (2018) Cultural diversity and mental health: considerations for policy and practice. *Frontiers in Public Health*, 6, doi: 10.3389/fpubh.2018.00179

Gordis, L. (2013) *Epidemiology*, 5th edn. London, Elsevier.

Gostin, L. O. (2017) 2016: the year of the soda tax. *The Milbank Quarterly*, 95(1), 19–23.

Gottwald, M. (2012) Developing skills. In M. Gottwald and J. Goodman-Brown, *A guide to practical health promotion*. Maidenhead, Open University Press.

Gottwald, M. and Goodman-Brown, J. (2012) An introduction to why health promotion is important. In M. Gottwald and J. Goodman-Brown, *A guide to practical health promotion*. Maidenhead, Open University Press.

Gover, A.R., MacKenzie, D.L. and Armstrong, G.S. (2000) Importation and deprivation explanations of juveniles' adjustment to correctional facilities. *International Journal of Offender Therapy and Comparative Criminology*, 44, 450–467.

Graham, H. (2007) *Unequal lives: health and socioeconomic inequalities*. London, McGraw-Hill Education.

Grant, A.M., Christianson, M.K. and Price, R.H. (2007) Happiness, health, or relationships? Managerial practices and employee well-being trade-offs. *Academy of Management Perspectives*, August, 51–63.

Green, J. (2004a) Health promotion – surviving in interesting times: Inaugural Lecture 18th May 2004. *International Journal of Health Promotion and Education*, 42, 68–77.

Green, J. (2004b) The power to choose. *Promotion & Education*, 11, 2–3.

Green, J. (2008) Health education – the case for rehabilitation. *Critical Public Health*, 18, 447–456.

Green, J., Ayrton, R., Woodall, J., Woodward, J., Newell, C., Cattan, M. and R.C. (2007) Child parent interaction in relation to road safety education. London, Department for Transport.

Green, J., Cross, R., Woodall, J. and Tones, K. (2019) *Health promotion: planning and strategies*, 4th edn. London, Sage.

Green, J. and South, J. (2006) *Evaluation*. Maidenhead, Open University Press.

Green, J., Steinbach, R. and Datta, J. (2012) The travelling citizen: emergent discourses of moral mobility in a study of cycling in London. *Sociology*, 46, 272–289.

Green, J. and Tones, K. (1999) Towards a secure evidence base for health promotion. *Journal of Public Health Medicine*, 21, 133–139.

Green, J., Tones, K., Cross, R. and Woodall, J. (2015) *Health promotion: planning and strategies*, 3rd edn. London, Sage.

Green, L.W., Poland, B.D. and Rootman, I. (2000) The settings approach to health promotion. In B.D. Poland, L.W. Green and I. Rootman (eds) *Settings for health promotion: linking theory and practice*. Thousand Oaks, CA, Sage.

Green, L.W. and Raeburn, J.M. (1988) Health promotion. What is it? What will it become? *Health Promotion*, 3, 151–159.

Greenhalgh, T. and Taylor, R. (1997) How to read a paper: papers that go beyond numbers (qualitative research). *BMJ*, 315, 740–743.

Gregg, J. and O'Hara, L. (2007a) The Red Lotus Health Promotion Model: a new model for holistic, ecological, salutogenic health promotion practice. *Health Promotion Journal of Australia*, 18 (1), 9–12.

Gregg, J. and O'Hara, L. (2007b) Values and principles evident in current health promotion practice. *Health Promotion Journal of Australia*, 18, 7–11.

Groff, P. and Goldberg, S. (2000) *Towards a new perspective on health policy*. Canada, Health Network.

Groot, E. (2011) Use of evidence in WHO health promotion declarations: overview, critical analysis, and personal reflection. *Reflective Practice*, 12, 507–513.

Grunseit, A.C., Rowbotham, S., Crane, M., Indig, D., Bauman, A.E. and Wilson, A. (2019) Nanny or canny? Community perceptions of government intervention for preventive health. *Critical Public Health*, 29, 274–289.

Gu, J., Strauss, C., Bond, R. and Cavanagh, K. (2015) How do mindfulness-based cognitive therapy and mindfulness-based reduction improve mental health and wellbeing? A systematic review and meta-analysis of mediation studies. *Clinical Psychology Review*, 37, 1–12.

Gustafson, T. (2011) *The civic duty to maintain health*. [Online] Available: www.citizenthink.net [Accessed 31 August 2020].

Hancock, T., Capon, A., Dooris, M. and Patrick, R. (2017) One planet regions: planetary health at the local level. *The Lancet Planetary Health*, 1, e92–e93.

Hann, A. and Peckham, S. (2010) Avoiding mixed messages: HPV vaccines and the 'cure' for cervical cancer. In S. Peckham and A. Hann, *Public health ethics and practice*. Bristol, Policy Press.

Hanson, A. (2007) *Workplace health promotion: a salutogenic approach*. Milton Keynes, Author-house.

Hardcastle, S.J., Hancox, J., Hatter, A. Maxwell-Smith, C., Thøgersen-Ntoumani, C. and Hagger, S. (2015) Motivating the unmotivated: how can health behaviour be changed in those unwilling to change? *Frontiers in Psychology*. 6, 835. 1 – 4. doi: 10.3389/fpsyg.2015.00835

Hardy, B., Hudson, B. and Waddington, E. (2000) *What makes a good partnership? A partnership assessment tool*. Leeds, Nuffield Institute for Health.

Harper, C.R., Steiner, R.J. and Brookmeyer, K.A. (2018) Using the social-ecological model to improve access to care for adolescents and young adults. *Journal of Adolescent Health*, 62, 641–642.

Hawkins, B. and McCambridge, J. (2020) Policy windows and multiple streams: an analysis of alcohol pricing policy in England. *Policy & Politics*, 48, 315–333.

Hayton, P., Caraher, M. and Harrison, D. (2000) Health promotion needs assessment for the Devon prisons cluster. Report to the Peninsular Health Authority, Devon.

Health Promotion Canada (2015) *The Pan-Canadian health promoter competencies and glossary*. Canada, Health Promotion Canada.

Health Promotion Forum of New Zealand (2012) Health promotion competencies for Aotearoa. Auckland, Health Promotion Forum of New Zealand.

Hechanova, R. and Waelde, L. (2017) The influence of culture on disaster mental health and psychosocial support interventions in Southeast Asia. *Mental Health, Religion & Culture*, 20, 31–44.

Heenan, D. (2004) A partnership approach to health promotion: a case study from Northern Ireland. *Health Promotion International*, 19, 105–113.

Hermens, N., Verkooijen, K. T. and Koelen, M. A. (2019) Associations between partnership characteristics and perceived success in Dutch sport-for-health partnerships. *Sport Management Review*, 22, 142–152.

Herrman, H., Stewart, D.E. and Diaz-Granados, N. (2011) What is resilience? *The Canadian Journal of Psychiatry*, doi:org/10.1177/070674371105600504

Hesman, A. (2014) Using health information and epidemiology. In J. Wills (ed.) *Fundamentals of health promotion for nurses*, 2nd edn. Oxford, Wiley.

Hill, A., Balanda, K., Galbraith, L., Greenacre, J. and Sinclair, D. (2010) Profiling health in the UK and Ireland. *Public Health*, 124 (5), 253–258.

HM Prison Service (2003) Prison Service Order (PSO) 3200 on health promotion. London, HM Prison Service.

Hobbs, M., Griffiths, C., Green, M.A., Jordan, H., Saunders, J. and McKenna, J. (2018) Associations between the combined physical activity environment, socioeconomic status, and obesity: a cross-sectional study. *Perspectives in Public Health*, 138 (3), 169–172.

Hobbs, M., Duncan, M.J., Collins, P., Mckenna, J., Schoeppe, S., Rebar, A.L., Alley, S., Short, C. and Vandelanotte, C. (2019) Clusters of health behaviours in Queensland adults are associated with different socio-demographic characteristics. *Journal of Public Health*, 41 (2), 268–277.

Hopper, E. (2019) Maslow's hierarchy of needs explained. [Online] Available: www.thoughtco.com [Accessed 29 June 2019].

Horton, R. (2014) Offline: why the sustainable development goals will fail. *The Lancet*, 383, 577–578.

Hsaio, Y., Chen, L., Whu, L., Chang, C. and Huang, S. (2010) Spiritual health, clinical practice stress, depressive tendency and health-promoting behaviours among student nurses. *Journal of Advanced Nursing*, 66 (7), 1612–1622.

Hu, S.C. and Kuo, H.-W. (2016) The development and achievement of a healthy cities network in Taiwan: sharing leadership and partnership building. *Global Health Promotion*, 23, 8–17.

Huber, M. (2011) How should we define health? *British Medical Journal, 343*, doi: https://doi.org/10.1136/bmj.d4163

Hubley, J. (2004) *Communicating health: an action guide to health education and health promotion*, 2nd edn. Oxford, Macmillan.

Hubley, J., Copeman, J. and Woodall, J. (2013) *Practical health promotion*. Cambridge, Polity Press.

Hubley, J., Copeman, J. and Woodall, J. (2021) *Practical health promotion*. Cambridge, Polity Press.

Huybregts, L., Becquey, E., Zongrone, A., Le Port, A., Khassanova, R., Coulibaly, L., Leroy, J.L., Rawat, R. and Ruel, M.T. (2017) The impact of integrated prevention and treatment on child malnutrition and health: the PROMIS project, a randomized control trial in Burkina Faso and Mali. *BMC Public Health*, 17: 237 doi: 10/1186/s12889-017-4146-6

Iacobucci, G. (2019) Life expectancy gap between rich and poor in England widens. *BMJ*, 364, l1492.

Iglehart, J. K. (1990) From the editor. *Health Affairs*, 9, 4–5.

International Institute for Global Health (2018) People, planet and participation: the Kuching statement on healthy, just and sustainable urban development. *Health Promotion International*, 33, 149–151.

Issel, L.M. (2014) *Health program planning and evaluation: a practical, systematic approach for community health*. 3rd edn. Burlington, MA, Jones & Bartlett Learning.

IUHPE (2016) Core competencies and professional standards for health promotion. International Union of Health Promotion and Education. Available: www.ukphr.org.

IUHPE (2018) Mission [Online]. Available: www.iuhpe.org/index.php/en/iuhpe-at-a-glance/mission [Accessed 12 February 2019].

Jaberi, A., Momennsab, M., Yetatalab, S., Ebadi, A. and Cheraghi, M.A. (2017) Spiritual health: a concept analysis. *Journal of Religion and Health*, doi:10.1007/s10942-017-0379-z

Jané-Llopis, E. and Barry, M.M. (2005) What makes mental health promotion effective? *Promotion & Education*, 12, 47–54.

Janz, N.K. and Becker, M.H. (1984) The health belief model: a decade later. *Health Education Quarterly*, 11, 1–47.

Jochelson, K. (2006) Nanny or steward? The role of government in public health. *Public Health*, 120, 1149–1155.

Johnson, A. and Baum, F. (2001) Health promoting hospitals: a typology of different organizational approaches to health promotion. *Health Promotion International*, 16, 281–287.

Johnson, D., Deterding, S., Kuhn, K., Staneva, A., Stoyanov, S. and Hides, S. (2016) Gamification for health and wellbeing: a systematic review of the literature. *Internet Interventions*, 6, 89–106.

Jones, J. and Barry, M.M. (2011) Exploring the relationship between synergy and partnership functioning factors in health promotion partnerships. *Health Promotion International*, 26, 408–420.

Jones, J. and Barry, M. M. (2018) Factors influencing trust and mistrust in health promotion partnerships. *Global Health Promotion*, 25, 16–24.

Kelly, M. P. and Barker, M. (2016) Why is changing health-related behaviour so difficult? *Public Health*, 136, 109–116.

Kelly, M. P. and Charlton, B. (1995) The modern and postmodern in health promotion. In R. Bunton, S. Nettleton and R. Burrows (eds) *The sociology of health promotion*. London, Routledge.

Kendall, J.M. (2003) Designing a research project: randomised controlled trials and their principles. *Emergency Medicine Journal*, 20, 164–168.

Khami, S., Moghaddam-Banaem, L., Mohamadi, E., Vedadhir, A.A. and Hajizadeh, E. (2018) Women's sexual and reproductive health care needs assessment: an Iranian perspective. *Eastern Mediterranean Health Journal*, 24 (7), 637–643.

Kickbusch, I. (1986) Issues in health promotion. *Health Promotion*, 1, 437–442.

Kilgarriff-Foster, A. and O'Cathain, A. (2015) Exploring the components and impact of social prescribing. *Journal of Public Mental Health*, 14, 127–134.

Koelen, M. A., Vaandrager, L. and Colomér, C. (2001) Health promotion research: dilemmas and challenges. *Journal of Epidemiology and Community Health*, 55, 257–262.

Kokko, S., Donaldson, A., Geidne, S., Seghers, J., Scheerder, J., Meganck, J., Lane, A., Kelly, B., Casey, M. and Eime, R. (2016) Piecing the puzzle together: case studies of international research in health-promoting sports clubs. *Global Health Promotion*, 23, 75–84.

Kokko, S., Green, L.W. and Kannas, L. (2014) A review of settings-based health promotion with applications to sports clubs. *Health Promotion International*, 29, 494–509.

Korda, H. and Itani, Z. (2013) Harnessing social media for health promotion and behavior change. *Health promotion practice*, 14, 15–23.

Korp, P. (2006) Health on the Internet: implications for health promotion. *Health Education Research*, 21, 78–86.

Korp, P. (2008) The symbolic power of 'healthy lifestyles'. *Health Sociology Review*, 1, 18–26.

Kubheka, B.Z., Carter, V. and Mwaura, J. (2020) Social media health promotion in South Africa: opportunities and challenges. *African Journal of Primary Health Care & Family Medicine*, 12, 2389.

Kumar, S. and Preetha, G. (2012) Health promotion: an effective tool for global health. *Indian Journal of Community Medicine*, 37, 5–12.

Kyoko, Y., Shiomi, M., Katayama, T., Hosoya, N. and Mariko, K. (2019) Effectiveness of an educational program for mid-level Japanese public health nurses to improve program planning competencies: a preliminary randomized control trial. *Public Health Nursing*, 36 (3), 388–400.

Lahtinen, E., Koskinen-Ollonqvist, P., Rouvinen-Wilenius, P., Tuominen, P. and Mittelmark, M.B. (2005) The development of quality criteria for research: a Finnish approach. *Health Promotion International*, 20, 306–315.

Lakerfeld, J. and Mackenbach, J. (2017) The upstream determinants of health. *Obesity Facts*, 10, 216–222.

Lalonde, M. (1974) A new perspective on the health of Canadians. Ottawa, Ministry of National Health and Welfare.

Lalot, F., Quiamzade, A. and Zerhouni, O. (2019) Regulatory focus and self-determination motives interact to predict students' nutrition-habit intentions. *Journal of Experimental Psychology: Applied*, 25 (3), 477–490.

Lane, A., Murphy, N., Donohoe, A. and Regan, C. (2017) Health promotion orientation of GAA sports clubs in Ireland. *Sport in Society*, 20, 235–243.

Laverack, G. (2004) *Health promotion practice: power and empowerment*. London, Sage.

Laverack, G. (2005) *Public health: Power, empowerment and professional practice*. Basingstoke, Palgrave.

Laverack, G. (2006) Improving health outcomes through community empowerment: a review of the literature. *Journal of Health, Population and Nutrition*, 24, 113–120.

Laverack, G. (2007) *Health promotion practice: building empowered communities*. Maidenhead, Open University Press.

Laverack, G. (2012) Where are the champions of global health promotion? *Global Health Promotion*, 19, 63–65.

Laverack, G. (2014a) *A–Z of health promotion*. Basingstoke, Palgrave Macmillan.

Laverack, G. (2014b) *The pocket guide to health promotion*. Maidenhead, Open University Press.

Laverack, G. (2017) *Health promotion in disease outbreaks and health emergencies*. London, CRC Press.

Laverack, G. and Manoncourt, E. (2016) Key experiences of community engagement and social mobilization in the Ebola response. *Global Health Promotion*, 23, 79–82.

Ledger, D. (2014) *Inside wearables – Part 2*, Cambridge MA, Endeavour Partners LLC.

Lee, M., Lee, H., Kim, Y., Kim, J., Cho, M., Jang, J. and Jang, H. (2018) Mobile app-based health promotion programs: a systematic review of the literature. *International Journal of Environmental Research and Public Health*, 15, 1–13.

Lester, C., Hamilton-Kirkwood, L. and Jones, N.K. (2003) Health indicators in a prison population: asking prisoners. *Health Education Journal*, 62, 341–349.

Levy, M. (2007) International public health and corrections: models of care and harm minimization. In R.B. Greifinger (ed.) *Public health behind bars: from prisons to communities*. New York: Springer.

Lidén, J. (2014) The World Health Organization and global health governance: post-1990. *Public Health*, 128, 141–147.

Lines, R. (2006) From equivalence of standards to equivalence of objectives: the entitlement of prisoners to health care standards higher than those outside prisons. *International Journal of Prisoner Health*, 2, 269–280.

Linsley, P. and Roll, C. (2020) *Health promotion for nursing students*. London, Sage.

Lookian, F., Ghadrdan, E. and Mousavi, M. (2019) Assessment of knowledge, attitude, and practice in the general population regarding hypertension: a cross-sectional study from Iran. *Journal of Pharmaceutical Care*, 6 (3–4), 62–67.

Loss, J., Lindacher, V. and Curbach, J. (2014) Online social networking sites – a novel setting for health promotion? *Health & Place*, 26, 161–170.

Lovatt, M., Eadie, D., Meier, P.S., Li, J., Bauld, L., Hastings, G. and Holmes, J. (2015) Lay epidemiology and the interpretation of low-risk drinking guidelines by adults in the United Kingdom. *Addiction*, 110 (12), 1912–1919.

Lowcock, D. and Cross, R.M. (2011) Health and health promotion. In P. Jones and G. Walker (eds) *Children's Rights in Practice*. London, Sage.

Lowenberg, J.S. (1995) Health promotion and the 'ideology of choice'. *Public Health Nursing*, 12, 319–323.

Lunyera, J., Kirenga, B., Stanifer, J.W., Kasozi, S., van der Molen, T., Katagira, W., Kamya, M.R. and Kalyesubula, R. (2018) Geographic differences in the prevalence of hypertension in Uganda: results of a national epidemiological study. *PloS One*, 13, e0201001.

Lupton, D. (1995) *The imperative of health: public health and the regulated body*. London, Sage.

Lupton, D. (2015) Health promotion in the digital era: a critical commentary. *Health Promotion International*, 30, 174–183.

Lupton, D. (2016) *The quantified self: a sociology of self-tracking*. Cambridge, Polity Press.

Lupton, D. (2020) 'Better understanding about what's going on': young Australians' use of digital technologies for health and fitness. *Sport, Education and Society*, 25 (1), 1–13.

Mabuza, M.P. (2018) *Health promotion: approaches, concepts, methods and critical perspectives*. Independently published.

MacDonald, M., Rabiee, F. and Weilandt, C. (2013) Health promotion and young prisoners: a European perspective. *International Journal of Prisoner Health*, 9, 151–164.

MacDonald, T.H. (1998) *Rethinking health promotion: a global approach*. London, Routledge.

Macias Balda, M. (2016) Complex needs or simplistic approaches? Homelessness services and people with complex needs in Edinburgh. *Social Inclusion*, 4, 28–38.

MacNamara, C. and Mannix-McNamara, P. (2014) Placing the promotion of health and well being on the Irish prison agenda – the complexity of health promotion in Irish prisons. *Irish Journal of Applied Social Studies*, 14, 49–59.

Mandal, A. (2019) *What is elephantiasis?* [Online] Available: www.news-medical.net [Accessed 23 July 2019].

Manstead, A.S.R. (2018) The psychology of social class: how socioeconomic status impacts thoughts, feelings, and behaviour. *British Journal of Social Psychology*, 57, 267–291.

Mantoura, P. and Potvin, L. (2013) A realist–constructionist perspective on participatory research in health promotion. *Health Promotion International*, 28, 61–72.

Marlow, L.A.V., Waller, J. and Wardle, J. (2015) Barriers to cervical cancer screening among ethnic minority women: a qualitative study. *Journal of Family Planning and Reproductive Health Care*, 41, 248–254.

Marmot, M. (2010) Fair society, healthy lives. The Marmot review. Strategic review of health inequalities in England post-2010. London, The Marmot Review.

Marmot, M., Allen, J., Boyce, T., Goldblatt, P. and Morrison, J. (2020) Health equity in England: The Marmot review 10 years on. London, Institute of Health Equity.

Marshall, L., Finch, D., Cairncross, L. and Bibby, J. (2019) Mortality and life expectancy trends in the UK: stalling progress. London, The Health Foundation.

Martin, T.G., Burgman, M. A., Fidler, F., Kuhnert, P.M., Low Choy, S., McBride, M. and Mengersen, K. (2012) Eliciting expert knowledge in conservation science. *Conservation Biology*, 26, 29–38.

Masse, R. and Williams-Jones, B. (2012) Ethical dilemmas in health promotion practice. In I. Rootman, A. Dupere, A. Pederson and M. O'Neill (eds) *Health promotion in Canada*, 3rd edn. Toronto, Canadian Scholars.

Mazzetti, G., Vignoli, M., Petruzziello, G. and Palareti, L. (2019) The hardier you are, the healthier you become: may hardiness and engagement explain the relationship between leadership and employees' health? *Frontiers in Psychology*, 9, 2784, 1–9, doi:10.3389/fpsyg.2018.02784

Mbuthia, F., Reid, M. and Fichardt, A. (2019) mHealth communication to strengthen postnatal care in rural areas: a systematic review. *BMC Pregnancy and Childbirth*, 19: 406. https://doi.org/10/1186/s12884-019-2531-0

McKee, M. and Raine, R. (2005) Choosing health? First choose your philosophy. *Lancet*, 365, 369–371.

McKelvey, K. and Halpern-Felsher, B. (2016) Adolescent cigarette smoking perceptions and behavior: tobacco control gains and gaps amidst the rapidly expanding tobacco products market from 2001 to 2015. *Journal of Adolescent Health*, 60 (2), 226–228.

McKibbon, K.A. and Marks, S. (1998) Searching for the best evidence. Part 1: where to look. *Evidence-Based Nursing*, 1, 68–70.

McKinlay, J.B. (1979) A case for refocusing upstream: the political economy of illness. In E.G. Jaco (ed.) *Patients, physicians, and illness*. 3rd edn. New York, The Free Press.

McLaughlin, H. (1969) SMOG grading – a new readability formula, *Journal of Reading*, 12 (8), 639–646.

McLeroy, K.R., Bibeau, D., Steckler, A. and Glanz, K. (1988) An ecological perspective on health promotion programs. *Health Education Quarterly*, 15, 351–377.

McMichael, A., Woodruff, R., Whetton, P., Hennessy, K., Nicholls, N., Hales, S., Woodward, A. and Kjellstrom, T. (2003) Human health and climate change in Oceania: a risk assessment. Canberra, Commonwealth Department of Health and Ageing.

McPhail-Bell, K., Fredericks, B. and Brough, M. (2013) Beyond the accolades: a postcolonial critique of the foundations of the Ottawa Charter. *Global Health Promotion*, 20, 22–29.

Mehtälä, M.A.K., Sääkslahti, A.K., Inkinen, M.E. and Poskiparta, M.E.H. (2014) A socio-ecological approach to physical activity interventions in childcare: a systematic review. *International Journal of Behavioral Nutrition and Physical Activity*, 11 (22), 1–12.

Mental Health Foundation. (2020) *Mental health statistics: poverty* [Online]. London: Mental Health Foundation. Available: www.mentalhealth.org.uk/statistics/mental-health-statistics-poverty#:~:text=A%20growing%20body%20of%20evidence,and%20experiencing%20mental%20health%20problems [Accessed 12 July 2020].

Mepham, D. (2014) Putting development to rights: integrating rights into a post-2015 agenda. *Rights Watch World Report 2014. Events of 2013*. US, Human Rights Watch.

Mereu, A., Sotgiu, A., Nuja, A., Casuccio, A., Cecconi, C., Fabiani, L., Guberti, E., Lorini, C., Mielli, L. Pocetta, G. and Contu, P. (2015) Professional competencies in health promotion and public health: what is common and what is specific? Review of the European debate and perspectives for professional development. *Epidemiologia e Prevenzione*, 39 (4), 33–38.

Micallef, R., Grewal, J.S., Khan, S., Wells, J. and Kayyali, R. (2019) Health champions in South London: evaluation of training and impact on public health. *International Journal of Pharmacy Practice*, 27, 71–79.

Michie, S., van Stralen, M.M. and West, R. (2011) The behaviour change wheel: a new method for characterising and designing behaviour change interventions. *Implementation Science*, 6, 42–53.

Milio, N. (1986) Promoting health through public policy. Ottawa, Canadian Public Health Association.

Millman, E., Lee, S. and Neimeyer, R. (2020) Social isolation and the mitigation of coronavirus anxiety: the mediating role of meaning. *Journal of Death Studies*, doi: 10.1080/07481187.2020.1775362

Minkler, M. (1999) Personal responsibility for health? A review of the arguments and the evidence at century's end. *Health Education & Behavior*, 26, 121–140.

Mittelmark, M.B. (2008) Health promotion: a professional community for social justice. *Promotion & Education*, 15, 3–5.

Mittelmark, M.B., Akerman, M., Gillis, D., Kosa, K., O'Neill, M., Piette, D., Restrepo, H., Rootman, I., Saan, H. and Springett, J. (2001) Mexico conference on health promotion: open letter to WHO Director General, Dr Gro Harlem Brundtland. 16, 3–4.

Moffatt, S., Steer, M., Lawson, S., Penn, L. and O'Brien, N. (2017) Link worker social prescribing to improve health and well-being for people with long-term conditions: qualitative study of service user perceptions. *BMJ Open*, 7, e015203.

Møller, L., Gatherer, A. and Dara, M. (2009) Barriers to implementation of effective tuberculosis control in prisons. *Public Health*, 123, 419–421.

Møller, L., Stöver, H., Jürgens, R., Gatherer, A. and Nikogosian, H. (2007) Health in prisons. Copenhagen: WHO.

Moon, G. and Gould, M. (2000) *Epidemiology: an introduction*. Buckingham, Open University Press.

Moorhead, S.A., Hazlett, D.E., Harrison, L., Carroll, J.K., Irwin, A. and Hoving, C. (2013) A new dimension of health care: systematic review of the uses, benefits, and limitations of social media for health communication. *Journal of Medical Internet Research*, 15, e85.

Moorley, C., Cahill, S. and Corcoran, N. (2016) Stroke among African-Caribbean women: lay beliefs of risks and causes. *Journal of Clinical Nursing*, 25, 403–411.

Morales, A. and Kettles, G. (2009) Healthy food outside: farmers' markets, taco trucks, and sidewalk fruit vendors. *Journal of Contemporary Health Law & Policy*, 26, 20–48.

Morgan, A. (2006) Needs assessment. In W. Macdowell, C. Bonell and M. Davies (eds) *Health promotion practice*. Maidenhead: Open University Press.

Morgan, A. and Ziglio, E. (2007) Revitalising the evidence base for public health: an assets model. *Promotion & Education*, 14, 17–22.

Morin, R.T., Galatzer-Levy, I.R., Maccallum, F. and Bonanno, G.A. (2017) Do multiple health events reduce resilience when compared with single events? *Health Psychology*, 36 (8), 721–728.

Morrison, V. and Bennett, P. (2016) *Introduction to health psychology*, 4th edn. London, Pearson.

Murphy, A., Chikovani, I., Uchaneishvilli, M., Makhashvili, N. and Roberts, B. (2018) Barrier to mental health care utilization among internally displaced persons in the Republic of Georgia: a rapid appraisal study. *BMC Public Health*, 18, 306–317.

Murphy, S. and Smith, C. (1993) Crutches, confetti or useful tools? Professionals, views on and use of health education leaflets. *Health Education Research*, 8, 205–215.

Murray, K.E., Eastman, A., Checkoway, H., Buul, A., Aden, R., Cavanaugh, A.M., Kidane, L. and Hussein, M. (2019) Occupational health risks and intervention strategies for US taxi drivers. *Health Promotion International*, 34 (2), 323–332.

Nagy, A., McMahon, A., Tapsell, L., Deane, F. and Arenson, D. (2018) Therapeutic alliance in dietetic practice for weight loss: insights from health coaching. *Nutrition & Dietetics*, 75, 250–255.

Nahr, N., Chaturvedi, S.K. and Nandan, D. (2011) Spiritual health scale 2011: defining and measuring 4th dimension of health. *Indian Journal of Community Medicine*, 36 (4), 275–282.

Naidoo, J. (1986) Limits to individualism. In S. Rodmell and A. Watt (eds) *The politics of health education: raising the issues*. London, Routledge & Kegan Paul.

Naidoo, J. and Wills, J. (2016) *Foundations for health promotion*. London, Elsevier.

Napier, D.A. (2017) *Culture matters: using a cultural contexts of health approach to enhance policy-making*. Geneva, WHO.

Ndomoto, L., Hibble, A., Obuzor, G., Nthusi, N., Quine, A., Chahal, P., Barasa, S.O., Newman-Taylor, K., Maguire, T. and Bowen, A. (2018) Why are we not measuring what matters in mental health in the UK? The case for routine use of recovery outcome measures. *Perspectives in Public Health*, 139 (4), 181–183.

Nettleton, S. (1995) *The sociology of health & illness*. Cambridge, Polity Press.

Nettleton, S. and Bunton, R. (1995) Sociological critiques of health promotion. In R. Bunton, S. Nettleton and R. Burrows (eds) *The sociology of health promotion*. London, Routledge.

Newton, J., Dooris, M. and Wills, J. (2016) Healthy universities: an example of a whole-system health-promoting setting. *Global Health Promotion*, 23, 57–65.

NHS Scotland (2019) Understanding needs. [Online] Available: www.healthscotland.scot [Accessed 30 June 2019].

NICE. (2019) Appraisal checklists, evidence tables, GRADE and economic profiles [Online]. London, NICE. Available: www.nice.org.uk/process/pmg20/resources/appendix-h-pdf-2549710190 [Accessed 10 February 2020].

Niveau, G. (2007) Relevance and limits of the principle of 'equivalence of care' in prison medicine. *Journal of Medical Ethics*, 33, 610–613.

Noble-Adams, R. (1999) Ethics and nursing research 1: development, theories and principles. *British Journal of Nursing*, 8, 888–892.

NOMS, HM Prison Service & Department of Health (2007) Prison health performance indicators. Guidance booklet. London, Offender Health.

Novilla, M.L.B., Barnes, M.D., Natalie, G., Williams, P.N. and Rogers, J. (2006) Public health perspectives on the family: an ecological approach to promoting health in the family and community. *Family & Community Health*, 29, 28–42.

Nuffield Council on Bioethics (2007) *Public health ethical issues*. London, Nuffield Council on Bioethics.

Nunes, S., Fernandes, H., Fisher, J. and Fernandes, M. (2018) Psychometric properties of the Brazilian version of the lived experiences component of the Spiritual Health and Life Orientation Measure (SHALOM). *Psicologia: Reflexão e Crítica*, 31 (2), doi: 10.1186/s4115-018-0083-2

Nutbeam, D. (2008) What would the Ottawa Charter look like if it were written today? *Critical Public Health*, 18, 435–441.

Nutbeam, D., Harris, E. and Wise, M. (2010) *Theory in a nutshell: a practical guide to health promotion theories*. London, McGraw Medical.

Nutbeam, D. and Kickbusch, I. (2000) Advancing health literacy: a global challenge for the 21st Century. *Health Promotion International*, 15 (3), 183–184.

Nutland, W. (2015) Using media to promote health: mass media, social media and social marketing. In W. Nutland and L. Cragg (eds) *Health promotion practice*, 2nd edn. Maidenhead, Open University Press.

Nyanja, N. and Tulinius, C. (2018) Understanding the fundamental elements of global health: using the Sen capability approach as the theoretical framework for a health needs assessment in deprived communities. *Education for Health*, 31, 43–47.

O'Neil, I. (2019) *Digital health promotion*. Cambridge, Polity.

Ofsted (2018) The annual report of Her Majesty's Chief Inspector of Education, Children's Services and Skills 2017/18. London, Crown.

Omonzejele, P.F. (2008) African concepts of health, disease and treatment: an ethical inquiry. *Explore*, 4, 120–126.

Orme, J., Powell, J., Taylor, P., Harrison, T. and Grey, M. (2003) *Public health for the 21st century*. Buckingham, Open University Press.

Ornell, F., Schuch, J., Sordi, A. and Kessler, F. (2020) 'Pandemic fear' and COVID-19: mental health burden and strategies. *Brazilian Journal of Psychiatry*, 42 (3), 232–235.

Owusu-Addo, E., Cross, R. and Sarfo-Mensah, P. (2017) Evidence-based practice in local public health service in Ghana. *Critical Public Health*, 27, 125–138.

Palfrey, C. (2018) *The future for health promotion*. London, The Policy Press.

Patrick, R. (2012) Work as a primary 'duty' of the responsible citizen: a critique of this work-centric approach. *People, Place and Policy*, 6, 5–15.

Patrick, R., Capetola, T., Townsend, M. and Nuttman, S. (2011) Health promotion and climate change: exploring the core competencies required for action. *Health Promotion International*, 27, 475–485.

Patwa, J. and Pandit, N. (2018) Open defecation-free India by 2019: how villages are progressing? *Indian Journal of Community Medicine*, 43 (3), 246–247.

Pedlar, M., Burgoyne, J. and Boydell, T. (1991) *The learning company: a strategy for sustainable development*. Maidenhead, McGraw Hill.

Perkins, N., Hunter, D.J., Visram, S., Finn, R., Gosling, J., Adams, L. and Forrest, A. (2020) Partnership or insanity: why do health partnerships do the same thing over and over again and expect a different result? *Journal of Health Services Research & Policy*, 25, 41–48.

Perkins, S., Simnett, I. and Wright, L. (1999) Creative tensions in evidence-based practice. In E.R. Perkins, I. Simnett and L. Wright (eds) *Evidence based health promotion*. Chichester, John Wiley & Sons.

Pescheny, J.V., Pappas, Y. and Randhawa, G. (2018) Facilitators and barriers of implementing and delivering social prescribing services: a systematic review. *BMC Health Services Research*, 18, 86, 1–14.

Peterson, A., Davis, M., Fraser, S. and Lindsay, J. (2010) Healthy living and citizenship: an overview. *Critical Public Health*, 20, 391–400.

Peterson, A. and Lupton, D. (1996) *The new public health: health and self in the age of risk*. St Leonards, Australia, Allen & Unwin.

Petticrew, M. and Roberts, H. (2003) Evidence, hierarchies, and typologies: horses for courses. *Journal of Epidemiology and Community Health*, 57, 527–529.

Philpott, M. (2018) *Serving of Alcohol at UEFA matches: Official Response from European Healthy Stadia Network [Online]*. Available: http://healthystadia.eu/serving-alcohol-uefa-matches/ [Accessed 21 December 2018].

Piper, S. (2009) *Health promotion for nurses: theory and practice*. Abingdon, Routledge.

Pittman, M. and Reich, B. (2016) Social media and loneliness: why an Instagram picture may be worth more than a thousand Twitter words. *Computers in Human Behavior*, 62, 155–167.

Poland, B. (2002) Transcription quality. In J.F. Gubrium and J.A. Holstein (eds) *Handbook of interview research: context and method*. Thousand Oaks, CA, Sage.

Poland, B. and Dooris, M. (2010) A green and healthy future: the settings approach to building health, equity and sustainability. *Critical Public Health*, 20, 281–298.

Poland, B.D., Green, L. W. and Rootman, I. (2000) Reflections on settings for health promotion. In B.D. Poland, L.W. Green and I. Rootman (eds) *Settings for health promotion: linking theory and practice*. Thousand Oaks, CA, Sage.

Poland, B., Krupa, G. and McCall, D. (2009) Settings for health promotion: an analytic framework to guide intervention design and implementation. *Health Promotion Practice*, 10, 505–516.

Pooley, J.A. and Cohen, L. (2010) Resilience: a definition in context. *Australian Community Psychologist*, 20 (1), 30–37.

Popay, J., Whitehead, M. and Hunter, D.J. (2010) Injustice is killing people on a large scale – but what is to be done about it? *Journal of Public Health*, 32, 148–149.

Popay, J., Williams, G., Thomas, C. and Gatrell, T. (2008) Theorising inequalities in health: the use of lay knowledge. *Sociology of Health and Illness*, 20 (5), 619–644.

Prince, M., Bryce, R., Albanese, E., Wimo, A., Ribeiro, W. and Ferri, C.P. (2013) The global prevalence of dementia: a systematic review and metaanalysis. *Alzheimer's & Dementia*, 9, 63–75.

Prince, M., Patel, V., Saena, S., Maj, M., Maselko, J., Phillips, M.R. and Rahman, A. (2007) No health without mental health. *The Lancet*, 370 (9590), 8–14.

Pringle, A., Zwolinsky, S., McKenna, J., Daly-Smith, A., Robertson, S. and White, A. (2013) Effect of a national programme of men's health delivered in English Premier League football clubs. *Public Health*, 127, 18–26.

Prochaska, J.O. and DiClemente, C.C. (1982) Transtheoretical therapy toward a more integrative model of change. *Psychotherapy: Theory, Research and Practice*, 19, 276–287.

Public Health England (2015) A Guide to Community-centred Approaches for Health and Wellbeing. London, Crown.

Public Health England (2018) Health profile for England: 2018. [Online] Available: www.gov.uk/government/publications [Accessed 21 August 2019].

Rabel, M., Laxy, M., Thorand, B., Peters, A., Schwettmann, L. and Mess, F. (2019) Clustering of health-related behavior patterns and demographics. Results from the population-based KORA S4/F4 cohort study. *Frontiers in Public Health*, 6, 387, 1–9. doi:10.3388/fpubh.2018.00387

Radzyminski, S. and Callister, L.C. (2016) Mother's beliefs, attitudes, and decision making related to infant feeding choices. *The Journal of Perinatal Education*, 25 (1), 18–28.

Raeburn, J. and MacFarlane, S. (2003) Putting the public into public health: towards a more people-centred approach. In R. Beaglehole (ed.) *Global public health: a new era*. Oxford, Oxford University Press.

Ramaswamy, M. and Freudenberg, N. (2007) Health promotion in jails and prisons: an alternative paradigm for correctional health services. In R.B. Greifinger, J. Bick and J. Goldenson (eds) *Public health behind bars: from prisons to communities*. New York, Springer.

Ramezani, M., Ahmadi, F., Mohammadi, E. and Kazemnejad, A. (2014) Spiritual care in nursing: a concept analysis. *Nursing Review*, 61 (2), 211–219.

Rankin, J. and Regan, S. (2004) *Meeting complex needs: the future of social care*. London: Turning Point.

Rendina, D., Campanozzi, A. and De Filippo, G. (2019) Methodological approach to the assessment of the obesogenic environment in children and adolescents: a review of the literature. *Nutrition, Metabolism & Cardiovascular Diseases*, 29 (6), 562–571.

Rhymer, W. and Speare, R. (2017) Countries' response to WHO's travel recommendations during the 2013–2016 Ebola outbreak. *Bulletin of the World Health Organization*.

Rich, E. and Evans, J. (2008) Learning to be healthy, dying to be thin: the representations of weight via body perfective codes in schools. In S. Riley, M. Burns, H. Frith, S. Wiggins and P. Markula (eds) *Representations, identities and practices of weight and body management*. Basingstoke, Palgrave Macmillan.

Rissel, C. (1994) Empowerment: the holy grail of health promotion? *Health Promotion International*, 9, 39–47.

Robbins, S. and Judge, T.A. (2014) *Essentials of organizational behaviour*, 12th edn. Boston, Pearson.

Robertson, S. (2006) Not living life in too much of an excess: lay men understanding health and well-being. *Health: An Interdisciplinary Journal for the Social Study of Health, Illness and Medicine*, 10, 175–189.

Robertson, S. and Williams, R. (2010) Men, public health and health promotion: towards a critically structural and embodied understanding. In B. Gough and S. Robertson (eds) *Men, masculinities and health: critical perspectives*. Basingstoke, Palgrave Macmillan.

Robertson, S., Woodall, J., Henry, H., Hanna, E., Rowlands, S., Horrocks, J., Livesley, J. and Long, T. (2018) Evaluating a community-led project for improving fathers' and children's wellbeing in England. *Health Promotion International*.

Robinson, T. (2008) Applying the socio-ecological model to improving fruit and vegetable intake among low-income African Americans. *Journal of Community Health*, 33 (6), 395–406.

Rodham, K. (2019) *Health psychology*, 2nd edn. London, Red Globe Press.

Rojatz, D., Merchant, A. and Nitsch, M. (2016) Factors influencing workplace health promotion intervention: a qualitative systematic review. *Health Promotion International*, 32, 831–839.

Rokeach, M. (1973) *The nature of human values*. New York, Free Press.

Root, M. (2019) The state of health coaching. *Fitness Journal*, 16 (5), 53–56.

Rose, N. (2000) Risk, trust and scepticism in the age of the new genetics. In B. Adam, U. Beck and J. Van Loon (eds) *The risk society and beyond: critical issues for social theory*. London, Sage.

Rosser, B. (2019) Intolerance of uncertainty as a transdiagnostic mechanism of psychological difficulties: a systematic review of evidence pertaining to causality and temporal precedence. *Cognitive Therapy and Research*, 43 (2), 438–463.

Rubin, H. J. and Rubin, I. S. (2005) *Qualitative interviewing*. Thousand Oaks, CA, Sage.

Rudd, R.E. (2015) The evolving concept of health literacy: new directions for health literacy studies. *Journal of Communication in Healthcare*, 8 (1), 7–9.

Ryan, G.W. and Bernard, H.R. (2003) Techniques to identify themes. *Field Methods*, 15, 85v109.

Salway, S., Carter, L., Powell, K., Turner, D., Mir, G. and Ellison, G. (2014) *Race equality and health inequalities: towards more integrated policy and practice*. London: Race Equality Foundation.

Santora, L., Arild Espnes, G. and Lillefjell, M. (2014) Health promotion and prison settings. *International Journal of Prisoner Health*, 10, 27–37.

Sarmiento, J.P. (2017) Healthy universities: mapping health-promotion interventions. *Health Education*, 117, 162–175.

Saunders, R.P., Evans, M.H. and Joshi, P. (2005) Developing a process-evaluation plan for assessing health promotion program implementation: a how-to guide. *Health Promotion Practice*, 6, 134–147.

Savage, M., Devine, F., Cunningham, N., Taylor, M., Li, Y., Hjellbrekke, J., Le Roux, B., Friedman, S. and Miles, A. (2013) A new model of social class? Findings from the BBC's Great British Class Survey experiment. *Sociology*, 47, 219–250.

Sayani, A. (2019) Social class and health inequalities. In T. Bryant, D. Raphael and M. Rioux (eds.) *Staying alive: critical perspectives on health, illness, and health care*. Toronto, Canadian Scholars.

Schneider, D. and Lilienfeld, D.E. (2015) *Lilienfeld's foundations of epidemiology*, 4th edn. Oxford, Oxford University Press.

Schudson, M. and Baykurt, B. (2016) How does a culture of health change? Lessons from the war on cigarettes. *Social Science and Medicine*, 165, 289–296.

Schwartz, B. (2004) *The paradox of choice*. New York, HarperCollins.

Schwartz, S.H. and Bilsky, W. (1987) Toward a universal psychological structure of human values. *Journal of Personality and Social Psychology*, 53 (3), 550–562.

Scottish Prison Service (2002) The health promoting prison: a framework for promoting health in the Scottish Prison Service. Edinburgh, Health Education Board for Scotland.

Scriven, A. (2017) *Ewles and Simnett's promoting health: a practical guide*, 7th edn. London, Elsevier.

Scriven, A. and Hodgins, M. (2012) *Health promotion settings: principles and practice*. London, Sage.

Seal, D.W., Belcher, L., Morrow, K., Eldridge, G., Binson, D., Kacanek, D., Margolis, A.D., McAuliffe, T. and Simms, R. (2004) A qualitative study of substance use and sexual behavior among 18- to 29-year-old men while incarcerated in the United States. *Health Education & Behavior*, 31, 775–789.

Seedhouse, D. (1997) *Health promotion: philosophy, prejudice and practice*. New York, John Wiley & Sons.

Senge, P. (1994) *The fifth discipline field book: strategies and tools for building a learning organization*. New York, DoubleDay.

Seppala, E., Rossomondo, T. and Doty, J.R. (2013) Social connection and compassion: important predictors of health and well-being. *Social Research: An International Quarterly*, 80 (2), 411–430.

Shah, G.H. (2018) Editorial: local health departments' role in non-profit hospitals' community health needs assessment. *American Journal of Public Health*, 108 (5), 595–597.

Shareck, M., Frohlich, K. L. and Poland, B. (2013) Reducing social inequities in health through settings-related interventions – a conceptual framework. *Global Health Promotion*, 20, 39–52.

Shaw, H.K. and Degazon, C. (2008) Integrating the core professional values of nursing: a profession, not just a career. *Journal of Cultural Diversity*, 15, 44–50.

Shaw, I. (2002) How lay are lay beliefs? *Health*, 6, 287–299.

Short, S.E. and Mollborn, S. (2015) Social determinants and health behaviors: conceptual frames and empirical advances. *Current Opinion in Psychology*, 5, 78–84.

Sidell, M. (2010) Older people's health: applying Antonovsky's salutogenic paradigm. In J. Douglas, S. Earle, S. Handsley, L. Jones, C. Lloyd and S. Spurr (eds) *A Reader in Promoting Public Health, Challenges and Controversy*, 2nd edn. London, Sage.

Sigler, R., Mahmoudi, L. and Graham, J.P. (2014) Analysis of behavioural change techniques in community-led total sanitation programs. *Health Promotion International*, 30 (1), 16–28.

Simbar, M., Aarabi, Z., Keshavarz, Z., Ramezani-Tehrani, F. and Baghestani, A.R. (2017) Promotion of physical activity of adolescents by skills-based health education. *Health Education*, 117 (2), 207–214.

Shimizu, K. (2020) 2019-nCoV, fake news, and racism. *The Lancet*, 395, 685–686.

Shultz, M. (2007) Comparing test searches in PubMed and Google Scholar. *Journal of the Medical Library Association: JMLA*, 95, 442.

Sibeon, R. (1999) Agency, structure, and social chance as cross-disciplinary concepts. *Politics*, 19, 139–144.

Sidel, V.W. and Levy, B.S. (2008) The health impact of war. *International Journal of Injury Control and Safety Promotion*, 15, 189–195.

Sim, J. (2002) The future of prison health care: a critical analysis. *Critical Social Policy*, 22, 300–323.

Small, R., Taft, A.J. and Brown, S. (2011) The power of social connection and support in improving health: lessons from social support interventions with childbearing women. *BMC Public Health*, 11 (Suppl. 5). https://doi.org/10.1186/1471-2458-11-S5-S4

Smith, C. (2000) Healthy prisons: a contradiction in terms? *The Howard Journal of Criminal Justice*, 39, 339–353.

Social Exclusion Unit (2002) *Reducing re-offending by ex-prisoners*. London, Crown.

Solar, O. and Irwin, A. (2010) *A conceptual framework for action on the social determinants of health*. Geneva, WHO.

Soubhi, H. and Potvin, L. (2000) Homes and families as health promotion settings. In B.D. Poland, L.W. Green and I. Rootman (eds) *Settings for health promotion: linking theory and practice*. Thousand Oaks, CA, Sage.

South, J., Bagnall, A.-M., Stansfield, J. A., Southby, K. J. and Mehta, P. (2019) An evidence-based framework on community-centred approaches for health: England, UK. *Health Promotion International*.

South, J., Bagnall, A. and Woodall, J. (2017) Developing a typology for peer education and peer support delivered by prisoners. *Journal of Correctional Health Care*, 23 (2), 214–229.

South, J., Higgins, T.J., Woodall, J. and White, S.M. (2008) Can social prescribing provide the missing link? *Primary Health Care Research & Development*, 9, 310–318.

South, J., Meah, A., Bagnall, A.-M., Kinsella, K., Branney, P., White, J. and Gamsu, M. (2010) People in Public health – a study of approaches to develop and support people in public health roles. Final report. London, NIHR Service Delivery and Organisation programme.

South, J. and Tilford, S. (2000) Perceptions of research and evaluation in health promotion practice and influences on activity. *Health Education Research*, 15, 729–741.

South, J. and Woodall, J. (2012) Planning and evaluating health promotion in settings. In A. Scriven and M. Hodgins (eds) *Health promotion settings: principles and practice*. London, Sage.

Southby, K. and Gamsu, M. (2018) Factors affecting general practice collaboration with voluntary and community sector organisations. *Health & Social Care in the Community*. 26 (3), e360-e369.

Southwick, S.M., Bonanno, G.A., Masten, A.S. Panter-Brick, C., Yehuda, R. (2014) Resilience definitions, theory, and challenges: interdisciplinary perspectives. *European Journal of Psychotraumatology*, 5 (1), https://doi.org/10.3402/ejpt.v5.25338

Sparks, M. (2010) News from Nairobi: politics, technology and mainstreaming. *Health Promotion Journal of Australia*, 21 (1), 3–4.

Squires, P. and Measor, L. (2001) 'Breaking in': partnership working, health promotion and prison walls. In D. Taylor (ed.) *Breaking down barriers: reviewing partnership practice*. Brighton, University of Brighton.

St Leger, L. (1997) Health promoting settings: from Ottawa to Jakarta. *Health Promotion International*, 12, 99–101.

Stainton-Rogers, W. (1991) *Explaining health and illness: an exploration of diversity*. London, Harvester/Wheatsheaf.

Staten, R., Miller, K., Noland, M.P. and Rayens, M.K. (2005) College students' physical activity: application of an ecological perspective. *American Journal of Health Studies*, 20, 58–65.

Stephenson, A., McDonough, S., Murphy, M.H., Nugent, C.D. and Mair, J.L. (2017) Using computer, mobile and wearable technology enhanced interventions to reduce sedentary behaviour: a systematic review and meta-analysis. *International Journal of Behavioural Nutrition and Physical Activity*, 14 (1), doi: 10.1186/s12966-017-0561-4

Steptoe, A., Shankar, A., Demakakos, P. and Wardle, J. (2013) Social isolation, loneliness, and all-cause mortality in older men and women. *PNAS: Proceedings of the National Academy of Sciences of the United States of America*, 100 (15), 5797–5801.

Stokols, D., Grzywacz, J.G., McMahan, S. and Phillips, K. (2003) Increasing the health promotive capacity of human environments. *American Journal of Health Promotion*, 18, 4–13.

Svalastog, A.L., Donev, D., Kristoffersen, N.J. and Gajović, S. (2017) Concepts and definitions of health and health-related values in the knowledge landscapes of the digital society. *Croatian Medical Journal*, 58 (6), 431–435.

Swain, R.B. (2017) A critical analysis of the sustainable development goals. In W. Leal Filho (ed.) *Handbook of Sustainability Science and Research*. Cham, Springer.

Sykes, S. (2014) Approaches to promoting health. In J. Wills (ed.) *Fundamentals of health promotion for nurses*, 2nd edn. Oxford, Wiley.

Szczekala, K., Kanadys, K., Wiktor, K. and Wiktor, H. (2018) Significance of motivational interviewing in public health. *Polish Journal of Public Health*, 128 (3), 128–131.

Tabreham, J.D. (2014) Prisoners' experience of healthcare in England: post-transfer to National Health Service responsibility: a case study. PhD, University of Lincoln.

Taj, F., Klein, M.C.A., Ribeiro, N. (2019) Digital health behavior change technology: bibliometric and scoping review of two decades of research. *JMIR Mhealth Uhealth*, 7 (12), doi: 10.2196/13311

Tannahill, A. (1985) What is health promotion? *Health Education Journal*, 44, 167–168.

Tannahill, A. (2009) Health promotion: the Tannahill model revisited. *Public Health*, 123, 369–399.

Taylor, P. (2007) The lay contribution to public health. In J. Orme, J. Powell, P. Taylor and M. Grey, *Public health in the 21st century: new perspectives on policy, participation and practice*. 2nd edn. Buckingham, Open University Press.

Tedeschi, B. (2017) Where a doctor saw a treatable cancer, a patient saw an evil spirit. [Online] Available: www.statnews.com [Accessed 22 July 2019].

Telford, L. (1998) Ethical dilemmas in health promotion. *Ontario Health Promotion E-Bulletin*, 79.

Tengland, P. (2016) Behavior change or empowerment: on the ethics of health promotion goals. *Health Care Analysis*, 24 (1), 24–46.

The Health Foundation. (2020) *Will COVID-19 be a watershed moment for health inequalities?* [Online]. London, The Health Foundation. Available: www.health.org.uk/publications/long-reads/will-covid-19-be-a-watershed-moment-for-health-inequalities [Accessed 12 July 2020].

Thomas, C. and Warwick-Booth, L. (2019) The state of women's health in Leeds: women's voices final report. Leeds, Leeds Beckett University.

Thompson, L. and Kumar, A. (2011) Responses to health promotion campaigns: resistance, denial and othering. *Critical Public Health*, 21, 105–117.

Thompson, S., Novak, C. and Thompson, K. (2014) Programme planning. In S.R. Thompson (ed.) *The essential guide to public health and health promotion*. London, Routledge.

Thorley, V. (2019) Is breastfeeding 'normal'? Using the right language for breastfeeding. *Midwifery*, 69, 39–44.

Tilford, S. (2016) President's Letter: Is there a future for the Ottawa Charter? *International Journal of Health Promotion and Education*, 54, 265–266.

Tilford, S., Green, J. and Tones, K. (2003) Values, health promotion and public health. Leeds: Centre for Health Promotion Research, Leeds Metropolitan University.

Toleikyte, L. and Salway, S. (2018) Local action on health inequalities: understanding and reducing ethnic inequalities in health. London: Public Health England.

Tones, B.K. (1986) Health education and the ideology of health promotion: a review of alternative approaches. *Health Education Research*, 1, 3–12.

Tones, K. (1998) Health promotion: empowering choice. In L.B. Myers and K. Midence (eds) *Adherence to treatment in medical conditions*. Amsterdam, Harwood Academic Publishers.

Tones, K. (2001) Health promotion: the empowerment imperative. In A. Scriven and J. Orme (eds) *Health promotion: professional perspectives*, 2nd edn. London, Palgrave.

Tones, K. and Tilford, S. (2001) *Health promotion: effectiveness, efficiency and equity*. Cheltenham, Nelson Thornes.

Torales, J., O'Higgins, M., Castadelli-Maia, J.M. and Ventriglio, A. (2020) The outbreak of coronavirus and the impact on global mental health. *International Journal of Social Psychiatry*, 66 (4), 317–320.

Torp, S., Kokko, S. and Ringsberg, K. C. (2014) *Promoting health in everyday settings: opportunities and challenges*. London, Sage.

Townsend, N. and Foster, C. (2011) Developing and applying a socio-ecological model to the promotion of healthy eating in the school. *Public Health Nutrition*, 16 (6), 1101–1108.

Tremblay, M.-C. (2019) The wicked interplay of hate rhetoric, politics and the internet: what can health promotion do to counter right-wing extremism? *Health Promotion International*, 35, 1–4.

Tsumori, H. (2018) No gender equality, no SDGs. [Online] Available: www.asia-pacific.undp.org/content/rbap/en/home/blog/2018/3/28/No-Gender-Equality-no-SDGs.html [Accessed 10 February 2019].

Tweed, E.J., Rodgers, M., Priyadarshi, S. and Crighton, E. (2018) 'Taking away the chaos': a health needs assessment for people who inject drugs in public places in Glasgow, Scotland. *BMC Public Health*, 18, 829–838.

Vader, J. (2006) Spiritual health: the next frontier. *European Journal of Public Health*, 16 (5), https://doi.org/10/1093/eurpub/ckl234

Van Den Broucke, S. (2018) Developing a core competencies framework for health promotion. *European Journal of Public Health*, 28 (Suppl. 4), 210–211.

Varea, V. and Underwood, M. (2016) 'You are just an idiot for not doing any physical activity right now': pre-service health and physical education teachers' constructions of fatness. *European Physical Education Review*, 22 (4), 465–478.

Verduyn, P., Ybarra, O., Résibois, M., Jonides, J. and Kross, E. (2017) Do social network sites enhance or undermine subjective well-being? A critical review. *Social Issues and Policy Review*, 11, 274–302.

Vujcich, D., Thomas, J., Crawford, K. and Ward, J. (2018) Indigenous youth peer-led health promotion in Canada, New Zealand, Australia, and the United States: a systematic review of the approaches, study designs, and effectiveness. *Frontiers in Public Health*, 6: 31, doi:10.3389/fpubh.2018.00031

Wallerstein, N. (2002) Empowerment to reduce health disparities. *Scandinavian Journal of Public Health*, 30, 72–77.

Wallerstein, N. (2006) What is the evidence on effectiveness of empowerment to improve health? *Report for the Health Evidence Network (HEN)*. Copenhagen: WHO Regional Office for Europe.

Ware, J.E. and Sherbourne, C.D. (1992) The MOS 36-item short-form health survey (SF-36): 1: conceptual framework and item selection. *Medical Care*, 30, 473–483.

Warwick-Booth, L. and Cross, R. (2018a) Evaluating a gender-specific intensive intervention programme: young women's voices and experiences. *Health Education Journal*.

Warwick-Booth, L. and Cross, R. (2018b) *Global health studies: a social determinants perspective*. Cambridge, Polity.

Warwick-Booth, L., Cross, R. and Lowcock, D. (2012) *Contemporary health studies: an introduction*. Cambridge, Polity Press.

Warwick-Booth, L., Cross, R. and Lowcock, D. (2021) *Contemporary health studies: an introduction*, 2nd edn. Cambridge, Polity Press.

Warwick-Booth, L., Cross, R., Woodall, J., Bagnall, A.-M. and South, J. (2018) Health promotion education in changing and challenging times: reflections from England. *Health Education Journal*, 78 (6), 692–704.

Watson, J. and Platt, S. (2000) Connecting policy and practice: the challenge for health promotion research. In J. Watson and S. Platt (eds) *Researching health promotion*. London, Routledge.

Wharf Higgins, J., Strange, K., Scarr, J., Pennock, M., Barr, V., Yew, A., Drummond, J. and Terpstra, J. (2011) 'It's a feel. That's what a lot of our evidence would consist of': public health practitioners' perspectives on evidence. *Evaluation & the Health Professions*, 34, 278–296.

Whitehead, D. (2006) The health promoting prison (HPP) and its imperative for nursing. *International Journal of Nursing Studies*, 43, 123–131.

Whitehead, D. (2010) A systematic approach to health promotion. In D. Whitehead and F. Irving (eds) *Health promotion & health education in nursing: a framework for practice*. Basingstoke, Palgrave Macmillan.

Whitehead, D. (2011) Before the cradle and beyond the grave: a lifespan/settings-based framework for health promotion. *Journal of Advanced Nursing*, 20, 2183–2194.

Whitehead, D., Taket, A. and Smith, P. (2003) Action research in health promotion. *Health Education Journal*, 62, 5–22.

Whitelaw, S., Baxendale, A., Bryce, C., Machardy, L., Young, I. and Witney, E. (2001) 'Settings' based health promotion: a review. *Health Promotion International*, 16, 339–352.

Whitsel, L.P. (2017) Government's role in promoting healthy living. *Progress in Cardiovascular Diseases*, 59, 492–497.

WHO (n.d.) Health education. [Online] Geneva, WHO. Available: who.int/topics/healtheducation [Accessed 10 August 2019].

WHO (1977) *World Health Assembly: Health for all by the year 2000*. Geneva, WHO.

WHO (1978) *Declaration of Alma Ata*. International Conference on Primary Health Care, 6–12 September, Alma Ata, Geneva, WHO.

WHO (1986) Ottawa Charter for health promotion. *Health Promotion*, 1, iii–v.

WHO (1988) *The Adelaide recommendations*. Geneva, WHO.

WHO (1991) *Sundsvall statement on supportive environments for health*. Geneva, WHO.

WHO (1995) Health in prisons. Health promotion in the prison setting. *Summary report on a WHO meeting, London*, 15–17 October 1995. Copenhagen, WHO.

WHO (1997a) *The Jakarta declaration on leading health promotion into the 21st century*. Geneva, WHO.

WHO (1997b) Report of a conference on intersectoral action for health: a cornerstone for health-for-all in the twenty-first century, 20–23 April 1997, Halifax, Nova Scotia, Canada. Geneva, WHO.

WHO (1998) *Health promotion glossary*. Geneva, WHO.

WHO (2000) *Mexico ministerial statement for the promotion of health: from ideas to action*. Geneva, WHO.

WHO (2003) *Healthy marketplaces: working towards ensuring the supply of safer food*. Cairo, WHO.

WHO (2005) *The Bangkok charter for health promotion in a globalized world*. Geneva, WHO.

WHO (2006) *Working together for health*. Geneva, WHO.

WHO (2009a) *Milestones in health promotion: statements from global conferences*. Geneva, WHO.

WHO (2009b) *Nairobi call to action*. Geneva, WHO.

WHO (2009c) *Zagreb declaration for healthy cities*. Copenhagen, WHO.

WHO (2011) *Adelaide statement on health in all policies*. Geneva, WHO.

WHO (2012) Water sanitation hygiene: fast facts [Online]. Available: www.who.int/water_sanitation_health [Accessed 25 February 2019].

WHO (2013) *The Helsinki statement on health in all policies*. Geneva, WHO.

WHO (2014) Mental health: a state of well-being. [Online]. Geneva, WHO. Available: www.who.int/features/factfiles/mental_health/en/ [Accessed 28 January 2018].

WHO (2016) Shanghai Declaration on promoting health in the 2030 Agenda for Sustainable Development [Online]. Geneva, WHO. Available: www.who.int/healthpromotion/conferences/9gchp/shanghai-declaration/en/ [Accessed 7 January 2018].

WHO (2017a) Shanghai declaration on promoting health in the 2030 agenda for sustainable development. *Health Promotion International*, 32 (1), 7–8.

WHO (2017b) *Dementia: a public health priority*. Geneva, WHO.

WHO (2018a) Road traffic injuries: key facts [Online]. Available: www.who.int/news-room/fact-sheets/detail/road-traffic-injuries [Accessed 4 March 2019].

WHO (2018b) Types of healthy settings [Online]. Geneva, WHO. Available: www.who.int/healthy_settings/types/cities/en/ [Accessed 7 January 2019].

WHO (2019a). Ten threats to global health in 2019 [Online]. Geneva: WHO. Available: www.who.int/emergencies/ten-threats-to-global-health-in-2019 [Accessed 2 May 2019].

WHO (2019b) *Universal health coverage for mental health*. Geneva, WHO.

WHO (2019c) Prevalence of tobacco smoking. Global Health Observatory Data. www.who.int/gho/tobacco/use/en [Accessed 31 July 2019].

WHO (2019d) *Infant mortality*. Geneva, WHO. Available: www.who.int [Accessed 5 August 2019].

WHO (2019e) Healthy markets [Online]. Geneva, WHO. Available: www.who.int/healthy_settings/types/markets/en/ [Accessed 20 February 2019].

WHO (2019f) School and youth health [Online]. Geneva, WHO. Available: www.who.int/school_youth_health/gshi/hps/en/ [Accessed 20 February 2019].

WHO (2019g) Workplace health promotion [Online]. Geneva, WHO. Available: www. who.int/occupational_health/topics/workplace/en/index1.html [Accessed 20 February 2019].

WHO (2020a) Depression [Online]. Geneva, WHO. Available: www.who.int/news-room/fact-sheets/detail/depression [Accessed 27 May 2019].

WHO (2020b) Global Health Observatory (GHO) data [Online]. Geneva, WHO. Available: www.who.int/gho/mortality_burden_disease/life_tables/situation_trends_text/en/ [Accessed 12 July 2020].

Wiggers, J. and Sanson-Fisher, R. (1998) Evidence-based health. In D. Scott and R. Weston (eds) *Evaluating health promotion*. Cheltenham, Nelson Thornes.

Wild, K. and McGrath, M. (2019) *Public Health and Health Promotion for Nurses at a Glance*. Oxford, John Wiley & Sons.

Wildridge, V., Childs, S., Cawthra, L. and Madge, B. (2004) How to create successful partnerships – a review of the literature. *Health Information & Libraries Journal*, 21, 3–19.

Wiles, R., Crow, G., Heath, S. and Charles, V. (2008) The management of confidentiality and anonymity in social research. *International Journal of Social Research Methodology*, 11, 417–428.

Wiley, L.F., Berman, M. L. and Blanke, D. (2013) Who's your nanny? Choice, paternalism and public health in the age of personal responsibility. *The Journal of Law, Medicine & Ethics*, 41, 88–91.

Wilkinson, R. and Pickett, K. (2009) *The Spirit Level*. London, Penguin.

Williams, G. (2014) Lay expertise. *Wiley Online Library*. [Online] Available: https://doi.org/10.1002/9781118410868.wbehibs555 [Accessed 31 July 2019].

Willig, C. (2001) *Introducing qualitative research in psychology: adventures in theory and method*. Buckingham, Open University Press.

Wills, J. and Jackson, L. (2014) Health promotion and public health. In J. Wills, (ed.) *Fundamentals of health promotion for nurses*, 2nd edn. Oxford, Wiley.

Wilson, J.S., Elborn, J.S. and Fitzsimons, D. (2011) 'It's not worth stopping now': why do smokers with chronic obstructive pulmonary disease continue to smoke? A qualitative study. *Journal of Clinical Nursing*, 20 (5–6), 819–827.

Winer, M. and Ray, K. (1994) *Collaboration handbook: creating, sustaining, and enjoying the journey*. Minnesota, Amherst H. Wilder Foundation.

Wise, S. (1995) Feminist ethics in practice. In R. Hugman and D. Smith (eds) *Ethical issues in social work*. London, Routledge.

Wong, T., Pharr, J.R., Bungum, T., Coughenour, C. and Lough, N.L. (2019) Effects of peer sexual health education on college campuses: a systematic review. *Health Promotion Practice*, 20 (5), 652–666.

Woodall, J. (2016) A critical examination of the health promoting prison two decades on. *Critical Public Health*, 26, 615–621.

Woodall, J. (2020a) COVID-19 and the role of health promoters and educators. *Emerald Open Research*, 2.

Woodall, J. (2020b) Health promotion co-existing in a high-security prison context: a documentary analysis. *International Journal of Prisoner Health*. 16 (3), 237–247.

Woodall, J. and Dixey, R. (2015) Advancing the health promoting prison: a call for global action. *Global Health Promotion*, 24, 58–61.

Woodall, J., Dixey, R. and South, J. (2013) Control and choice in English prisons: developing health-promoting prisons. *Health Promotion International*, 29, 474–482.

Woodall, J. and Freeman, C. (2019) Promoting health and well-being in prisons: an analysis of one year's prison inspection reports. *Critical Public Health*, 30 (5), 555–566.

Woodall, J., Raine, G., South, J. and Warwick-Booth, L. (2010) Empowerment & health and well-being: evidence review. Leeds, Centre for Health Promotion Research, Leeds Metropolitan University.

Woodall, J. and Rowlands, S. (2021) Professional practice. In R. Cross, L. Warwick-Booth, S. Rowlands, J. Woodall, I. O'Neil and S. Foster (eds) *Health promotion: global principles and practice*, 2nd edn. London, CABI.

Woodall, J. and South, J. (2012) Health promoting prisons: dilemmas and challenges. In A. Scriven and M. Hodgins (eds) *Health promotion settings: principles and practice*. London, Sage.

Woodall, J., South, J., Dixey, R., de Viggiani, N. and Penson, W. (2015) Expert views of peer-based interventions for prisoner health. *International Journal of Prisoner Health*, 11, 87–97.

Woodall, J., Trigwell, J., Bunyan, A., Raine, G., Eaton, V., Davis, J., Hancock, L., Cunningham, M. and Wilkinson, S. (2018) Understanding outcomes and processes of a social prescribing service: a mixed method analysis. *BMC Health Services Research*. 18 (604), 1–12.

Woodall, J., Warwick-Booth, L. and Cross, R. (2012) Has empowerment lost its power? *Health Education Research*, 27, 742–745.

Woodall, J., Warwick-Booth, L., South, J. and Cross, R. (2018) What makes health promotion distinct? *Scandinavian Journal of Public Health*, 46, 118–122.

Woodall, J., Woodward, J., Witty, K. and McCulloch, S. (2014) An evaluation of a toothbrushing programme in schools. *Health Education*, 114, 414–434.

World Economic Forum (2015) How should we measure wellbeing? [Online] Available: www.weforum.org [Accessed 3 February 2019].

Worley, C.G. and Jules, C. (2020) COVID-19's uncomfortable revelations about agile and sustainable organizations in a VUCA world. *The Journal of Applied Behavioral Science*, 56, 279–283.

Wright, J., O'Flynn, G. and Macdonald, D. (2006) Being fit and looking healthy: women's and men's constructions of health and fitness. *Sex Roles*, 4 (9–10), 707–716.

Wright, J., Small, N., Raynor, P., Tuffnell, D., Bhopal, R., Cameron, N., Fairley, L., Lawlor, D.A., Parslow, R., Petherick, E.S., Pickett, K.E. and Waiblinger, D. (2013) Cohort profile: the born in Bradford multi-ethnic family cohort study. *International Journal of Epidemiology*, 42 (4), 978–991.

Wright, L. (1999) Doing things right. In E.R. Perkins, I. Simnett and L. Wright (eds) *Evidence based health promotion*. Chichester: John Wiley & Sons.

Wright, M.T., Roche, B., von Unger, H., Block, M. and Gardner, B. (2010) A call for an international collaboration on participatory research for health. *Health Promotion International*, 25, 115–122.

Yamey, G., Sridhar, D. and Abbasi, K. (2018) The extricable links between health, wealth, and profits. *BMJ*, 363: k4418 doi: 10.1136/bmj.k4418

Yiengprugsawan, V., Somboonsook, B., Seubsman, S. and Sleigh, A.C. (2012) Happiness, mental health, and socio-demographic associations among a national cohort of Thai adults. *Journal of Happiness Studies*, 13 (6), 1019–1029.

Yosef, Z., Lelisa, S. and Tamrat, S. (2019) Knowledge, attitude, practice, and associated factors of breast cancer self-examination among urban health extension workers in Addis Ababa, central Ethiopia. *Journal of Midwifery & Reproductive Health*, 7 (2), 1662–1671.

Zalmanovitch, Y. and Cohen, N. (2013) The pursuit of political will: politicians' motivation and health promotion. *The International Journal of Health Planning and Management*, DOI: 10.1002/hpm.2203.

Zeleke, D.A., Gelaye, K.A. and Mekonnen, F.A. (2019) Community-led total sanitation and the rate of latrine ownership. *BMC Research Notes*, 12 (14). https://doi.org/10.1186/s13104-019-4066-x

Zosel, R. (2014) 10 tips for using social media to promote health: reflections from fertility week [Online]. Available: blogs.crikey.com.au/croakey/2014/11/20/10-tips-for-using-social-media-to-promote-health-reflections-from-fertility-week/ [Accessed 12 July 2020].

INDEX